Anaesthesia in Laparoscopic Surgery

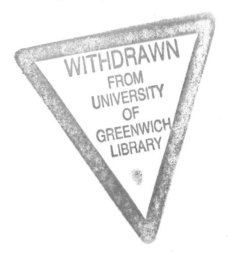

Anaesthesia in Laparoscopic Surgery

Editors

Jayashree Sood MD, FFARCS, PGDHHM
Chairperson
Dept. of Anaesthesiology,
Pain and Perioperative Medicine
Sir Ganga Ram Hospital, New Delhi, India

Anil Kumar Jain MD
Senior Consultant
Dept. of Anaesthesiology,
Pain and Perioperative Medicine
Sir Ganga Ram Hospital, New Delhi, India

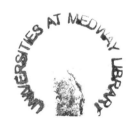

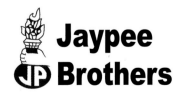
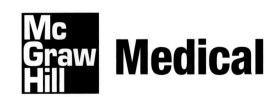

First published in India in 2009 by

Jaypee Brothers Medical Publishers (P) Ltd

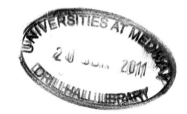

Corporate Office
4838/24 Ansari Road, Daryaganj, **New Delhi** - 110002, India, +91-11-43574357

Registered Office
B-3 EMCA House, 23/23B Ansari Road, Daryaganj, **New Delhi** 110 002, India
Phones: +91-11-23272143, +91-11-23272703, +91-11-23282021,
+91-11-23245672, Rel: +91-11-32558559 Fax: +91-11-23276490, +91-11-23245683
e-mail: jaypee@jaypeebrothers.com, Website: www.jaypeebrothers.com

First published in USA by The McGraw-Hill Companies, 2 Penn Plaza, New York, NY 10121.
Exclusively worldwide distributor except South Asia (India, Nepal, Sri Lanka, Bhutan, Pakistan, Bangladesh,
Malaysia).

ISBN-13: 978-0-07-163320-8
ISBN-10: 0-07-163320-0

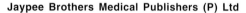

Contributors

Amitabh Dutta MD
Junior Consultant

Anil Kumar Jain MD
Senior Consultant

Anjeleena Kumar Gupta DA, FRCA
Junior Consultant

Annu Sarin Jolly MD, DIP
Junior Consultant

Aparna Sinha MD
Associate Consultant

Archna Koul MD
Junior Consultant

Bimla Sharma MD, DGO
Senior Consultant

Chand Sahai MD, DA
Senior Consultant

Chandan Marwah MD, DNB
Junior Consultant

Deepanjali Pant MD
Junior Consultant

Jayashree Sood MD, FFARCS, PGDHHM
Chairperson

Lakshmi Jayaraman DA, DNB
Junior Consultant

Naresh Dua MD
Junior Consultant

Pradeep Jain MD
Senior Consultant

Rashmi Jain DNB
Junior Consultant

Shikha Sharma MD
Associate Consultant

Subhash Gupta MD
Senior Consultant

Vijay Vohra MD, FRCA
Senior Consultant, Vice Chairperson

All Contributors from:
Department of Anaesthesiology,
Pain and Perioperative Medicine
Sir Ganga Ram Hospital, New Delhi, India

Foreword

The past decade has witnessed an immense and spectacular development in the field of laparoscopic surgery and anaesthesia both in terms of technical development and the better knowledge regarding the management of the patients. The spectrum of laparoscopic surgery has now been extended from simple abdominal surgery to complex thoracic surgery. The laparoscopic surgery is now performed in all types of patients, i.e. neonate, pregnant, morbidly obese, trauma victims and other patients with co-morbid medical condition.

A need for a specialized textbook to address the special issues pertaining to anaesthesia in laparoscopy was long overdue. The present textbook will definitely take care of that gap appropriately. The book will be of immense help for all the anaesthesiologists and surgeons practising laparoscopy. The book has been well written and illustrated with updated information. The chapters have been cleverly thought and arranged covering all the aspects of perioperative management in laparoscopic surgery. The language of the book is very lucid and can be easily understood by the readers.

The efforts of the editors J Sood and AK Jain in unifying all the aspects of the topic are commendable. Contributions by different experts who are actively practising the speciality further increase the credibility of the book. I sincerely believe that this book will find a permanent place in the mind and heart of all the medical fraternity in general and anaesthesiologists in particular.

BK Rao
Chairman
Board of Management
Sir Ganga Ram Hospital
New Delhi, India

Comments:
A Surgeon's Perspective

The Department of Anaesthesiology at Sir Ganga Ram Hospital, New Delhi is a center of excellence having been at the forefront of the technological revolution and advances in patient care and management over the decades. Sir Ganga Ram Hospital today is globally recognized as a leading center for services in laparoscopy and minimal access surgery. More than thirty thousand laparoscopic procedures have been performed till date.

The introduction of laparoscopy two decades ago was one of the most significant advances in modern medicine. There has been a sweeping revolution in surgical practice ever since that has radically altered the performance and delivery of surgical care to patients. In tandem with this surgical revolution, there has been subtle yet very significant progress in anaesthesia care and management. The introduction of laparoscopy and carboperitoneum result in an altered physiologic milieu in the patient intraoperatively, which leads to altered responses that need to be recognized and managed by the supervising anaesthesiologist. Thus, the advent of laparoscopy has presented anaesthesiologists with a novel, yet peculiar, set of patient circumstances and challenges that need to be addressed and managed for optimal patient outcomes.

Anaesthesia in laparoscopic surgery has been elaborated in great detail and chapters have been written by experts in the field within the department with many years of insight and experience. I am aware that anaesthesia protocols within the department are continuously refined and updated, commensurate with growing awareness and increasing expertise. Professional expertise has been accumulated over sixteen years and thirty thousand operations. This is reflected in the lucid prose and comprehensive attention to detail in this book. This book promises to be a veritable treatise on the subject. As a practicing surgeon, I wholeheartedly endorse the concept of this book, as well as the final product.

It is my sincere desire that anaesthesiologists everywhere are able to benefit and gain from the numerous insights and tips provided in these chapters. These would necessarily lead to greater surgeon comfort and ultimately better patient care and improved patient outcome, which is a common endeavour of healthcare professionals around the world.

Pradeep Chowbey
Chairman
Minimal Access and Bariatric Surgery Centre
Sir Ganga Ram Hospital, New Delhi, India

Preface

Over the past decade, laparoscopic surgery has become a widely accepted form of healthcare tool for millions of people. With explosive growth in laparoscopic surgery, both practitioners and medical organizations have recognized the need for improved care of this increasing patient population. *Anaesthesia in Laparoscopic Surgery* focusses on all the issues involved in laparoscopy and highlights the pathophysiology of pneumoperitoneum. This book is intended as a resource for anaesthesiologists, both in practice and training, as well as other healthcare professionals involved in laparoscopic surgery.

A committed work space of five operation theatres, with appropriate equipment and state-of-the-art monitors together with a dedicated team of anaesthesiologists, nurses and technical staff handle the 20 to 25 odd patients coming for laparoscopic procedures each operation theatre day. These procedures, ranging from cholecystectomy, bariatric surgery, thoracoscopy to removal of pheochromocytomas; in patients of ASA grades I to III/IV, for more than a decade has given considerable experience to our team, all of whom have had a hand in the creation of this book.

Though the term 'laparoscopy' was initially coined for the examination of the abdominal organs, nowadays, it is loosely used for extraperitoneal procedures (TEP inguinal hernia repair) as well as extra-abdominal procedures such as thoracoscopy.

The contributors, authorities in their respective fields, explore a variety of important issues in laparoscopic anaesthesia and surgery, including preoperative assessment, choice of anaesthesia, intraoperative monitoring, pain management and postoperative complications. Duplication of specific issues is inevitable and unavoidable in a multiauthored text.

Jayashree Sood
Anil Kumar Jain

Acknowledgements

I am highly indebted to Dr VP Kumra, Emeritus Consultant, Department of Anaesthesiology, Pain and Perioperative Medicine, Sir Ganga Ram Hospital whose guidance has enabled me to complete this book. I am grateful to Dr BK Rao, Chairman, Board of Management, Sir Ganga Ram Hospital, for his continuous support and guidance. Dr Pradeep Chowbey was first to establish the department of Minimal Access Surgery in India and devote himself fully for the laparoscopic surgery. I am grateful to him for providing clinical material and inspiration. My thanks are due to Dr Anil Jain for co-editing and to Dr Girish Joshi for introducing the book. I am obliged to all my colleagues who have contributed to this book.

A special thanks is due to Mrs Silvi Philip and Mr Prakash Bisht for their secretarial help.

This book would not have been possible without the constant inspiration and support of my husband, Dr Subhash Sood and my blue eyed children Rahul, Ruchi and Dheeraj, and my grand daughter 'Ayra'.

Jayashree Sood

Acknowledgements

I am grateful to Dr BK Rao, Chairman, Board of Management, Sir Ganga Ram Hospital, who has always been a pillar of support and inspiration. I thank Dr Jayashree Sood, Chairperson, Department of Anaesthesiology, for her constant guidance. I express my deep sense of gratitude to Dr Pradeep Chowbey, Chairman, Department of Minimal Access Surgery, who has always been a source of inspiration and advice. Special thanks are due to Dr Pradeep Jain for moral support and helpful suggestions.

I gratefully acknowledge the constant support and professional expertise of all the contributors from the Department of Anaesthesiology, Sir Ganga Ram Hospital, New Delhi. This book saw the light of day due to their hard work and expertise.

Sincere appreciation also goes to our secretary Ms Silvi Philip and Mr Subrato Adhikary of M/s Jaypee Brothers Medical Publishers (P) Ltd, New Delhi for their support of this project.

I also wish to express my appreciation for the cooperation of my wife, Dr Sandhya Jain, in making this venture a success.

Anil Kumar Jain

Contents

Introduction

It is a great honor and pleasure for me to introduce to this book on anesthesia for laparoscopic and thoracoscopic surgery. Minimally invasive surgery (also referred to as minimal access surgery) has become routine for patients undergoing abdominal and thoracic surgery. Extensive laparoscopic and thoracoscopic procedures are now being performed in patients of all ages (young and old) and in those with significant comorbidities as well as the obese and pregnant patients. There is increasing evidence that the endoscopic approach facilitates postoperative recovery and improves outcome beyond the intraoperative period. However, these procedures present intraoperative challenges usually not seen with the traditional "open" approach.

Although there are numerous review articles and monographs written on the anesthetic management of patients undergoing laparoscopic and thoracoscopic procedures, Jayshree Sood and her colleagues have presented a comprehensive book that covers all aspects of these procedures in great depth. This book is easy to read with excellent illustrations and figures, as well as tables that allow rapid access to essential information. It is obvious that in addition to reviewing the published information the authors have written from first-hand observations and experience. The section on "clinical pearls" provides practical information. As with all such efforts, there is some overlap of information, which should help to reinforce the important aspects of anesthetic management for these endoscopic procedures. This book succeeds in transmitting information about anesthesia for laparoscopy and thoracoscopy in an effective manner.

I am sure that this extremely important book will be a source of up-to-date knowledge and practical advice that will greatly increase the expertise of the anesthesia practitioner for patients undergoing laparoscopy and thoracoscopy. I commend the editors and the authors for creating a valuable resource for the readers that will improve patient care and perioperative outcome.

Girish P Joshi, MBBS, MD, FFARCSI
Professor of Anesthesiology and Pain Management
Director of Perioperative Medicine and Ambulatory Anesthesia
University of Texas, Southwestern Medical Center, Dallas, Texas, USA

CHAPTER 1

History of Laparoscopic Procedures

"The cleaner and gentler the act of operation, the less pain the patient suffers, the smoother and quicker the convalescence, the more exquisite his healed wound, the happier his memory of the whole incident"
—Lord Moynihar (1920)

INTRODUCTION

The rising popularity of laparoscopic surgery is one of the most spectacular events in modern surgical history putting an end to the era of 'Big surgeons Big incisions'.

The history of laparoscopic revolution is quite intriguing and can be traced back to the tenth century AD. The Arabian physician Abulkasim (936-1013) is often credited with being the first to use reflected light to inspect an internal organ, the cervix.

Other investigators subsequently developed instruments to examine the nasal recesses and urinary bladder with artificial light and mirror. However, these interventions were associated with thermal tissue injury caused by the illuminating light source. This was probably the reason that cystoscopy which was developed in the nineteenth century preceded other forms of endoscopy, because of the coolant effect of water on the distal light source. The early pioneers introduced the trocars and cystoscopes directly into the peritoneal cavity.[1] At the turn of the 20th Century, Georg Kelling of Dresden (Fig. 1.1) used a cystoscope to observe the abdominal organs of dogs. He realized that pneumoperitoneum was very important for exposure and therefore used room air for insufflation of the peritoneal cavity. He, then, coined the term "celioscopy" to describe this technique.

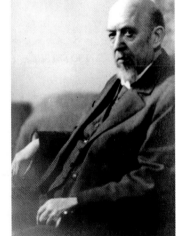

Fig. 1.1: Georg Kelling

The importance of photography to record the endoscopic findings was also recognized early and by 1874 Steen had modified existing cameras to record images of bladder pathology.

The first report of using this procedure in man was by the Swedish physician Hans Christian Jacobaeus in 1910 (Fig. 1.2). He is also credited with coining the term "laparoscopy".

These early procedures were entirely diagnostic in nature; the exposure obtained and the instruments available then did not permit any operative intervention.

Goetz and later Veress developed a spring loaded insufflation needle for the safe introduction of gas into the abdomen (pneumoperitoneum), which is used till today.[1]

One of the most important aspects of laparoscopy is the use of an optimal insufflating gas. The ideal gas for pneumoperitoneum should be non-toxic, inexpensive, colourless, nonflammable, readily soluble in blood and easily ventilated through the lungs.

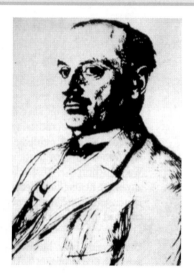

Fig. 1.2: Hans Christian Jacobaeus

Air was the first gas to be used for pneumoperitoneum and for several decades it was the insufflating gas of choice. It was cheap and easily available. Later oxygen was also used for a long time. However, both these gases support combustion and have a potential for gas embolism because they have a poor Ostwald's blood gas solubility coefficient (0.006, 0.013).

In the 1970s, nitrous oxide (N_2O) emerged as the gas preferred by gynaecologists because of its low cost and high turnover. However, it supports combustion, if mixed with methane (from the bowel).

In 1924, Richard Zollikofer of Switzerland promoted the use of CO_2 as the insufflating gas for pneumoperitoneum rather than filtered air or nitrogen, and which has now become the standard gas for pneumoperitoneum. It is relatively inert, permitting the use of electrocoagulation, and is readily absorbed by the peritoneal membrane (blood/gas solubility 0.48) and is readily exhaled via the lung. Previously, industrial impure CO_2 was employed, which led to arrhythmias. Nowadays with the availability of pure CO_2, these problems have been overcome.

Other alternative gases like helium, argon and xenon are inert but expensive and have a very low blood gas solubility (0.00018), and therefore, have high chances of gas embolism if accidental injection in to a blood vessel occurs.

Raoul Palmer in Paris (1944) (Fig. 1.3) stressed the importance of monitoring intra-abdominal pressure. It was another 20 years, however, before Kurt Semm in Kiel, Germany, developed an automatic insufflation device that monitored intra-abdominal pressure and gas flow. Prior to this time air was introduced into the peritoneal cavity by means of a syringe.[2]

With the development of safer insufflation needles as well as instruments for controlling gas flow during pneumoperitoneum, complications such as bowel perforations and injuries to retroperitoneal vessels were significantly reduced. Nevertheless, because laparoscopy was considered a "blind" procedure with an inherent risk of injury to intraperitoneal structures, acceptance was slow throughout Europe and North America.

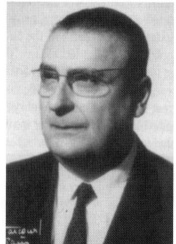

Fig. 1.3: Raoul Palmer

One of the most significant advances in rigid endoscopy was the development of the rod lens system in 1966 by the British optical physicist Hopkins. His design resulted in vastly improved image, brightness and clarity. These same principles are still utilized in laparoscopes today. The introduction of fiberoptic (cold) light sources in the early 1960s eliminated the risk of bowel burns caused by incandescent lighting.

Laparoscopic visualization of the abdominal cavity was once restricted to the individual directing the operative procedure and participation by other members of the surgical team was limited. Therefore, surgery was generally cumbersome and tedious because of the inability of the assistant(s) to effectively interact with the surgeon.

The development of a computer chip TV camera attached to the laparoscope in 1986 solved this problem and changed the face of surgery. It facilitated the extension of laparoscopic surgical techniques to more complicated procedures and also aided in training programmes. Easy documentation of the procedures became possible in videotapes.

Laparoscopic cholecystectomy for the purpose of removing gallstones in pigs was performed by Frimdberg in 1978 (personal communication, 1990).

Although in 1985, Erich Muhe of Germany (Fig. 1.4) described his technique of laparoscopic cholecystectomy in humans using the galloscope, it was in 1987 that the complete removal of a diseased gall bladder in a patient was performed by Mouret in Lyon, France. Interest in these procedures grew almost exponentially, largely fuelled by patient demands.[2]

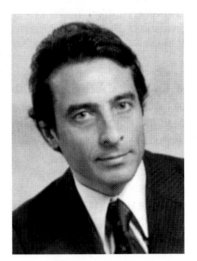

Fig. 1.4: Erich Muhe

Public awareness that endoscopic surgery is associated with diminished pain and cosmetic disfigurement as well as quicker resumption of normal activities accelerated its acceptance so much that all wanted the 'pin hole' surgery.[3]

Initially laparoscopic surgery was confined to short diagnostic gynaecological procedures, which were conducted on young healthy females. However, now they are conducted on older and high risk patients who were earlier considered unfit for laparotomy. Nowadays, more and more patients are being referred for surgery as soon as the diagnosis has been established, relegating medical treatment.

After the acceptance of laparoscopic procedures like cholecystectomy and appendicectomy, which are intraperitoneal procedures, there was a surge for extraperitoneal surgery which included inguinal hernia repair, adrenalectomy and nephrectomy including donor nephrectomy. These procedures necessitate extraperitoneal insufflation of gas with the attendant risk of increased CO_2 absorption.

It has become the standard surgical approach for gastroesophageal reflux disease (GERD), donor nephrectomy, adrenal tumours and morbid obesity. In fact, nowadays, there is hardly any absolute contraindication for a procedure to be performed laparoscopically, since the postoperative benefits far exceed the stress of intraoperative pathophysiological changes.[3]

The rapid development in the field of laparoscopic surgery, its increasing list of procedures and the inclusion of high risk patients would not have been possible without concurrent advancements in anaesthetic techniques. The anaesthesiologist has constantly strived to provide safe anaesthesia for these "minimal access" surgeries where there is "maximal trespass" of normal homeostasis. Extremes of patient positioning, insufflation of exogenous gases and increased intra-abdominal pressure (IAP) pose a severe strain on the patient's physiology. The anaesthesiologist, should be aware of these changes and the possible complications during the various procedures, so that early detection and prompt treatment may be instituted. The initial learning curve for a new procedure may be quite long and anaesthesiologists have patiently cooperated and encouraged their surgical colleagues till the surgical technique could be mastered.

Robotic systems for videoscopic surgery were introduced in the late 1990s to enhance manoeuvrability, visualization and ergonomics for minimally invasive thoracoscopic and laparoscopic surgery (Figs 1.5A and B).

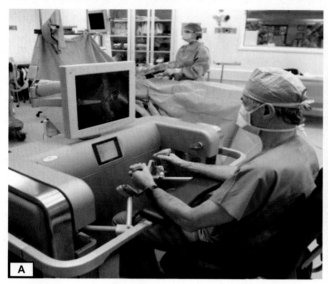
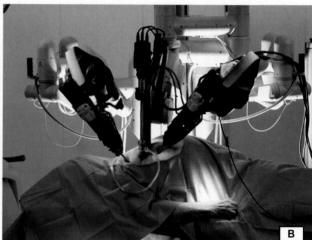

Figs 1.5A and B: Robotic surgery

The robot can reproduce a surgeon's movements rapidly, precisely and without tremor of the human hand or fatigue. They may be useful teaching modalities and might offer potential benefits in decreasing learning curves and increasing safety in a teaching environment. It allows the tutor to take over at any desired moment or to literally take the resident by the hand to guide him in videoscopic manoeuvres.

CONCLUSION

To conclude, advances in laparoscopic surgery have been associated with parallel development in anaesthetic approaches and a team approach among the surgeon, anaesthesiologist and theatre staff has been pivotal in its development. It is a challenging anaesthesia speciality and the anaesthesiologist must constantly improvise and evolve his approach in the face of an ever expanding domain of laparoscopic surgery.

REFERENCES

1. Grzegorz S. Litynski. Highlights in the History of Laparoscopy, 1996.
2. Karl A. Zucker. Surgical Laparoscopy, 1991.
3. Jayashree Sood, Lakshmi Jayaraman, V.P. Kumra. Endoscopic Surgery- Anaesthetic Challenges – A Historical Review. Indian J Anaesth 2006; 50(3): 178-82.

Gases Used in Laparoscopic Surgery

INTRODUCTION

In the past decade, the concept of minimal access surgery has changed the management of surgical patients and now almost every abdominal surgery is being performed laparoscopically.

One of the most important aspects of laparoscopy is the use of an optimal insufflating gas to create adequate space for the surgery. The ideal insufflating gas for pneumoperitoneum should be nontoxic, colourless, readily soluble in blood, easily ventilated through the lungs, nonflammable and inexpensive. Various gases that have been used in laparoscopic surgery are air, O_2, N_2O, N_2, CO_2, Argon and Helium.[1,2] (Table 2.1)

In the early days of laparoscopy, pneumoperitoneum was established by using room air or oxygen. The main consideration in choosing a gas is its solubility and its support to combustion. The more soluble a gas, a greater volume of it can be tolerated in case of embolism (Fig. 2.1).[3,4]

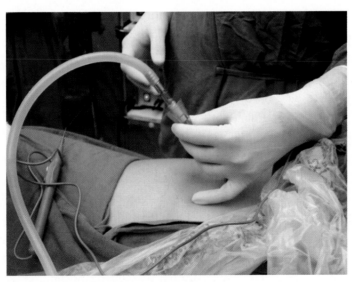

Fig. 2.1: Insufflation of gas

Table 2.1: Physical properties of common insufflation gases

Gas	Inert gas valency	Solubility (ml/100ml H_2O) 0°C	Combustion suppression
Air	-	2.92	-
N_2	3,5	2.3	+ + +
N_2O	-	130	-
CO_2	-	171	+ + +
He	0	0.97	+ + +
Ar	0	5.6	+ + +

AIR

Air is composed of various gases. Some of its constituents are constant (N_2-78%, O_2-21%, Ar-0.9%) while some change according to temperature and humidity (H_2O vapour 0-7% and CO_2 0.01-0.1%). It is colourless, odourless, tasteless and because it contains oxygen, it supports combustion. It was the first gas to be used for pneumoperitoneum, but because of low Ostwald's blood gas solubility coefficient (0.017) there were high chances of fatal venous air embolism if there was an inadvertent air entry into a blood vessel, and therefore, was withdrawn.[1,5]

OXYGEN

Like air, it is colourless, odourless and easily available gas. But since it supports combustion and has low blood gas solubility coefficient (0.036) it has been abandoned as an insufflating gas.

NITROGEN

Nitrogen is colourless, odourless, tasteless and an inert gas. It constitutes more than 78 per cent of atmospheric air. Rutherford discovered it in 1772. The greatest risk with N_2 is a fatal outcome in case of embolism.

NITROUS OXIDE (FIG. 2.2)

Colton was the first to administer N_2O in 1844 and in 1879 Paul Bert demonstrated its ability to cause general anaesthesia when administered under hyperbaric conditions.

It is a colourless, odourless and nonirritating gas with relatively low solubility in blood (0.42). At room temperature, it is very stable and inert chemically.

N_2O has no effect on pH and acid base changes, unlike CO_2.[6] It has no effect on MAP and pulse rate but causes a slight decrease in cardiac output. Pulmonary artery hypertension is not noted with N_2O pneumoperitoneum unlike with CO_2. It causes elevated plasma catecholamines. The effect of N_2O on hepatoportal circulation is negligible. It increases intracranial pressure, although it is less than that with CO_2. There is no difference in promotion of port-site tumour growth, when N_2O was used as insufflating gas, as compared with CO_2[7,8] (Table 2.2).

The transfer rate of N_2O into peritoneal cavity, after the creation of pneumoperitoneum with air, has been reported to be very rapid,[9] since it is 34 times more soluble than air. Although it is nonflammable, it may support combustion as actively as oxygen when present in proper concentration with flammable gases. Explosions have been reported with N_2O and methane (obtained from bowel) during intestinal surgery. If bowel perforation is recognized during laparoscopy, the peritoneal cavity should be vented and purged with CO_2, and N_2O removed from anaesthetic mixture.[10] These disadvantages led to renunciation of N_2O in favour of CO_2. However, diagnostic

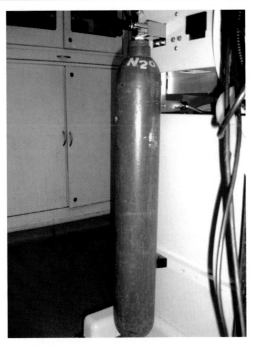

Fig. 2.2: Nitrous oxide cylinder

endoscopists prefer N_2O as an alternative gas for diagnostic laparoscopy under local anaesthesia, since it produces less peritoneal irritation and less pain, permitting laparoscopy in awake patients. Since electrocautery is not used under these circumstances, the risk of explosion is slight.[11,12]

CARBON DIOXIDE

CO_2 is the insufflating gas of choice as it is relatively inert, readily absorbed, does not support combustion and therefore, permits the use of electrocautery.[1,2]

It is highly soluble in blood with a solubility coefficient of 0.49 at 37°C. It is used from the central pipeline system or cylinders. It is carried in blood in three forms (Figs 2.3 and 2.4):

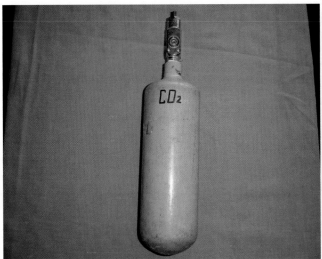

Fig. 2.3: Carbon dioxide cylinder

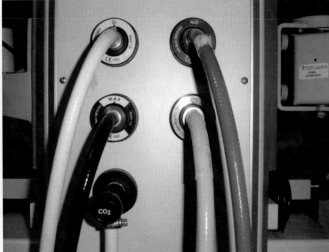

Fig. 2.4: Piped gas system

A great bulk in the form of bicarbonate (90%), a small amount is dissolved in plasma (5-10%) and rest is combined with protein, mainly haemoglobin.[13]

The CO_2 dissociation curve is steeper and more linear than oxyhaemoglobin dissociation curve, therefore, rise in partial pressure of CO_2 will cause a rise in the CO_2 carried by the blood to the lungs.[14,15]

Absorption of CO_2 during carboperitoneum causes minimal hypercarbia and acidaemia. Mild hypercarbia ($PaCO_2$ of 45-50 mmHg) has little impact on haemodynamic function while severe hypercarbia($PaCO_2$ 50-60 mmHg) alters cardiovascular function by stimulating the sympathetic nervous system with elevation in plasma catecholamines, which cause vasoconstriction, rise in heart rate, blood pressure and even dysrhythmias. The elevation of plasma cataecholamines has been largely attributed to an increase in IAP,[16-18] which is the most important factor responsible for the pathophysiological changes occurring during laparoscopy.

Marathe demonstrated that despite significant and large increases in the arterial $PaCO_2$ beginning at the intraabdominal pressure of 5 mmHg, haemodynamic alterations only occurred when the $PaCO_2$ increased by 33 per cent and no change in the mean arterial pressure was observed despite significant alterations in arterial $PaCO_2$ and increased intraabdominal pressure. This discrepancy suggests that deleterious effects in haemodynamic and cardiovascular function are due to both, long duration of CO_2 insufflation and high intraabdominal pressure.[14,17,18]

The increase in partial pressure of CO_2 in arterial blood ($PaCO_2$) during laparoscopic surgery was first described in 1969 in 15 patients who underwent pelvic laparoscopy using insufflation of CO_2 under halothane anaesthesia with a volume-limited constant minute-volume ventilation.[14] This effect is not seen with other insufflating gases and therefore, assumed to be a result of CO_2 absorption by peritoneum. CO_2 is then transported to the lungs where it is eliminated by ventilation.

In healthy individuals, the rise in pCO_2 and the concomitant drop in pH is clinically insignificant because of buffering systems and quick elimination by the lungs. During carboperitoneum, total body CO_2 excretion is increased, but O_2 consumption remains stable indicating that the source of CO_2 elevation is not due to hypermetabolism.[11,15]

Accumulation of CO_2 is associated with increase in pulmonary arterial pressure. In animal models, carboperitoneum causes pulmonary artery hypertension.[18]

CO_2 has least effect on hepatic blood flow. Renal blood flow has not been shown to be influenced by the type of insufflating gas.[19,20]

While the initial rise in ICP is due to mechanical factors of an increase in IAP, the rise in late stages (chemical) is due to the effects of hypercapnia which produces a reflex vasodilatation of CNS vasculature and increases ICP.[21-23]

Pilper suggested that the rate limiting factor for CO_2 absorption was local perfusion, but surface area also plays a role.[23] There is sufficient evidence in literature supporting a direct effect of elevated $PaCO_2$ on ICP.[22]

Westlate et al and Newton et al found that emphysematous patients with high $PaCO_2$ had elevated(CSF pressure and exhibited signs and symptoms of elevated ICP (headache, blurring of vision and papilledema).[23]

Fuji et al concluded that creation of CO_2 pneumoperitoneum in patients undergoing laparoscopic cholecystectomy produces hypercapnia and reflex vasodilatation of the CNS with increased flow through middle cerebral artery. They also showed that cerebral blood flow increased 10 min after peritoneal insufflation, parallel to the rise in $PaCO_2$. Likewise, 10 min after peritoneal deflation the blood flow and $PaCO_2$ returned to the baseline value. These observations were confirmed by Liu et al in a similar study. Some authors, have therefore, suggested that CO_2 pneumoperitoneum should be avoided in patients with intracranial lesion or head trauma[22] (Table 2.2).

Table 2.2: Clinical properties of laparoscopic insufflation gases

Gas	CO	PR	MAP	Pul. HTN	ICP	Hepatic flow	Renal flow	Venous emboli	Port-site metastasis
Air	↓	↔	↔	↔	–	–	–	–	–
N_2	↔	–	↔	↔	–	–	–	–	–
N_2O	↓	↔	↔	–	↑	–	–	–	↔
CO_2	↔↓	↔↓	↔↑	↓	↑	↓	↔	↔↑	↑
He	↔↓	↔↑	↔↑	↔↑	↑	↓	↓	↔	↔
Ar	↔↓	↔	↔	↔↑	–	↓	↓	↔	–

↔ No change
↓ Decrease
↑ Increase
- Not applicable

COMPLICATIONS DUE TO INSUFFLATION OF CO_2

- Pain in abdomen – peritoneal irritant
- Shoulder pain – due to carbonic acid
- Lowering the threshold for arrhythmias in the presence of halogenated hydrocarbons specially halothane.
- Venous gas embolism
- Promotion of port site tumour growth

Gas embolism: It is a rare but potentially lethal complication of laparoscopic surgery. The consequences of venous gas embolism is dependent on blood gas solubility coefficient, i.e. Oswald's number of the gas. The mechanism and true incidence of gas embolism during laparoscopy is unknown. Philips reported 15 instances of gas embolism during 523 gynaecologic laparoscopies.[24] Multiple cases of significant gas embolism during gynaecologic laparoscopy, and cases of fatal CO_2 gas embolism during laparoscopic upper abdominal surgery including cholecystectomy have been reported.[5,24,25]

The outcome depends on both the type and quantity of gas used. Since CO_2 is more soluble in blood than N_2O or air, a greater volume of CO_2 embolism can be tolerated when compared with N_2O or air embolism. The complication occurs when the venous pressure is lower than the atmospheric pressure (i.e. during neurological and gynaecologic procedures) or when gas is forced inadvertently under pressure during laparoscopic procedures. The gas entering the vein may occlude the right ventricle, causing right cardiac failure, PAH and collapse of systemic arterial pressure.[25]

If gas embolus is suspected the surgeon is alerted, insufflation stopped and insufflation gas released, 100 per cent oxygen supplied, the patient should be placed in left lateral, head down position(Durant's), if possible, Dysrhythmias managed and closed chest compressions are initiated if necessary. Venous catheters may be placed for superior vena cava (SVC), right atrial, ventricle and outflow tract gas aspiration. The administration of N_2O as an anesthetic agent should be stopped since it rapidly enters the gas space containing CO_2, thus adding to the gas volume.

PROMOTION OF PORT-SITE TUMOUR GROWTH

The mechanism by which intra-abdominal insufflation promotes port-site malignant cell growth is not completely understood. The actual reported incidence ranges from 1 to 11 per cent,[24] The various theories proposed are:
1. The degree of tumour manipulation and the technical skills of surgeon, both leading to mechanical implantation (as during retrieval of a specimen through the trocar).

2. Specific properties of the tumour : stage and aggressiveness.

3. Components of laparoscopic technique: high IAP and gas turbulence produce a spray effect (which explains the finding of metastases in port sites not used during manipulation of tumour) and type of gas used.

Carboperitoneum has been implicated in port-site metastasis because the immune response is suppressed in malignancy and inflammatory mediators are released by the peritoneum.

Growth of tumour at port-sites is stimulated more by carboperitoneum than by gasless laparoscopy[27] or laparotomy although this was not a universal finding. One study has found that air promotes intraperitoneal growth, whereas CO_2 was associated with subcutaneous growth.[26,27,28]

HELIUM

In 1886, helium was discovered in the gaseous atmosphere surrounding the Sun by the French astronomer Pierre Jansen, who detected a bright yellow line in the spectrum of the solar chromosphere during an eclipse.

The second lightest element (after hydrogen), helium is a colourless, odourless and tasteless gas that changes to a liquid at -268.90°C (-4520F).[29,30] Chemically inert, group O (noble gases), helium has low density, low solubility (0.00098) and high thermal conductivity. In dry air, it is present in a concentration of 5.24 ppm and in atmosphere in approximately 1 part per 2,00,000.[29,30]

As an insufflating gas, helium causes minimal hypercarbia and changes in pH during laparoscopy. A decrease in base excess[15,31] is seen which is probably related more to the IAP than to the pharmacologic properties of the gas. Helium has minor effects on the cardiovascular status.[18] There is minimal increase in pulse rate and mean arterial pressure and mean pulmonary artery wedge pressure.[32]

Insufflation with helium does not result in an increase in ventilation requirement although it is associated with a mean rise in peak airway pressure. Therefore, helium pneumoperitoneum is not associated with significant hypercarbia, respiratory acidosis or increased pulmonary artery pressure[2] (Table 2.2).

Elevated plasma catecholamines have been documented during pneumoperitoneum with helium although to a slightly lesser degree but more comparative studies are required. Helium has no effect on renal blood flow but slightly decreases the hepatic blood flow.[7] Helium produces a small increase in intracranial pressure.[33]

Due to its very low blood gas solubility venous gas emboli have a greater haemodynamic aftermath with helium than with CO_2 or N_2O. Nevertheless, helium is more diffusible than CO_2 because of its low density and this may aid in the dissolution of small helium emboli in the blood to a degree approaching that of CO_2.[25] Emboli due to CO_2 and helium do not cause bronchoconstriction. Helium emboli may therefore, behave in a similar manner to CO_2 because of rapid diffusibility and minimal effects on pulmonary mechanics.

No promotion of port-site tumour growth has been suggested with helium.[8,28]

Therefore, to maintain the established benefits of minimal access surgery in high risk patients, use of helium has been suggested for creating pneumoperitoneum. The absence of hypercarbia, acidemia and pulmonary hypertension that characterize carboperitoneum suggests that helium may be the insufflating agent of choice in patients with significant cardiopulmonary disease.

ARGON

A colourless, odourless, tasteless, monoatomic gas of group O(61), Argon (Ar) accounts for 0.94 per cent of air. Its presence in air was suspected by Cavendish in 1785 and confirmed by Lord Rayleigh and Sir William Ramsay in 1894. It was first of the noble gases discovered on earth. Argon is 2.5 times as soluble in water as

Table 2.3: Summary of major characteristics of common insufflation gases

Gas	Major advantage	Major disadvantage	Suggested application
Air	Acid-base and haemodynamic changes (+).	Dissolves slowly in case of emboli. Promotes port-site tumour growth.	- Only in research protocol studies
N_2	Acid-base and haemodynamic changes(+).	Dissolves slowly in case of emboli.	- Only in research protocol studies
N_2O	Applicable with LA/RA. Acid-base & haemodynamic changes(+)	Support combustion with methane.	- LA/RA cases - Cases without electrocautery
CO_2	Dissolves quickly in case of emboli. Solubility coefficient 0.48	Peritoneal irritation, acidemia, ↑ ICP, port-site metastasis(+)	- Most laparoscopic surgeries
He	Acid-base & haemodynamic changes(+) Port-site tumour growth (-).	Dissolves slowly in case of emboli. High thermal conductivity.	- Only in research protocol studies - To preserve hepatic blood flow - Laparoscopic cancer cases
Ar	Acid-base and haemodynamic changes (+).	Dissolves slowly in case of emboli. ↓ Liver blood flow.	- Only in research protocol studies

N_2 and approximately as soluble as O_2. The outermost shell of argon has eight electrons making it exceedingly stable and thus, chemically inert.

Argon has no effect on pH or acid-base status.[31] Pneumoperitoneum with argon increases vascular resistance and mean arterial pressure more than carboperitoneum and reduces the stroke volume. It does not cause pulmonary arterial hypertension. Argon does not increase the ICP. Argon induces maximum decrease in hepatic blood flow as compared with other insufflatory gases. Renal blood flow is not influenced. Argon emboli have greater haemodynamic aftermath than more soluble gases (Table 2.2). Due to decreased solubility in blood there is rapid respiratory and metabolic acidosis resulting in death in most cases.[31] Increased incidence of port-site metastasis has been reported with argon insufflation although no viable mechanism has been contributed to it and therefore more comparative studies with other insufflating gases are required.[7,8]

CONCLUSIONS

Therefore, an ideal laparoscopic insufflation gas should be readily available, relatively inexpensive, colourless, highly soluble in plasma and suitable for use in most patients and procedures. It should be chemically stable, physiologically inert and non explosive.

Because CO_2 possesses many of the preceding characteristics, it is the most widely used gas for insufflation. Hb has more affinity for CO_2 than for other gases, adding a higher safety margin in the rare event of gas embolism.

N_2O is not a part of acid-base buffer system and has only weak haemodynamic effects. The main drawback with N_2O is the ability to cause combustion.

Helium has minimum physiologic and respiratory effects, but its low water and plasma solubility makes it dangerous in the event of gas emboli.

In conclusion, CO_2 maintains its dominant role as the primary insufflating gas in laparoscopy. It has been shown to be good and safe choice. N_2O can be used when general anaesthesia is unwarranted or acid-base changes are a primary consideration. He, Ar, Air and N_2 should be used only in protocol studies mainly because of their potential of gas emboli and their lack of significant benefit over CO_2 or N_2O (Table 2.3).

REFERENCES

1. Menes T, Spivak H. Laparoscopy: searching for the proper insufflation gas. Surg Endosc 2000;14(1l): 1050-6. Review.

2. Neuhaus SJ, Gupta A, Watson DI. Heiium and other alternative insufflation gases for laparoscopy. Surg Endosc 2001;15(6): 553-60. Epub 2001 Apr 3. Review.

3. Khan M, Alkalay I, Stein M. Acute changes in lung mechanics following pulmonary emboli of various gases in dogs. J Appl Physiol 1972;33:774-7.

4. Roberts M, Mathiesen K, Wolfe B. Venous gas embolization model for laparoscopic surgery. Surg Endosc 1995; 9: A210.

5. Graff TD, Arbegast NR, Phillips DC, Harris LC, et al. Gas embolism: a comparative study of air and carbon dioxide as embolic agents in the systemic venous system. Am J Obstet Gynecol 1959;78:259-63.

6. Magno R, Medegard A, Bengtsson R, Tronstad SE. Acid-base balance during laparoscopy. Acta Obstet Gynaecol Scand 1979;58:81.

7. Gupta A, Watson DI, Ellis T, Jamieson GG. Tumour implantation, following laparoscopy using different insufflation gases. ANZ J Surg 2002;72(4):254-7.

8. Hopkins MP, von Gruenigen V, Haller NA, Holda S. The effect of various insufflation gases on tumor Implantation in an animal model. Am J Obstet Gynecol 2002;187(4):994-6.

9. Brodsky JB, Lemmens HJ, Collins JS, Morton JM, et al. Nitrous oxide and laparoscopic bariatric surgery. Obes Surg 2005; 15(4):494-6.

10. Aitola P, Airo I, Kaukinen S, Ylitalo P. Comparison of N_2O and CO_2 pneumoperitoneums during laparoscopic cholecystectomy with special reference to postoperative pain. Surg Laparosc Endosc. 1998;8(2):140-4.

11. El-Kady A, Abd-El-Razek M. Intraperitoneal explosion during female sterilization by laparoscopic electrocoagulation. Int J Gynaecol Obstet 1976;14:487-8.

12. Gunatilake D. Fatal intraperitoneal explosion during electrocoagulation via laparoscopy. Int J Gnaecol Obstet 1978;15: 353-7.

13. Brackman MR, Finelli FC, Light T, Llorente O, et al. Helium pneumoperitoneum ameliorates hypercarbia and acidosis associated ith carbon dioxide insufflation during laparoscopic gastric bypass in pigs. Obes Surg 2003;13(5):768-71.

14. Holthausen UH, Nagelschmidt M, Troidl H. CO_2 pneumoperitonieum: what we know and what we need to know. World J Surg. 1999;23(8):794-800. (Review)

15. Magno R, Medegard A, Bengtsson R, Tronstad SE. Acid-base balance during laparoscopy. Acta Obstet Gynecol Scand 1979; 58:81-6.

16. De Waal EE, Kalkman CJ. Haemodynamic changes during low-pressure carbon dioxide pneumoperitoneum in young children. Paediatr Anaesth 2003;13(1):18-25.

17. Gutt CN, Oniu T, Mehrabi A, Schemmer P, et al. Circulatory and respiratory complications of carbon dioxide insufflation. Dig Surg. 2004; 21(2): 95-105. Epub 2004 Feb 27. Review.

18. Hazebroek EJ, Haitsma JJ, Lachmann B, Steyerberg EW, et al. Impact of carbon dioxide and helium insufflation on cardiorespiratory function during prolonged pneumoperitoneum in an experimental rat model. . Surg Endosc 2002;16(7): 1073-8. Epub 2002 Apr 9.

19. Hazebroek EJ, de Bruin RW, Bouvy ND, van Duikeren S, et al. Short-term impact of carbon dioxide, helium, and gasless laparoscopic donor nephrectomy on renal function and histomorphology in donor and recipient. Surg Endosc 2002;16(2): 245-51. Epub 2001 Nov 16.

20. Meierhenrich R, Gauss A, Vandenesch P, Georgieff M, et al. The effects of intraabdominally insufflated carbon dioxide on hepatic blood flow during laparoscopic surgery assessed by transesophageai echocardiography. Anesth Analg 2005;100(2): 340-7.

21. Halverson A, Buchanan R, Jacobs L, Shayani V, et al. Evaluation of mechanism of increased intracranial pressure with insufflation. Surg Endosc 1998;12(3):266-9.

22. Mobbs RJ, Yang MO. The dangers of diagnostic laparoscopy in the head injured patient. J Clin Neurosci 2002; 9(5): 592-3.

23. Moncure M, Salem R, Moncure K, Testaiuti M, et al. Central nervous system metabolic and physiologic effects of laparoscopy. Am Surg 1999;65(2):168-72.

24. Kama NA. Influence of nitrous oxide anesthesia on venous gas embolism with carbon dioxide and helium during pneumoperitoneum. Surg Endose 2001;15(10):1237-8.

25. Lantz PE, Smith JD. Fatal carbon dioxide embolism complicating attempted laparoscopic cholecystectomy – case report and literature review. J Forensic Sci 1994;39(6):1468-80. Review.

26. Curet MJ. Port site metastases. Am J Surg. 2004;187(6):705-12. Review.

27. Bouvy ND, Giuffrida MC, Tseng LN, Steyerberg EW, et al. Effects of carbon dioxide pneumoperitoneum, air pneumoperitoneum, and gasless laparoscopy on body weight and tumor growth. Arch Surg 1998; 133(6):632-6.

28. Neuhaus SJ, Watson DI, Ellis T, Rowland R, et al. Wound metastasis after laparoscopy with different insufflation gases. Surgery 1998; 123(5): 579-83.

29. Handbook of Chemistry and Physics, 78th Edn 1997-1998. The Chemical rubber Co, Cleveland, Ohio. pp 4-20, 6-201.

30. The Merck Index; 11th Edn 1989; pp 123-24, 274.

31. Kuntz C, Wunsch A, Bodeker C, Bay F, et al. Effect of pressure and gastype on intraabdominal, subcutaneous, and blood pH in laparoscopy. Surg Endosc 2000;14(4):361-71.

32. McMahon AJ, Baxter JN, Murray W, Imrie CW, et al. Helium pneumoperitoneum for laparoscopic cholecystectomy: ventilatory and blood gas changes. Br J Surg 1994;81(7):1033-6.

33. Schob OM, Allen DC, Benzel E, Curet MJ, et al. A comparison of the pathophysiologic effects of carbon dioxide, nitrous oxide; and helium pneumoperitoneum on intracranial pressure. Am J Surg 1996;172(3):248-53.

CHAPTER 3

Ideal IAP during Laparoscopy

INTRODUCTION

Endoscopy has been used for examination of organs since 912-1013 A.D.[1] In 1901, Kelling performed abdominal endoscopy on a dog using air to fill the abdominal cavity.[2] He coined the term 'Celioscopy' for this technique. Swedish physician Jacobaeus,[3] in 1910 then used this procedure for the first time in human beings.

The early pioneers introduced the trocars and cystoscopes directly into the peritoneal cavity. It was another 30 years before pneumoperitoneum was used prior to insertion of the first cannula. Goetz (1981)[1] and later Veress (1938) developed the automatic insufflating needle to establish pneumoperitoneum. In 1944, Raoul Palmer advocated the importance of monitoring intra-abdominal pressure (IAP).[4] 20 years later, Kurt Semm in Kiel, Germany developed an automatic insufflation (Fig. 3.1) device that monitored abdominal pressure and gas flow.[4]

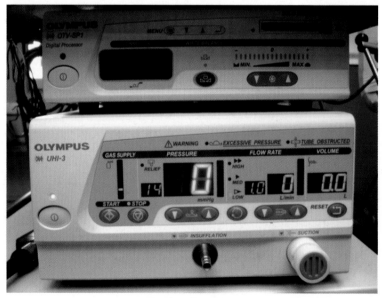

Fig. 3.1: Insufflator

Laparoscopic procedures represent a new and exciting development in the management of several surgical problems. This technique avoids large abdominal incisions which are associated with postoperative pain, shortens hospital stay and results in minimal morbidity and mortality. Laparoscopy requires the establishment of pneumoperitoneum. Air, oxygen, nitrous oxide, helium have all been used for this purpose but none of them have been proved to be ideal. Carbon dioxide though not physiologically inert, is the most common gas used to induce pneumoperitoneum. The insufflation of the gas (Fig. 3.2) into the peritoneal cavity results in the rise of intra-abdominal pressure and leads to complex physiological changes affecting a number of homeostatic systems.

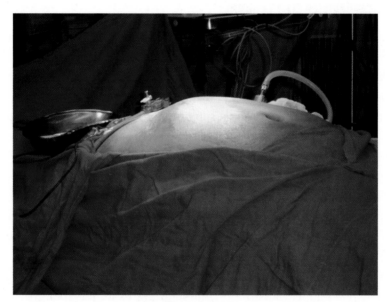

Fig. 3.2: Pneumoperitoneum

WHAT IS THE INTRA-ABDOMINAL PRESSURE?

Abdomen is a closed cavity consisting of a movable diaphragm, costal arch, contracting abdominal muscles and the intestines. The intra-abdominal pressure (IAP) is the steady pressure within this closed cavity and it varies with respiration. The normal values of IAP are 0-5 mmHg, with values >12 mmHg are considered to be increased.[5] Raised IAP has deleterious effects which have now been demonstrated in numerous human and animal studies.[6,7]

The physiological changes observed during pneumoperitoneum are related to patient position (degree of Trendelenburg or reverse Trendelenburg used), biochemical changes caused by introduction of insufflating gas (CO_2) and mechanical changes caused by raised intraabdominal pressure. Several pathophysiological changes are seen on different systems of the body depending on the level of intra-abdominal pressure. The effects can be summarized as that of low (7-11 mmHg), standard (12-15 mmHg) or high (>15 mmHg) IAP.

PHYSIOLOGICAL EFFECTS AT LOW IAP (7-10 mmHG)

Although very few studies have investigated the effect of low intraabdominal pressure on homeostatic mechanisms but some studies[8] demonstrate fewer adverse haemodynamic effects with low intraabdominal pressure. Haemodynamic changes occurring from raised IAP are variable and unpredictable. Upto 10 mmHg IAP, the haemodynamic and metabolic parameters do not change significantly.[6] Hepatic blood flow, hepatic arterial, portal and microvascular perfusion are all affected with a significant reduction in flow occurring with intraabdominal pressures as low as 10 mmHg.[9] Liver dysfunction as evidenced by raised liver enzymes following pneumoperitoneum has been suggested at standard intraabdominal pressure. Low intraabdominal pressure has been shown to result in significant decrease in postoperative changes in liver function tests.[10] Barczynski et al[11] demonstrated in their study lower pain scores, lower incidence of shoulder tip pain and better quality of life within 7 days following laparoscopic surgery, keeping intra-abdominal pressure as low as 7 mmHg. They also demonstrated less postoperative nausea and vomiting in low pressure group compared to standard pressure.

PHYSIOLOGICAL EFFECTS AT STANDARD IAP (12-15 mmHG)

Studies have demonstrated that upto IAP 15 mmHg the cardiac output does not change although the dp/dt values get significantly reduced.[6] There is a reduction in the stroke volume due to the depressant effect of carbon dioxide on the myocardial contractility and rise in the afterload. At standard IAP there is compression of the capacitance vessels as opposed to collapse resulting in relative increase in venous return.[12] The blood flow velocity in the femoral vein gets reduced during laparoscopic surgery at 14 mmHg IAP, which can disturb venous return and stagnate blood flow predisposing to thromboembolism.[13] Mean arterial blood pressure may rise initially till an IAP 15 mmHg[6,14] due to shunting of blood away from the abdominal cavity but thereafter normalises or decreases. Heart rate may rise transiently in response to increase in systemic vascular resistance and arterial blood pressure to maintain cardiac output but most studies have reported no significant long term changes in heart rate with laparoscopy.[15] Joris et al[16] observed a significant increase in mean arterial pressure (35%) after peritoneal insufflation along with an increase of systemic vascular resistance (65%) and pulmonary vascular resistance (90%) and a decrease in cardiac index (20%) while the pulmonary capillary wedge pressure and central venous pressure increased. In a small subset (0.5%) of otherwise healthy patients, however, bradycardia and asystole can occur during CO_2 insufflation and pneumoperitoneum.[17-19] Although the exact mechanism is not clear, it is believed that direct pressure on the vagus nerve causes a stimulatory parasympathetic effect that leads to a drop in heart rate.[20]

Pneumoperitoneum leads to cephalad shift of the diaphragm, reduced lung expansion, reduced diaphragmatic excursion causing pattern of restrictive lung disease. There is a fall in functional residual capacity, tidal volume and minute ventilation.[5,21-24] Pulmonary vascular resistance increases, uneven distribution of ventilation to non dependent parts of the lungs produces ventilation perfusion mismatch, hypoxia and hypercarbia.[25] An IAP of 15 mmHg also raises the $PaCO_2$ by 10 mmHg and decreases lung compliance by 25 per cent.[26]

Oliguria (urine output <0.5 ml/kg/hr) has been usually seen during laparoscopy.[27] As IAP increases, the renal dysfunction occurs attributable to compression on the renal vasculature, the renal parenchyma and the inferior vena cava leading to decreasing renal blood flow (RBF), cortical and medullary perfusion and renal venous outflow.[28] As IAP approaches 15 mmHg there is a pressure dependent reduction in the glomerular filtration rate (GFR), RBF, creatinine clearance, sodium excretion and urine output.[29,30] At IAP 15 mmHg, urine output decreases by as much as 63 per cent, GFR by 21 per cent and RBF by 26 per cent.[31,32] At all levels of increasing IAP the serum potassium level rises.[30] Apart from renal compression there is a release of neurohormonal factors as renin, aldosterone, endothelin and antidiuretic hormone resulting in systemic vasoconstriction and fluid retention.[15,32-34] Regional blood flow to all intra-abdominal organs including hepatic, mesenteric, intestinal mucosa, stomach, duodenum, pancreas and spleen is reduced as IAP approaches 15 mmHg. However, the blood flow to adrenal glands is preserved. The reduction in blood flow results in tissue hypoxia and intestinal swelling.[21-24] Hepatic perfusion has a unique autoregulatory mechanism known as "hepatic arterial buffer response (HABR).[35] Richter et al[36] demonstrated loss of this response at an intra-abdominal pressure of 12-15 mmHg. Hypertension induced hepatic ischaemia secondary to raised intra-abdominal pressure appears to be the cause. Jakimowicz et al also demonstrated a significant reduction in portal venous flow using a Laser-Doppler technique.[37] A few studies have demonstrated increased levels of aminotransferase (ALT and AST), alcohol dehydrogenase and glutathione S-transferase. However, this phenomenon is transient with these enzymes returning to normal values within 1-3 days.[38-40] Impairment of microcirculation occurs with pressures as low as 15 mmHg and within a short time interval (60 minutes).[41] Hence, increasing IAP may result in visceral hypoperfusion, secondary bacterial translocation as well as impaired wound healing.[42-44]

Rise in intra-abdominal pressure compresses inferior vena cava and increases lumbar spinal pressure by reducing drainage from the lumbar plexus, thereby increasing intracranial pressure and intraocular pressure.[45] Raised intra-abdominal pressure (15 mmHg) results in increased cerebral blood flow.[6] Hypercapnia associated with laparoscopy further produces reflex vasodilatation in the central nervous system attributing to increase in the intracranial pressure.[46]

PHYSIOLOGICAL EFFECTS AT HIGH IAP (>15mmHG)

Studies demonstrate enhanced physiological changes with rising intra-abdominal pressure. At 20 mmHg the cardiac output decreases and the systemic vascular resistance increases due to the collapse of the capacitance vessels. There is decrease in blood flow due to compression of the inferior vena cava[7,47] as IAP approaches 20 mmHg, resulting in hypotension which is a serious complication in upto 13 per cent of laparoscopies. High intrathoracic pressure during intermittent positive pressure ventilation further impairs venous return and cardiac output particularly if positive end expiratory pressure is also applied. Pulmonary capillary wedge pressure, CVP, right and left side cardiac filling pressures usually increase with IAP >20 mmHg.[6,15,21-24] Studies have shown that cardiac output changes during raised intra-abdominal pressure depend on the intravascular volume.[48] An IAP of 40 mmHg results in 53 per cent decrease in cardiac output in hypovolemic animals, 17 per cent decrease in normovolemic animals and 50 per cent decrease in hypervolemic animals.

A deterioration in myocardial contractility is associated with a defect in cardiac metabolism. A metabolically stable heart is able to consume more oxygen when exposed to any stress, indicating that it increases myocardial oxygen consumption and oxygen extraction with less lactate accumulation in the myocardium. During the occurrence of any shift to anaerobic metabolism, myocardial oxygen extraction and myocardial lactate extraction decrease. As a result of these changes myocardial tissue lactate increases and tissue ATP decreases. At IAP >15 mmHg myocardial oxygen consumption has shown to be reduced,[6] as seen by the decrease in the ATP in the myocardial tissue. A drop in the ATP impairs relaxation of the heart.

Pneumoperitoneum associated with IAP of 15-20 mmHg is associated with increase in the peak and plateau alveolar pressures as much as 50 and 81 per cent respectively.[15,49] Decreased functional residual capacity promotes ventilation perfusion mismatch and an intrapulmonary shunting which may lead to hypoxemia, this however, rarely occurs in patients with normal preoperative pulmonary function. Ventilation with positive end-expiratory pressure (PEEP) significantly improves pulmonary gas exchange and preserves arterial oxygenation during prolonged pneumoperitoneum,[50] but PEEP in presence of elevated intra-abdominal pressure increases intrathoracic pressure and produces marked reduction in cardiac output. Therefore, it should be applied cautiously. A modern ventilation technique is the 'alveolar recruitment strategy' consisting of manual ventilation to an airway pressure of 40 cm H_2O for 10 breaths over 1 min., followed by usual mechanical ventilation with mild positive end-expiratory pressure (5 cm H_2O). This improves arterial oxygenation without cardiovascular compromise or respiratory complications.[51]

A 60 per cent decrease in portal venous blood flow is seen with IAP > 20 mmHg resulting in liver dysfunction.[52] Prolonged renal hypoperfusion as evidenced by raised IAP carries the risk of acute tubular necrosis (ATN). Renal dysfunction with resulting anuria has been reported with IAP of 20-25 mmHg,[5,21-24] although in patients with preexisting renal disease changes secondary to raised IAP have not been associated with renal failure as a long term effect.[32,33,53,54] The rise in serum potassium levels is pronounced with IAP > 15 mmHg but the values do not reach levels that would be considered clinically harmful.[30] Renal compression and neuroendocrine response associated with raised IAP makes fluid management controversial in laparoscopic live donor nephrectomy. In order to maintain renal perfusion and avoid deleterious effects on graft function, some investigators have suggested the use of isotonic and hypertonic intravascular volume expansion for transplant cases.[52] An alternative to volume expansion is to decrease IAP as much as visualisation will allow.

Some prophylactic measures have also been suggested at low dose dopamine 2 mcg/kg/min to prevent ATN following long lasting pneumoperitoneum.[55] Warm insufflation of CO_2 has been associated with local renal vasodilation resulting in higher urine output such that it may be beneficial to patients with borderline renal function. Esmolol inhibits release of renin and blunts the pressor response to induction and maintenance of pneumoperitoneum. Therefore, it may protect the kidneys against renal ischaemia during laparoscopy.[56]

DISADVANTAGES OF HIGH IAP

Each laparoscopic surgical procedure requires establishment of an appropriately large working space in the abdominal cavity to allow safe access to the abdominal organs. This working space is mostly created by creating a pneumoperitoneum. It is commonly believed that a higher intra-abdominal pressure of pneumoperitoneum results in better exposure of the surgical field, better access to the abdominal contents providing a safe surgical approach. But, this pressure can cause adverse haemodynamic consequences, pulmonary and hepatorenal dysfunction. Patients are liable to develop thrombosis secondary to venous stasis. Incidence of nausea and vomiting is greater as well as the use of analgesic in the postoperative period is higher. The increased morbidity in terms of delayed return to normal activities stresses the importance of limiting the raised intra-abdominal pressure.

ADVANTAGES OF LOW IAP

Barcynski et al hypothesised that largest volume of gas is pumped into the peritoneal cavity until the IAP value of 7-8 mmHg is achieved. A further increase of pressure leads to a geometrically decreasing increment of pneumoperitoneum volume. At this value of IAP the adverse haemodynamic effects are low. It has also been demonstrated that this pressure is associated with less postoperative pain, less shoulder tip pain and a better quality of life after 7 days. Patients with cardiorespiratory embarrassment, hepatorenal compromise and the elderly would be specially benefited by limiting the IAP.

In order to limit these problems especially in elderly patients with chronic conditions of cardiorespiratory dysfunctions another method of creating working space was developed in which the abdominal integument is lifted (e.g. **laparolift, laparotensor**) without the need for employing any gas. In this technique, working space is established by elevating the anterior part of the abdominal wall 10-15 cm by a mechanical retractor and no gas is used. The intra-abdominal pressure remains normal and hence the adverse effects of increased IAP and absorbed CO_2 are avoided. Studies[57] support lower changes in heart rate, mean arterial pressure, airway pressure and arterial PCO_2 with the gasless technique. This technique has negligible effect on urine output.[30] This may center clinical benefits on patients with severe comorbidity who present for laparoscopic surgery. Some operators employ 4 mmHg pneumoperitoneum additionally combined with abdominal integument lifting. However, the marked increased technical difficulty of laparoscopy using gasless technique, increased operating time and lack of clinical benefit with regard to postoperative pain and nausea makes laparoscopy with CO_2 a preferable technique over gasless method.

CONCLUSIONS

Thus, in view of the adverse effects as described herein by maintaining increased intra-abdominal pressure over prolonged periods such as cardiorespiratory compromise, renal and hepatic dysfunction, it is advisable to limit the intra-abdominal pressure to around 12 mmHg as much as a good exposure would allow. Each laparoscopic procedure has to be individualised, a single value of intra-abdominal pressure for all cases cannot be ascertained.

CLINICAL PEARLS

1. IAP that has minimal effects on haemodynamics ≤ 12 mmHg
2. Limit IAP in elderly, patients with cardiorespiratory compromise, hepatorenal dysfunction.
3. Less postoperative pain and better quality of life after 7 days of surgery by limiting IAP.
4. Low pressure pneumoperitoneum is superior to laparolift.

REFERENCES

1. Vitale GC, Sanfllippo JS, Penissat J. Kurt Semm. The history of Endoscopy Laparoscopic surgery. An atlas for general surgeons 1995; 3-11.
2. Kelling G. Uber Oesophagoskopie, Gastroskopie and Colioskopie. Munch Med Wochenschr 1901; 49: 21-24.
3. Jacobaeus HC, Über die Möglichkeit, die Zystoskopic bei Untersuchung seroser Hohlungen anzuwenden. Munch Med Wochenschr 1910; 57: 2090-92.
4. Filipi CJ, Fitzgibbons Jr. RJ, Salerno GM. Historical Review: Diagnostic laparoscopy to laparoscopic cholecystectomy and beyond. Surgical Laparoscopy ed. Karl A. Zucker. 1991; 3-21.
5. Malbrain MLNG. Intra-abdominal pressure in the ICU: clinical tool or toy? In: Vincent JL (ed) Year Book of Intensive Care and Emergency Medicine. Springer-Verlag, Berlin. 2001; 547-85.
6. Katraoglu SF, Atalay F, Keskin A, et al. Myocardial hemodynamic and metabolic changes during abdominal insufflation with carbon dioxide. Eur Surg Res 1998; 30: 205-13.
7. Ivankovich AD, Miletich DJ, Albrecht RF, et al. Cardiovascular effects of intraperitoneal insufflation with carbon dioxide and nitrous oxide in the dog. Anesthesiology 1975; 42: 281-87.
8. Davides D, Birbas K, Vezakis A, McMahon MJ. Routine low-pressure pneumoperitoneum during laparoscopic cholecystectomy. Surg Endosc 1999; 13: 887-9.
9. Diebel LN, Wilson FR, Dulchavski SA, Saxe J. Effects of increased blood flow. J Trauma 1992; 33: 279-83.
10. Hasukie S. Postoperative changes in liver function tests: a randomised comparison of low and high pressure laparoscopic cholecystectomy: Surg Endosc 2005;19:1451-5.
11. Barczynski M, Herman RM. A prospective randomized trial on comparison of low-pressure (LP) and standard-pressure (SP) pneumoperitoneum for laparoscopic cholecystectomy. Surg Endosc 2003;17(4)533-8.
12. Wolf JS Jr, Stoller ML. The physiology of laparoscopy: basic principles, complications and other considerations. J Urol 1994; 152: 294-302.
13. Goodwin AT, Swift RI, Smart P, Chadwick SJD. Effects of pneumoperitoneum and position of patient on femoral vein hemodynamics during laparoscopic surgery. Minim Invasive Ther 1994; 3: 337-39.

14. Ho SA, Gunther RA, Wolfe BM. Intraperitoneal carbon dioxide insufflation and cardiopulmonary functions. Arch Surg 1992; 127: 928-33.

15. O'Malley C, Cunningham AJ. Physiologic changes during laparoscopy. Anesthesiol Clin N Am 2001; 19(1): 1-19.

16. Joris JL, Noirot DP, Legrand MJ, Jacquet NJ, et al. Hemodynamic changes during laparoscopic cholecystectomy. Anesth Analg 1993; 75: 1067-71.

17. McKenzie R, Wadhwa RK, Bedger RC. Noninvasive measurement of cardiac output during laparoscopy. J Reprod Med 1980; 24:247-50.

18. Reed DN Jr, Nourse P. Untoward cardiac changes during CO_2 insufflation in laparoscopic cholecystectomies in low risk patients. J Laparo Endosc Adv Surg tech A. 1998; 8(2): 109-14.

19. Reed DN Jr, Duff JL. Persistent occurrence of bradycardia during laparoscopic cholecystectomies in low risk patients. Dig Surg 2000; 15(5): 513-17.

20. Wolf JS Jr, Stoller ML, eds. Laparoscopic Surgery. In: Tanagho EA, Mc Aninch JW. Smith's General Urology, 16th ed New York, NY: Lange Medical books / McGraw- Hill Companies, Inc: 2004; 140-62.

21. Sugrue M, Hilman KM. Intra-abdominal hypertension and intensive care. In: Vincent JL (ed) Year Book of Intensive Care and Emergency Medicine. Springer-Verlag, Berlin. 1998; 667-76.

22. Sugrue M. Intra-abdominal pressure. Clin Int Care 1995; 6: 76-79.

23. Schein M, Wittmann DH, Aprahamian CC, Condon RE. The abdominal compartment syndrome: the physiological and clinical consequences of elevated intra-abdominal pressure. J Am Coll Surg 1995; 180: 745-53.

24. Malbrain MLNG. Abdominal pressure in the critically ill. Cur Opinion Crit Care 2000; 6: 17-29.

25. Wittgen CM, Andrus CH, Fitzgerald SD, Baudendistel LJ, et al. Analysis of the haemodynamic and ventilatory effects of laparoscopic cholecystectomy. Arch Surg 1991; 126: 997-1001.

26. Versichelen L, Serreyn R, Rolly G, Vanderkerckhove D. Physiological changes during anaesthesia administration for gynaecological laparoscopy. J. Reprod Med 1984; 29: 697-700.

27. Keith LL, Thomas HS. Physiologic response to laparoscopic surgery: practical considerations. Healing well.com (2004).

28. Richards W, Scovill W, Shin B, Reed W. Acute renal failure asociated with increased intra-abdominal pressure. Ann Surg 1983; 197: 183-7.

29. Venkatesh R, Landman J, Sundaram CP, et al. Prevention, recognition and management of laparoscopic complications in urologic surgery. AUA update 2003; 22:322-32.

30. McDougall EM, Monk TG, Wolf JS Jr., et al. The effect of prolonged pneumoperitoneum on renal function in an animal model. J Am Coll Surg 1996; 182(4): 317-28.

31. Razvi HA, Fields D, Vargas JC, et al. Oliguria during laparoscopic surgery: evidence for direct renal parenchymal compression as an etiologic factor. J. Endourol 1996; 10(1):1-4.

32. Nguyen NT, Perez RY, Fleming M, et al. Effect of prolonged pneumoperitoneum on intraoperative urine output during laparoscopic gastric bypass. J Am Coll Surg 2002; 195(4): 476-83.

33. Seiba M, Schulsinger D, SoSa RE. The renal physiology of laparoscopic surgery. AUA update 2000; 19: 178-83.

34. O'leary E, Hubbard K, Tormey W, Cunningham J. Laparoscopic cholecystectomy: haemodynamic and neuroendocrine responses after pneumoperitoneum and changes in position. Br J Anaesth 1996; 76: 640-4.

35. Lautt WW. Mechanism and role of intrinsic regulation of hepatic arterial blood flow: hepatic arterial buffer response. Am J Physiol 1985; 245 (5 pt 1): 4549-56.

36. Richter S, Olinger A, Hildebrandt U, Menger MD, et al. Loss of physiologic hepatic blood flow control ("hepatic arterial buffer response") during CO_2 pneumoperitoneum in the rat. Anesth Analg 2001; 93: 872-7.

37. Jakimowicz J, Stultiens G, Smulders F. Laparoscopic insufflation of the abdomen reduces portal venous flow. Surg Endosc 1998; 12: 129-32.

38. Andrei VE, Schein M, Margolis M, Rucinski JC, et al. Liver enzymes are commonly elevated following laparoscopic cholecystectomy: is elevated intraabdominal pressure the cause? Dig Surg 1998; 15: 256-9.

39. Morino M, Giraudo G, Festa V. Alterations in hepatic function during laparoscopic surgery: an experimental clinical study. Surg Endosc 1998; 12: 968-72.

40. Saber AA, Laraja RD, Nalbandian HI, Pablos-Mendez A, et al. Changes in liver function tests after laparoscopic cholecystectomy: not so rare, not always ominous. Am Surg 2000; 66: 699-702.

41. Malbrain M. Intra-abdominal pressure in ICU: pathophysiological and clinical insights. Europ Society of Anaesth Refresher Courses 2002.

42. Diebel LN, Dulchavsky SA, Wilson RF. Effect of increased intra-abdominal pressure on mesenteric arterial and intestinal mucosal blood flow. J Trauma 1992; 33: 45-49.

43. Diebel LN, Dulchavsky SA, Brown WJ. Splanchnic ischaemic and bacterial translocation in the abdominal compartment syndrome. J Trauma 1997; 43: 852-55.

44. Windberger UB, Auer R, Keplinger F, Langle F, et al. The role of intra-abdominal pressure on splanchnic and pulmonary hemodynamic and metabolic changes during carbon dioxide pneumoperitoneum. Gastrointest Endosc 1999;49:84-91.

45. Halverson AL, Barret WL, Iglesias AR, Lee WT, et al. Decreased cerebrospinal fluid absorption during abdominal insufflation. Surg Endosc 1999; 13: 797-800.

46. Fuji Y, Tanaka H, Tsurukoa H, Amaha K. Middle cerebral arterial blood flow velocity increases during laparoscopic cholecystectomy. Anesth Analg 1994; 78: 80-83.

47. Diament M, Benumof JL, Saidman LJ. Hemodynamics of increased intra-abdominal pressure. Anesthesiology 1978; 48: 23-27.

48. Kashtan J, Green JF, Parson EQ, Holcroft JW. Hemodynamic effects of increased abdominal pressure. J Surg Res 1981; 30: 249-55.

49. Bardoczky GI, Engelman E, Levarlet M, et al. Ventilatory effects of pneumoperitoneum monitored with continuous spirometry. Anesthesia 1993, 48(4): 309-11.

50. Hazebrock EJ, Haitsma JJ, Lachmann B, Bonjer HJ. Mechanical ventilation with positive end-expiratory pressure preserves arterial oxygenation during prolonged pneumoperitoneum. Surg Endosc 2002; 16: 685-9.

51. Pang CK, Yap J, Chen PP. The effect of an alveolar recruitment strategy on oxygenation during laparoscopic cholecystectomy. Anaesth Intens Care 2003; 31: 176-80.

52. London ET, Ho HS, Neuhaus AM, et al. Effect of intravascular volume expansion on renal function during prolonged CO_2 pneumoperitoneum. Ann Surg 2000; 231(2): 195-201.

53. Dunn MD, McDougall EM. Renal Physiology, laparoscopic considerations. Urol Clin N Am 2000; 27(4): 609-14.

54. Cisek LJ, Gobet RM, Peters CA. Pneumoperitoneum produces reversible renal dysfunction in animals with normal and chronically reduced renal function. J Endourol 1998; 12(1): 95-100.

55. Perez J, Taura P, Ruedaj, Balust J. Role of dopamine in renal dysfunction during laparoscopic surgery. Surg Endosc 2002; 1297-1301.

56. Colome M, Chiu JW, White PF. The use of esmolol as an alternative to remifentanil during desflurane anaesthesia for fast-track outpatient gynecologic laparoscopic surgery. Anesth Analg 2001; 92: 352-7.

57. Johnson PL, Sibert KS. Laparoscopy, Gasless vs CO_2 pneumoperitoneum. J Reprod Med 1991; 42: 255-59.

CHAPTER 4

Haemodynamic Effects of Pneumoperitoneum

INTRODUCTION

Laparoscopic abdominal surgery has been used increasingly over the past 10 years, thus becoming the preferred technique for the treatment of several intra-abdominal diseases.[1] Laparoscopic methods depend essentially on the establishment of an intraperitoneal space.[2] A pneumoperitoneum using carbon dioxide (CO_2) therefore is routinely induced to give the region of interest a good exposure.[3] Although CO_2 pneumoperitoneum (PP) has been proved safe and effective, a number of clinical and experimental studies have demonstrated that PP may be detrimental to cardiopulmonary performance.[4,5] Significant complications have been reported with laparoscopic cholecystectomy including myocardial infarction, pulmonary edema, and congestive heart failure. There is clearly a subset of patients who are at risk for adverse events during laparoscopic surgery, however, the risk has not been quantified, nor has the specific group of patients been clearly identified. Such risk quantification is even more required in aging surgical population with associated medical diseases.[6,7] Therefore, it is important to establish the true effects of pneumoperitoneum on the cardiovascular function and other physiological functions.[8]

CARDIOVASCULAR EFFECTS

The extent of cardiovascular changes depend on the interaction of several patients and surgical factors including intra-abdominal pressure (IAP), patient position, CO_2 absorption, ventilatory strategy and surgical technique, and the nature and duration of the procedure. The patient's intravascular volume, pre-existing cardiopulmonary status, depth of anesthesia, anaesthetic agent used, neurohormonal factors and perhaps patient medication all can influence the cardiovascular responses to the creation of pneumoperitoneum and laparoscopy. Combined effect of all these factors manifest in a given patient. In general intraperitoneal pressure and nature of insufflating gas has dominant effect on CVS, anaesthesia and patient position modulate this effect.

Cardiovascular changes are proportional to intra-abdominal pressure generated. In an experimental model Ishizaki[9] et al investigated the safe upper limit of intra-abdominal pressure following insufflation. The threshold pressure that had minimal effect on haemodynamics function was 12 mm of Hg. Some of the pneumoperitoneum related changes in haemodynamic parameters include increased systemic arterial and central venous pressure, increased vascular resistance and decrease cardiac output. Other major alterations such as central hypertension, arrhythmia, decreased mesenteric blood flow, hypercarbia, acidosis and increased vasopressin release have all been documented.[10-17]

It is difficult to separate haemodynamic changes caused by nature of insufflating gas from that by increased intra-peritoneal pressure. Most authors conclude that haemodynamic effects are the result of coupling an increased intra abdominal pressure with the use of carbon dioxide as the insufflation gas. In a study Marathe demonstrated that despite significant and large increase in the arterial $PaCO_2$ beginning at the intra-abdominal pressure of 8 mm of Hg, hemodynamic alterations only occurred when the $PaCO_2$ increased by 33 per cent and no change in mean arterial pressure was observed despite significant alterations in the arterial $PaCO_2$ and increased intra-abdominal pressure.[18] Incidentally it was thought that there were negligible systemic effects from intra-abdominal insufflation of CO_2.

There have been several studies attempting to separate the pneumoperitoneum effects of hypercapnia from increased intra-abdominal pressure. In a canine chronic obstructive pulmonary disease model, it was concluded that the hemodynamic changes were due to increased abdominal pressure as the changes were similar with both CO_2 and helium insufflation.[19] However, in a pig model where CO_2 insufflation was also compared to helium insufflation, the CO_2 pneumoperitoneum produced an elevated systolic blood pressure, a slight increase in heart rate and a decrease in cardiac output, when compared to the effects of the helium pneumoperitoneum.[20] These changes were attributed to CO_2 absorption from the peritoneal surface, as they were not seen in the helium insufflation.

HO, Saunders et al[21] in a pig model, where they compared CO_2 with nitrogen insufflation, concluded that haemodynamic effects were entirely due to CO_2 absorption as no haemodynamic changes were observed in the nitrogen group. There are many examples of studies in which haemodynamic changes are seen in CO_2 insufflation, however, they cannot be attributed to either CO_2 absorption or intra-abdominal pressure independently as there were no appropriate comparisons performed (Table 4.1). The information obtained from animal studies would suggest that in normal patients the haemodynamic effects of laparoscopy with CO_2 insufflation were primarily due to CO_2 absorption and the resultant serum acid-base changes.

CHANGES IN CARDIOVASCULAR FUNCTION

Induction of pneumoperitoneum causes significant circulatory changes. The filling pressure of the heart, pulmonary artery occlusion (wedge) pressure (PAOP) and central venous pressure (CVP), which are marginally reduced by the induction and by positioning in reverse Trendelenburg (rT) increase when CO_2 insufflation starts.[15,22-24]

Table 4.1: The cardiovascular responses to pneumoperitoneum

Method of Measurement	HR	CVP	PCWP	MAP	SVR	CI/CO	Reference
ED	↔			↑	↑	↓	Elliot S et al[41]
TEE	↔			↑	↑	↓	Dorsay DA et al[42]
PAC	↔	↑	↑	↑	↑	↓ occ. ↑	Zollinger A et al[39], Hein HA[51]
TBC	↔			↑	↑	↓ or ↔	Koksoy C et al[36], Walder AD et al[37]

HR: heart rate; **CVP:** central venous pressure; **PCWP:** pulmonary capillary wedge pressure; **MAP:** mean arterial pressure; **SVR:** systemic vascular resistance; **CI/CO:** cardiac index/cardiac output; **ED:** esophageal Doppler probe; **TEE:** transesophageal echocardiography; **PAC:** pulmonary artery catheter; **TBC:** transthoracic bioimpedence cardiography; ↑: increase; ↓: decrease; ↔: no change.

The increase in filling pressure is not associated with increase in LVEDA or LVESA, as measured by transesophageal echocardiography. Most studies reported an increase in mean arterial pressure (MABP) during the insufflation.[14,22,23,25] The increase in MABP represents increased afterload[26] and is associated with an increase in left ventricular wall stress.[27] Calculated systemic vascular resistance (SVR) increases markedly[15,22,23,25,28-32,65] particularly during early phase of insufflation, with partial restoration starting 10-15 min after the creation of the pneumoperitoneum. Some authors have demonstrated increase in LVEDA by TEE, indicating that pneumoperitoneum causes an increased EDV.[30,33] The effect of insufflation on CI (or cardiac output) is less consistent. Both invasive and non invasive techniques have been used to measure the haemodynamic effects of PPN. Investigators have used transthoracic bio-impedence,[34-39] esophageal doppler probe,[40,41] transesophageal echocardiography[32,42,43] or pulmonary artery catheter[3,22,23,39,51,64] for studying hemodynamic effects of PPN. As shown above, majority of studies show similar trends with increased central filling pressure, increased MABP and increased SVR. The effect on cardiac output differs. Several authors have reported consistent decrease in CI related to pneumoperitoneum.[31,35,44-46] Many of these have been as great as 30 per cent. In Zuckerman et al study CI fell 27.2 per cent from a patient awake state to the lowest recorded value of the pneumoperitoneum. The CI decreased by 10.6 per cent when base line was used as reading after induction of anaesthesia. Mc Laughlin et al[43] reported a reduction of 30 per cent. The clearest picture of the pattern of haemodynamic changes is from a study reporting serial CI determinations in 15 healthy adults.[23] Induction of anaesthesia and positioning in rT prior to insufflation caused a 35 to 40 per cent reduction in CI. A further reduction to 50 per cent of awake values occurred during the initial phase of CO_2 insufflation in rT.

Other studies have shown no change in cardiac output. Trans thoracic impedance cardiography has produced an inconsistent result. Some studies showed a 30 per cent reduction in CI, but others have shown no significant change.[15,44,47] Dorsay et al found no differences in cardiac output (CO) with pneumoperitoneum. More recently, when both the thermodilution technique and the transesophageal techniques were used in the same patient the results showed no significant changes in cardiac output.[31,48,49] These studies show that pulmonary capillary wedge pressure (PCWP) increases consistently with pneumoperitoneum, but both impedence and measures by TEE do not show a corresponding change in left ventricular volume. This might indicate that the pressure increases are due to the direct pressure effects of the pneumoperitoneum rather than any change in the preload. Myre et al,[31] simultaneously studied invasive haemodynamic and transesophageal measurement of cardiac volume during pneumoperitoneum, they found no change in CI during pneumoperitoneum. Anderson et al also showed no change in cardiac output by PPN.[50]

PHASIC NATURE

The haemodynamic changes associated with pneumoperitoneum appear to be phasic in nature. Joris and colleagues observed a fall in CI coincident with a rise in SVR and MAP after induction of anaesthesia and reverse Trendelenburg positioning. There followed a further reduction of CI to 50 per cent of its preoperative value 5 minutes after the beginning of carbon dioxide (CO_2) insufflation.[23] Finally, the CI gradually increased and SVR reduced after 10 minutes of CO_2 insufflation.

Other studies support this phasic change in haemodynamic function.[15,51,52]

PATIENT POSITION

Laparoscopic surgery has three potential causes of major physiological changes in the anaesthetized patient: Patient position, creation of the pneumoperitoneum and potential for systemic absorption (systemic effect) of insufflating gas.[27] Maximum haemodynamic changes are observed when the pneumoperitoneum created with patients in the reverse Trendelenburg position. Joris[23] and colleagues documented a decline in CI to 50% of baseline following insufflation of the abdomen in the head up position, whereas no changes were observed in cardiac index or ejection fraction with insufflation in supine position. The CVP and PCWP are also influenced by patient posture.

Using TEE, Dorsay et al looked at the haemodynamic effects of both position and pneumoperitoneum in patients undergoing, laparoscopic cholecystectomy. The CI was not affected by pneumoperitoneum but the reverse Trendelenburg position resulted in an 11 per cent reduction in cardiac output.[42,30] Zuckerman et al[54] using impedence cardiography showed that change of position to reverse Trendelenburg after insufflation, had no effect on their measured haemodynamic parameters. They also stated that the effects of insufflation and position are short lived and all the haemodynamic parameters returned toward the baseline over time. To further test the effect of position the patient was again placed in the flat position and then in the reverse Trendelenburg position without any effect on the CI, SV or LVEDV.

CAUSES OF HAEMODYNAMIC CHANGES (FIG. 4.1)

Several factors have been proposed as contributory to the circulatory changes induced by pneumoperitoneum. A light level of general anaesthesia could be responsible for an increased afterload at the onset of pneumoperitoneum. Although stability of heart rate was not sufficient to ascertain a stable or adequate level of anaesthesia, the haemodynamic response would have been observed soon after introduction of the 10 mm trocar by an open technique, and not only after insufflation, if nociceptive stimulation was the cause of the circulatory changes. There is stimulation of the sympathetic nervous system caused by an elevated $PaCO_2$ value after the absorption of the CO_2 gas through the peritoneum.[53,55,56] Although the increase in $EtCO_2$ was delayed in relation to that of the systolic arterial pressure, an increase in alveolo-arterial gradient in carbon dioxide after peritonal insufflation has been described by Harris et al.[57] Arterial CO_2 changes could therefore, have occurred sooner than $EtCO_2$ changes and could have been a causal factor for insufflation-induced circulatory changes. A causal role of carbon dioxide is however, unlikely because haemodynamic values returned to pre insufflation values despite a sustained increase in $EtCO_2$. Elevated splanchnic and peripheral resistance under pneumoperitoneum,[30] the compression of the intra abdominal venous system[58,59] and increase in intra-aortic pressure and afterload imposed on the left ventricle[60] are other factors likely to be involved in the haemodynamic events after pneumoperitoneum. These intra-peritoneal pressure effects on loading conditions are usually superimposed on those of mild postural changes such as 10° head up tilt. The latter effects are usually reported as insufficient or absent in patient with normal left ventricular function.[14,27,30] Finally, humoral factors may be involved in the increase in left ventricular loading conditions. Catecholamine and other humoral factors have, infact, been shown to increase after onset of pneumoperitoneum.[23,61] There is a marked increase in plasma vasopressin concentration in patients undergoing laparoscopic cholecystectomy, immediately after the pneumoperitoneum was formed and reduced soon after the pneumoperitoneum was released. Vasopressin released may be triggered by circulatory changes such as decrease in transmural atrial pressure [62] or by neurogenic stimuli arising from the pneumoperitoneum due to increased intra-abdominal pressure, peritoneal distension or chemical stimulation due to the presence of carbon dioxide.[11,63] It can be speculated that these potential causal factors may dissipate during sustained pneumoperitoneum.

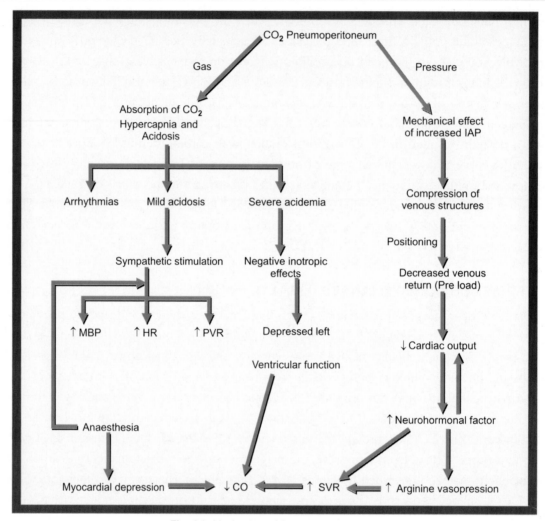

Fig. 4.1: Mechanism of fall in cardiac output

SGRH EXPERIENCE

Over 20,000 laparoscopic procedures have been performed in SGRH hospital. Most were under general anaesthesia. Monitoring included non-invasive automatic blood pressure, electrocardiography, pulse oximetry, capnography and multi gas analysis of inspired and exhaled gases. Haemodynamic responses observed were dependent on anaesthetic technique. Narcotic base anaesthetic technique produced hypertension, mild tachycardia in most patients. Most patients required treatment for high blood pressure. Esmolol IV, nifedipine sublingual (S/L) or intranasal or sorbitrate was used, to treat hypertensive responses.

Sevoflurane 2-3 per cent or isoflurane 1-1.5 per cent in N_2O, fentanyl and relaxant technique attenuated hypertensive responses. Bradycardia was common. Some patients required maintenance of blood pressure with fluid and inotropes.

TIVA with propofol, fentanyl and relaxant also produced stable haemodynamic conditions, except bradycardia. Before surgical stimulation, an epoch of hypotension were common.

It appears because of depth of anaesthesia and vasodilation produced by isoflurane, sevoflurane and propofol, hypertension responses were minimized. In comparison, narcotic based technique had hypertensive response because of lack of depth in anaesthesia.

PATIENTS WITH CARDIAC DISEASE

Patients undergoing laparoscopic cholecystectomy experiences significant haemodynamic depression. Decreases in cardiac output as great as 30 per cent have been reported during laparoscopic surgery. In young adults significant complications have been reported with laparoscopic cholecystectomy, including myocardial infarction, pulmonary edema and congestive heart failure. There is clearly a subset of patients who are at risk for adverse events during laparoscopic cholecystectomy.

Haemodynamic changes in cardiac patients or patients with impaired cardiac functions were investigated by some investigators. Fumihiro et al [49] and Uchikoshi have shown that pattern of haemodynamic changes in these patients are similar to that seen in patients without cardiac diseases. Specifically, HR, MAP and CI did not change and CVP, mPAP and PCWP increased under pneumoperitoneum. They noted that CVP and PCWP had sufficiently higher value in the cardiac diseases group than in the control group. The increased mPAP and PCWP might be critical factors for patients with pulmonary hypertension or impaired cardiac function. Iwase et al [24] reported significantly decreased urine output under PPN in patients with cardiac diseases and observed lung edema and heart failure in one patient who needed intensive post operative care. Uchikoshi et al commented that patients with cardiac diseases seem to be in danger of cardiac failure during laparoscopic cholecystectomy whenever PPN is used for long time.

REFERENCES

1. McDermott JP, Regan MC, Page R, Stokes MA, Barry D, Moriarty DC. Cardiovascular effects of laparoscopy with and without gas insufflation. Arch. Surg. 1995;130:984-88.
2. Gutt CN, Daume J, Schaeff B, Paolucci V. Systems and instruments for laparoscopic surgery without pneumoperitoneum. Surg Endose 1997;11:868-74.
3. Feig BW, Burger DH, Dougherty TB et al: Pharmacological interventions can reestablish baseline haemodynamic parameters during laparoscopic surgery. 1994;166:733.
4. Ogihera Y, Isshiki A, Kindscher JD, Goto H: Abdominal wall lifting versus CO2 insufflation for laparoscopic resection of ovarian tumors. J. Clin Anesth. 1999;11:406-412.
5. Wooley DS, Puglisi RN, Bilgrami S, Quinn JV, Slotman GJ Comparison of the haemodynamic effects of gasless abdominal distension and CO2 pneumoperitoneum during incremental positive end expiratory pressure. J. Surg. Res 1995;58:75-80.
6. Horvath KD, Whelan RL, Lier B, Viseomi S, Barry L, Buck K, The effects of elevated intra abdominal pressure, hypercarbia and positioning on the haemodynamic responses to laparoscopic colostomy in pigs, Surg. Endose 1998;12:107-14.
7. Kawamura YJ, Sawada T, Sunami E, Saito Y, Watanake T, Masaki T, Muto T Gasless laparoscopically assisted colomic surgery. Ann. J. Surg. 1999;177:515-17.
8. Tagaki S, Hepatic and portal vein blood flow during carbon dioxide pneumoperitoneum for laparoscopic hepatectomy. Surg. Endose 1998;12:427-431.
9. Ishizaki Y. Bandai Y, Shimomura K. et al. Safe intra abdominal pressure of CO_2 pneumoperitoneum during laparoscopic surgery. Surgery 1993;114:549.
10. Kleinhaus S, Sanmartand R, Boleys, Effects of laparoscopy on messenteric blood flow. Arch. Surgery, 1978;113:867-69.
11. Melville R, Frizis H, Forsling M, Lequeshe1. - The stimulation for vasopressin release during laparoscopy. Survey gynacol abstract 1985; 161: 253-56.
12. Witten CM, Andrus C, Fitzgerald S, Baundendistal L, Dahms T, Karminski D, Prospective analysis of haemodynamics and ventilatory effects of laparoscopic cholecystectomy. Arch. Surg. 1991;126:997-1001.
13. Myles P, Brady arrhythmias and laparoscopy: A prospective study of heart rate changes with laparoscopy. Aust N2 J Obstat Gynarcol 1991;31:171-73.
14. Liu SY, Leighton T, Davis J, Kleix S. Lippmann N, Bongard F. Prospective analysis of cardiovascular responses to laparoscopic cholecystectomy. J. Laparoscopic endose surg. 1991;5:241-46.
15. Westerband A, Van Dc Water, Amzallag M, Lebowitz P, Cardiovascular Changes during Laparoscopic Cholecystectomy. Surg Gynecol Obstect 1992; 175: 535-38.

16. Ho H, Glinther R, Wolf B. Intra peritoneal carbon dioxide insufflation and cardio pulmonary functions. Arch. Surg 1992;127:92 8-933.

17. Diebel L, Dulcharsky S, Wilson R. Effects of increased intra-abdominal pressure on mesenteric arterial and intestinal mucosal blood flow. J. Trauma 1992;33:45-49.

18. Marathe V, Lily R, Silvestry S, Gower DD. Alterations in haemodynamics and left ventricular contractility during carbon dioxide pneumoperitoneum. Surg Endosc 1996;10:974-978.

19. Fitzgerald SD, Andras CH, Baridendistal L.J., Dalims TE, Kaminski DL. Hypercarbia during carbon dioxide pneumoperitoneum. Ann. J. Surg. 1992;163:186-190.

20. Leighton T, Pianim M, Liu A, Kono M, Klein S, Bongard F. Effects of hypercarbia during experimental pneumoperitoneum. Ann. J. Surg. 1992; 58: 717-721.

21. Hashimoto S, Hashikura Y, Munnakata Y, Kawaski S, Makuchi P. Changes in cardiovascular and respiratory system during laparoscopic cholecystectomy. J. Laparoendosc Surg. 1993; 3 (6): 535-39.

22. Safran D, Sagambati S, Orlando R Laparoscopy in high risk patients cardiac patients. Surg. Gynecol Obstat 1993;176:548-554.

23. Joris J, Letouse D, Horiora P, Lainy M. Ventilatory effects of CO_2 insufflation during laparoscopy cholecystectomy. Anesthesiology 1991:75 (Suppl) 7121.

24. Iwase K, Takenake H, Yogura A, Ishizaka T, Oshima S. Haemodynamic alterations during laparoscopic cholecystectomy. A comparison with mini-laparoscopic cholecystectomy. Dig Surg. 1993;10:5-9.

25. Fox I.G, Hein HAT, Gawey RJ, Hellman CI, Ramsay MAZ. Physiological alteration during laparoscopic cholecystectomy in ASA III and IV pts. Anesthesiology 1993;79:A 55.

26. Breton G, Poulin E, Fortin C, Mamazza J, Robert J. Evaluation clinique et haemodynamique des cholecytatomics par vote laparoscopique. Ann Chir 1991;45:783-90.

27. Cunningham AJ, Turner J, Rosen baum S, Rafferty T Transesophageal echocardiographic assessment of hemodynamic function during laparoscopic cholecystectomy. Br. J anaesth 1993; 70:C21.

28. Kubota K, Kajivara N, Toruya M, Ishihera T et al. Alterations in respiratory function and haemodynamics during laparoscopic cholecystectomy under pneumoperitoneum. Surg Endosc 1993; 7:500- 04.

29. Odeberg S, Ljungqvist O, Svenberg T, et al. Haemodynamic effects of pneumoperitoneum and the influence of posture during anesthesia for laparoscopic surgery. Acta Anesthesiol Scand. 1996; 38:276-83.

30. Gannedahl P, Odieberg S, Bredin L, Sollari A. Effect of posture and pneumoperitoneum during anesthesia on the indices of left ventricular filling-Acta Anesthesiol Scand 1996; 40:160-6.

31. Myre K, Bnanes T, Smith G, Stokeland O. Simultaneous haemodynamic and echo cardiographic changes during abdominal gas insufflation. Surg. Laparosc Endosc 1997;7:415-419 (1997).

32. Myre K, Rostrup M, Buanes T, Stokland O, Plasma catecholamines and haemodynamic changes during pneumoperitoneum. Acta Anesthesiol Scand 1998; 42:343-47.

33. Monk TG, Despotis GJ, Hogne CW, Lappas DG. Haemodynamic and echocardiograhic alterations during laparoscopic surgery. Anesthesiology 1993;79:54.

34. Johanssen G, Anderson M, Juhi B. The effects of general anesthesia on the haemodynamic events during laparoscopy with CO2 insufflation. Acta. Anesthesiol Scand 1989;33:132-6.

35. Crithchley LAH, Critchley JAJH, Gin T: Haemodynamic changes in patients undergoing laparoscopic cholecystectomy: measurement of transthoracic electric bio impedance. Br. J. Anesth. 1993;70:681.

36. Koksoy C, Kuzu MA, Kurti et al: Haemodynamic effects of pneumoperitoneum during laparoscopic cholecystectomy: A prospective comparative study using bio impedance cardiography: Br. J. Surg. 1995;82:972.

37. Walder AD, Aitkenrihead AR: Role of vasopression in the haemodynamic responses to laparoscopic cholecystectomy. Br. J. Anesth. 1997;78:264.

38. Dhoste K, Lacoste I, Karayan J, et al. Haemodynamic and ventilatory change during laparoscopic cholecystectomy elderly ASA III patients. Can J. Anesth 1996;42:783.

39. Zollinger A, Krayer S, Singer T et al: Haemodynamic effects of pneumoperitoneum in elderly patients with an increased cardiac risk. Ecur. J. Anesthesiol 1997; 14: 266.

40. Haxby EJ, Gray MR, Rodriguez C, et al. Assessment of cardiovascular changes during laparoscopic hernia repair using esophageal Doppler. Br. J. Anesth. 1997;78:515.

41. Elliot S, Savill P, Eckersall S: Cardiovascular changes during laparoscopic cholecystectomy. A study using transoesophageal Doppler. Eur. J Anesthesiol 1998;15:50.

42. Dorsay DA, Greene FI, Baysinger CI: Haemodynamic changes during laparoscopic cholecystectomy monitored with transoesophageal echocardiography. Surg. Endose 1995; 9: 128.

43. Mclaughlin JG, Scheeras DE, Dean RJ, Bonnel BW (1995). The adverse haemodynamics effects of laparoscopic cholecystectomy. Surg. Endosc. 9:121-124.

44. Lenz R, Thomas T, Wilkins D (1976). Cardiovascular changes during laparoscopy using impedance cardiography. Anesthesiology 31:4-12(1976).

45. Davidson BS, Cromeens DM, Feig BW. Alternative methods of exposure minimize cardiopulmonary risk in experimental animals during minimally invasive surgery. Surg Endosc 1996;10(3):301-4.

46. Hirvonen EA, Poikolainen EO, Paakkonen ME et al. The adverse affects of anesthesia, head up tilt and CO_2 pneumoperitoneum during laparoscopic cholecystectomy. Surg Endosc 2000;14:272-77.

47. E K Man L, Abrahamson J, Biber B. Haemodynamic changes during laparoscopy with positive and expiratory pressure ventilation. Acta Anesthesiol Scand 1988;32:447-453.

48. D'Angelo AJ, Kline RG, Chen MHM, Halpern, Cohen JT. Utility of trans esophageal echocardiography end pulmonary artery catheterization during laparoscopic assisted abdominal aortic aneurysm repair. Surg Endosc 1997;11:1099-1101.

49. Uchikoshi F, Kamiike W, Iwase K, Ito T, Nezu R, Nishida T. Laparoscopic cholecystectomy in patients with cardiac disease: Haemodynamic advantage of the abdominal wall retraction method. Surg. Laparosc Endosc 1997;3:196-201.

50. Anderson L, Wallin CJ, Sollevi A, Odeburg W.S. Pneumoperitoneum in healthy humans do not affect central blood volume or cardiac output. Acta Anesthesiol Scand 1998;43:809-14.

51. Hein HA, Joshi GP, Ramsay et al. Haemodynamic changes during laparoscopic cholecystectomy in patients with severe cardiac diseases. J. Clin Anesth. 1997;9:261.

52. Branche PE, Duperret ST, Sagnard PE, et al: Left ventricular loading modifications induced by pneumoperitoneum: A time course echo cardiographic study. Anesth. Analg 1998;86: 482.

53. Alexander G, Brown E. Physiological alterations during pelvic laparoscopy. Ann, J Obstet. Gynecol 1969:105:1078-81.

54. R Zuckerman, M Gold, P Jenkins, LA Rauseher, M Jons, S Heneghass. Surg Endosc 2001; 15: 561-565. The effects of pneumoperitoneum and patient position on haemodynamics during laparoscopic cholecystectomy.

55. Richardson D, Wassermen A, Patterson J: General and regional circulatory responses to changes in blood Ph and carbon dioxide tension. J. Clin. Invest 1961; 40:31-43.

56. Mullet CE, Viale JP, Sognert PE et al. Pulmonary CO_2 elimination during surgical procedures using intra- or extra peritoneal CO_2 insufflation. Anesth. Analg. 1993; 76: 622-6.

57. Harris S, Baltan tyne G, Luther M, Perrino A. Alteration of cardiovascular performance during laparoscopic colostomy: a combined haemodynamic and echo cardiographic analysis. Anesth. Analg. 1996; 83: 482-7.

58. Toomesian J, Glavinovich G, Johnson MN, Gazzaniza AB. Haemodynamic change following pneumoperitoneum and graded Haemorrhage in the dog. Surg forum 1978; 29: 32-3.

59. Ivankovich AD, Miletich DJ, Albrecht RF et al. Cardiovascular effects of intra peritoneal insufflation with carbon dioxide and nitrous oxide in the dog. Anesthesiology 1975; 42:281-7.

60. Robotham JL, Wise RA, Bromberger-Barnea B. Effects of changes in abdominal pressure on left ventricular performance and regional blood flow. Crit Care Med 1985; 13(10):803-9.

61. O'Leary E, Hubband K, Tormey W, Cunnigham A. Laparoscopic cholecystectomy: Haemodynamic neuro endurine responses after pneumoperitoneum and changes in position. Br. J.A. 1996; 76:640-6.

62. Robertson G. Regulation of vasopressure secretion-lri: Seldin D, Giebisch G, etc. Clinical disturbance of water metabolism. New York: Raven press, 1993; 102-11.

63. Punnonen R, Viinamaki O. Vasopressin release during laparoscopy: role of increased intra-abdominal pressure. Lancert 1982; 1:176-6.

64. Horvonem EA, Nuutineum LS, Kareko M: Haemodynamic changes due to trendelenburg positioning and pneumoperitoneum during laparoscopic hysterectomy. Acta. Anesthesiol Scand 1995;39:949.

65. Kelman GR, Swapp GH, Smith I et al. cardiac output and arterial blood gas tension during laparoscopy. Br. J. Anesth. 1972; 44:155-62.

CHAPTER 5

Effect of Pneumoperitoneum on Respiratory System

INTRODUCTION

Laparoscopic surgery has greatly expanded in scope and volume over the last two decades. Laparoscopic surgery is an increasingly used surgical technique, mainly due to claims of minimal postoperative morbidity and markedly reduced hospital stay.[1] It is well recognised that abdominal insufflation with carbon dioxide and the Trendelenburg position during laparoscopy, even if maintained for a short period of time, can cause serious physiological changes in respiratory mechanics, lung volume and gas exchange with a consequent risk to the patient.[2-4] Pneumoperitoneum and the position of the patient required for laparoscopy produce multiple pathophysiologic changes, which though well tolerated by young and healthy patients, could be devastating in elderly and sick patients.

RESPIRATORY CHANGES DURING LAPAROSCOPY

During laparoscopy, various physiological changes in respiratory system can occur. These are discussed as follows:
1. Ventilatory changes
2. Increase in $PaCO_2$
3. Physiologic effects of carbon dioxide
4. Patient position
5. Influence of anaesthesia

VENTILATORY CHANGES

Pneumoperitoneum produces significant respiratory changes involving lung and chest wall mechanics, pulmonary volumes and gas exchange. With abdominal insufflation, intra-abdominal pressure (IAP) increases, mainly upto 12-15 mmHg, which results in cephalad displacement of the diaphragm, limitation of diaphragmatic and anterior abdominal wall movement, decreased lung volumes, atelectasis and increase in peak inspiratory pressure (PIP), shunt fraction and dead space ventilation.[1,2]

Functional residual capacity (FRC), already reduced by induction of general anaesthesia, decreases even further, by 20 to 25 per cent, 5 min after abdominal insufflation. Respiratory compliance decreases by 30 to 50% in healthy patients. The reduction in respiratory compliance is due to decreases in lung (upto 38 per cent) and chest wall compliance (upto 45 per cent).[5,6] The respiratory resistance increases as much as 79 per cent, 5 min after abdominal insufflation due to a marked increase in lung and chest wall resistance. In contrast, airway resistance is not significantly affected by abdominal insufflation. The duration of pneumoperitoneum has no significant effect on pulmonary mechanics unless complications such as bronchospasm or subcutaneous emphysema occur. Approximately 15 min after abdominal deflation, respiratory compliance and resistance return to preinsufflation level.[5-11]

Healthy patients tolerate pneumoperitoneum well, despite the respiratory changes. Various studies suggest that there are no clinically significant changes in shunt fraction or dead space ventilation even in a 10° to 20° head up or head down position. Oxygen saturation remains stable, and PaO_2 /PAO_2 as well as $EtCO_2$/$PaCO_2$ gradients are not significantly affected.[5-7,13,14]

Abdominal insufflation may also cause changes in lung space and distortion of the lung, as the pressure generated by the abdominal insufflation is unlikely to be applied uniformly to the lung surface and this may partly be responsible for the decreased lung compliance.[5,15] When there is a base line decrease in lung volumes and low respiratory compliance, as is often seen in obese, ASA III to IV patients and patients with pulmonary disease, superimposed pneumoperitoneum could produce dramatic changes in pulmonary mechanics by shifting the lungs to a flat, noncompliant portion of the pressure-volume curve. Ventilation-perfusion (V-Q) mismatch, high peak inspiratory pressure (PIP), and increased physiologic dead space make adequate ventilation and elimination of carbon dioxide difficult.[17,18] Hypoventilation, combined with increased intrathoracic pressure and decreased cardiac output, might result in inadequate oxygenation.

Abdominal wall lift (AWL), a technique utilizing a fan retractor, was proposed for use during laparoscopic procedures to reduce the haemodynamic and respiratory effects of abdominal insufflation. This technique allows a decrease in the IAP of more than 50 per cent. Application of AWL during laparoscopic cholecystectomy significantly improves peak airway pressure and total resistance of the respiratory system. However, the elastance of the respiratory system remains elevated, probably due to an AWL-induced impairment of anterior abdominal wall and diaphragmatic mechanics.[12]

INCREASE IN PaCO₂

Carbon dioxide is the gas most commonly used for pneumoperitoneum since it does not support combustion, is readily available, is relatively inexpensive and its high solubility minimizes the risk of fatal gas embolism. The CO_2 is absorbed from the peritoneal cavity and carried by blood through the systemic and portal veins and excreted via the lungs. Hence, the pulmonary excretion of CO_2 (VCO_2) and $PaCO_2$ increase.[5,6]

In patients under general anaesthesia and controlled mechanical ventilation, $PaCO_2$ progressively increases and reaches a plateau 15 to 30 min after beginning of CO_2 insufflation.[5,6,18-21]

The rate of absorption of a gas depends on its solubility in tissue, pressure gradients across membrane containing the gas, the absorption area and the diffusion constant of the gas. Carbon dioxide is much more soluble in body fluids than oxygen (ratio 23:1) or nitrogen (ratio 35:1). During laparoscopy $PaCO_2$ values may increase despite continued hyperventilation due to absorption of a large amount of carbon dioxide.[21-23] Hypercarbia was not observed when helium or N_2O was used for insufflation.[24-26] The level of $PaCO_2$ reflects the balance between production, endogenous (metabolism) and exogenous (absorption) utilization and elimination. This balance is controlled primarily via the lungs (Table 5.1).

Table 5.1: Factors affecting $PaCO_2$

Increase in production	Decrease in elimination
Endogenous CO_2 production • Metabolic state • Light anaesthesia (incomplete muscle relaxation) *Absorption of exogenous CO_2* • Level of intra-abdominal pressure • Extent of dissection • CO_2 subcutaneous emphysema • CO_2 pneumothorax	• Changes in pulmonary mechanics • V-Q mismatch • Increased dead space ventilation • Inadequate mechanical ventilation • Inadequate muscle relaxation • Reduced cardiac output • Respiratory depression during spontaneous ventilation

Theoretically high increase in VCO_2 and $PaCO_2$ are expected but it does not happen clinically because of impaired peritoneal perfusion due to haemodynamic changes and enormous buffering capacity of the blood.

The increase in intra-abdominal pressure produces cephalad shift of the diaphragm resulting in reduction of functional residual capacity (FRC), total lung volume (TLV) and pulmonary compliance. If FRC decreases below the closing volume, atelectasis and intrapulmonary shunting may occur, resulting in hypoxaemia. These changes produce ventilation perfusion (V/Q) mismatch with increased physiological dead space, which is evident by increased arterial to alveolar gradient for partial pressure of CO_2 [(a-A) DCO_2].[27-28] The increase in (a-A) D CO_2 can also be due to reduced cardiac output associated with laparoscopy and this is exaggerated in patients with pulmonary or cardiovascular disease. The ventilatory function is further deteriorated by Trendelenburg position with resultant cephalad shift of carina which may result in endobronchial movement of endotracheal tube and one lung ventilation leading to hypoxia and hypercarbia.

Although permissive hypercarbia has become an accepted approach to treatment of certain medical conditions, one should make a reasonable attempt to maintain normocapnia during laparoscopic procedures.

PHYSIOLOGICAL EFFECTS OF CARBON DIOXIDE

Hypercarbia produces considerable physiological changes. In awake, healthy individuals, breathing a gas mixture containing 3 per cent CO_2 produces a feeling of discomfort. Breathing 5 to 7 per cent CO_2 causes acute distress with disorientation, dyspnea and anxiety.[29] Narcosis occurs with a $PaCO_2$ greater than 90 mmHg. Hypercarbia causes a predictable increase in cerebral blood flow (CBF). For each 1mmHg increase in $PaCO_2$, CBF increases 1.8ml/100g/min and cerebral blood volume increases 0.04ml/100gm. As $PaCO_2$ increases from 40 to 80 mmHg, CBF doubles. In patients with intracranial lesions and increased intracracnial pressure, these changes in CBF and cerebral blood volume could be disastrous.

The enzyme system of the body requires tight control of acid base balance for proper function. Under normal circumstances, a narrow range of pH 7.36 to 7.44 is maintained despite a wide variation in acid production. The Henderson-Hasselbach equation defines the relationship between pH, PCO_2 and HCO_3

$$pH = 6.1 + \log [HCO_3^-] / 0.0301 \times PCO_2$$

In the acute situation, as seen with CO_2 pneumoperitoneum, for every 10 mmHg change in $PaCO_2$ the pH will change 0.08 units in the opposite direction.[30,31] The $PaCO_2$ level has the major regulatory effect on ventilation via central mechanisms, and to a much lesser degree via stimulation of peripheral chemoreceptors in the carotid and aortic bodies. The chemosensitive area, located in the ventral surface of the medulla, is extremely sensitive to hydrogen ions. However, the blood-brain barrier is relatively impermeable to hydrogen ions. Thus CO_2, which easily crosses the blood-brain barrier, indirectly controls this region by formation of carbonic acid, which dissociates to produce HCO_3^- and H^+. The activation of receptors in the chemosensitive area results in stimulation of the inspiratory center and increase in the rate of respiration. The maximal stimulation is attained at a $PaCO_2$ level of about 100 mmHg. Any further increase results in respiratory depression.[32] Many anaesthetic drugs cause respiratory depression by altering the ventilatory response to CO_2. Volatile agents and sedatives or hypnotic drugs decrease the slope of the CO_2 response curve, while all opioids produce a dose dependant respiratory depression by shifting the CO_2 response curve to the right and resetting the respiratory centres to respond to a higher level of $PaCO_2$. Apart from ventilatory effects, hypercarbia influences pulmonary circulation. It increases pulmonary vascular resistance and locally augments hypoxic pulmonary vasoconstriction, probably by causing acidosis. In a case of pre-existing pulmonary hypertension, superimposed pulmonary vasoconstriction from a high level of CO_2 causes an additional stress on the right ventricle, which potentially could lead to a right ventricular failure in a poorly compensated heart. CO_2 produces excitation of the sympathetic nervous system and provokes multiple responses. Many of the sympathetic effects of CO_2 are directly related to stimulation of the medullary vasomotor centres. In addition, stimulation of chemoreceptor areas of the carotid and aortic bodies trigger sympathetic responses. High levels of CO_2 influence the release of catecholamines from the adrenal medulla. The plasma concentrations of norepinephrine and epinephrine may rise two to three fold. The mechanism is unclear, but both decreased pH and increased $PaCO_2$ have been implicated.[33,34] The cardiovascular effects of hypercarbia are the result of a balance between the direct cardiodepressant effect of CO_2 and the increased activity of the sympathetic nervous system. The depressant effect of CO_2 is possibly secondary to pH changes.[35] Activation of the sympathetic nervous system by CO_2 in healthy individuals overcompensates for direct cardiodepression. When CO_2 is added to a breathing gas mixture under controlled conditions to produce a $PaCO_2$ in the range of 39 to 50 mmHg, there is a significant increase in cardiac output, cardiac index, heart rate, stroke volume and myocardial contractility. Left ventricular work and myocardial oxygen consumption are increased upto 20 per cent.[36] Coronary blood flow is autoregulated to match metabolic requirements.

Although the threshold level of $PaCO_2$ that produces cardiac arrhythmias is high even then there is an increased risk of arrhythmias when hypercarbia is accompanied by electrolyte imbalance or superimposed on pre-existing cardiac conduction abnormalities. Scott reported arrhythmias in upto 27 per cent of patients undergoing spontaneous ventilation during laparoscopy.[43] Vasodilatation produced by CO_2 results in a 14 per cent fall of the peripheral vascular resistance with a 10 mmHg increase in $PaCO_2$.[36] The effect on systemic blood pressure is the result of a balance between increased cardiac output and decreased peripheral resistance. The usual effect is a mild to moderate increase in mean blood pressure, but the response may vary from slight hypotension to marked hypertension.

PATIENT POSITION

It is a common practice to alter the patient's position to facilitate surgical exposure during laparoscopy. The Trendelenburg position is generally used for pelvic laparoscopy, while the head-up position is routine for upper abdominal surgery. In addition, the lithotomy position and right or left tilt can be utilized for several laparoscopic procedures. The Trendelenburg position reduces FRC, TLV and pulmonary compliance facilitating atelectasis. This can be minimised by judicial application of positive end-expiratory pressure (PEEP). These changes are more marked in morbidly obese, elderly and debilitated patients. The position of the endotracheal tube should be checked after the change of patient position. The reverse Trendelenburg position improves respiratory function; hence, it is the most preferred position as far as the respiratory system is concerned. The steepness of the tilt, associated cardiac disease, anaesthetic drugs and the patient's intravascular volume status have a major effect on the magnitude of these changes. The effect of position is more marked in obese, elderly and sick patients.[42]

INFLUENCE OF ANAESTHESIA

Laparoscopic surgery can be performed under local or regional anaesthesia, general anaesthesia with spontaneous breathing or controlled ventilation. Under local or regional anaesthesia, $PaCO_2$ is unaltered by pneumoperitoneum because of significantly increased spontaneous minute ventilation.[27] The awake patient undergoing discomfort produced by the pneumoperitoneum may require a high level of sedation, which can result in respiratory depression, an unpredictable rise of $PaCO_2$ and a fall in oxygen saturation.[32]

In spontaneously breathing patients under general anaesthesia, intraperitoneal insufflation of CO_2 increases minute ventilation, but this increase is not sufficient enough to keep $PaCO_2$ within normal limits. Rise in $PaCO_2$ upto 60.8 ± 10.9 mmHg has been reported.[37] This is related to the ventilatory depressant effect of the general anaesthetic agents that blunt the ventilatory response to hypercapnia and increased intra abdominal pressure (IAP). General anaesthesia with mechanical ventilation allows relatively easy control of the elimination of CO_2 in healthy patients under normal circumstances. A 20 to 30 per cent increase in minute ventilation is usually sufficient to compensate for CO_2 absorption.[21-23] Hyperventilation should be achieved by increasing the respiratory rate rather than the tidal volume.[21-23] An increase in tidal volume might produce a significant increase in peak inspiratory pressure (PIP) due to high IAP and changes in pulmonary mechanics. The desire to maintain relatively normal CO_2 values should be weighed against the potential risks of significantly increasing airway pressure. Dramatic changes in pulmonary mechanics in patients with obesity and some pulmonary disease could make hyperventilation almost impossible. So, moderate hypercarbia is acceptable in these patients.[21,22] Intermittent decompression of the abdomen will allow reasonable control of $PaCO_2$. PEEP of 5 to 10 cm of H_2O is advocated by many to prevent atelectasis, increase FRC, and improve oxygenation.[23,37]

MONITORING OF PaCO₂ AND EtCO₂

Capnography provides valuable information about changes in $PaCO_2$. Although the $PaCO_2$ / $EtCO_2$ gradient increases during laparoscopy, it does not change significantly in healthy patients.[5,6,13,18,19,38] However, in morbidly obese ASA III and IV patients with haemodynamic instability, and patients breathing spontaneously, under general anaesthesia end tidal CO_2 might not be a reliable indicator of $PaCO_2$.[17,39-41] Increased dead space ventilation, as is often seen in pulmonary disease such as emphysema or conditions associated with decreased cardiac output, results in an increased $PaCO_2$ /$EtCO_2$ gradient. Low or normal $EtCO_2$ could be an indicator of difficulty in elimination of CO_2 rather than a reflection of actual $PaCO_2$ levels. A sudden drop in $EtCO_2$ might reflect a dramatic fall in cardiac output, as seen in pulmonary embolism. In these situations, frequent arterial blood gas sampling is required to accurately assess $PaCO_2$.

If capnography is not available or not functioning properly then clinical signs like tachycardia, increase in blood pressure, sweating, soda lime colour changes in case of closed circuit, and increase in oozing of blood from capillaries at surgical site has to be constantly observed throughout the procedure.[39-42]

SUMMARY

Laparoscopy has become one of the most common surgical interventions. Although it has multiple postoperative benefits as less trauma, less pain, less postoperative ileus, less postoperative pulmonary dysfunction, quick recovery, short hospital stay and cosmetic acceptability. It presents a significant challenge in high risk patients. Pneumoperitoneum and altered patient position result in complex pathophysiologic changes that may cause cardiovascular and respiratory decompensation.

CLINICAL PEARLS

1. Thorough preoperative evaluation, optimization of the patient's medical condition, careful monitoring, understanding and appropriate management of cardiopulmonary disturbances are essential for successful management of patients who undergo laparoscopic surgery.
2. General anaesthesia with muscle relaxation and endotracheal intubation remains the most commonly used technique for laparoscopic procedures.
3. Local, regional, or general anaesthesia with LMA, may be an acceptable alternative in selected cases.

REFERENCES

1. The Southern Surgeons Club: A prospective analysis of 1518 laparoscopic cholecystectomies. New Engl J Med 1991; 324: 1073-8.
2. Cunningham AJ. Laparoscopic cholecystectomy: anesthetic implications: Anesth Analg 1993; 76: 1120-3.
3. Drummond GB, Martin LVH. Pressure-volume relationships in the lung during laparoscopy. Br J Anaesth 1978; 50: 261-70.
4. Puri GD, Singh H. Ventilatory effects of laparoscopy under general anaesthesia. Br J Anaesth 1992; 68: 211-3.
5. Pelosi P, Foti G, Cereda M, et al. Effects of carbon dioxide insufflation for laparoscopic cholecystectomy on the respiratory system. Anaesthesia 1996; 51: 744-9.
6. Koivusalo AM, Lindgren L. Respiratory mechanics during laparoscopic cholecystectomy. Anesth Analg 1999; 89: 800.
7. Hirvonen EA, Nuutinen LS, Kauko M. Ventilatory effects, blood gas changes and oxygen consumption during laparoscopic hysterectomy. Anesth Analg 1995; 80: 961.
8. Kendall AP, Bhatt S, Oh TE. Pulmonary consequences of carbon dioxide insufflation for laparoscopic cholecystectomies. Anaesthesia 1995; 50: 286.
9. Obeid F, Saba A, Fath J, et al. Increase in intra-abdominal pressure affects pulmonary compliance. Arch Surg 1995; 130: 544.
10. Fahy BG, Barnas GM, Flowers JL, et al. The effects of increased abdominal pressure on lung and chest wall mechanics during laparoscopic surgery. Anesth Analg 1995; 81: 744.
11. Oikkonen M, Tallgren M. Changes in respiratory compliance at laparoscopy: Measurements using side stream spirometry. Can J Anesth 1995; 42: 495.
12. Carry PY, Gallet D, Francois Y, et al. Respiratory mechanics during laproscopic cholecystectomy. The effects of the abdominal wall lift. Anesth Analg 1998; 87: 1393.
13. Bures E, Fusiciardi J, Lanquetot H, et al. Ventilatory effects of laparoscopic cholecystectomy. Acta Anesthesiol Scand 1996; 40: 566.
14. Tan PL, Lee TL, Tweed WA. Carbon dioxide absorption and gas exchange during pelvic laparoscopy. Can J Anesth 1992; 39: 677.
15. Klineberg PL, Rheder K, Hyatt RE. Pulmonary mechanics and gas exchange in seated normal man with chest restriction. Journal of Applied Physiology 1981; 51: 26-32.
16. Yasinski P, Joris J, Desaive C, et al. Respiratory changes during CO_2 pneumoperitoneum in morbidly obese patients. Acta Anaesthesiol Belg 1995; 46: P189.
17. Domsky M, Wilson RF, Heins J. Intraoperative end-tidal Carbon dioxide values and derived calculations correlated with outcome: prognosis and capnography. Crit Care Med 1995; 23:1497.
18. Baraka A, Jabbour S, Hammound R, et al. End tidal carbon dioxide tension during laparoscopic cholecystectomy. Anaesthesia 1994; 49:304.

19. Nyarwaya JB, Mazoit JX, Samii K. Are pulse oximetry and end-tidal carbon dioxide tension monitoring reliable during laparoscopic Surgery? Anaesthesia 1994; 49:775.
20. Mullet CE, Viale JP, Saguard PE, et al. Pulmonary CO_2 elimination during Surgical procedures using intra or extraperitoneal CO_2 insufflation. Anesth Analg 1993; 76: 22.
21. Wabba RW, Mamazza J. Ventilatory requirements during Laparoscopic Cholecystectomy. Can J Anesth 1993; 40: 206.
22. McMahon AJ, Baxter JN, Kenny G, et al. Ventilatory and blood gas changes during laparoscopic cholecystectomy. Br J Surg 1993; 80:1252.
23. Hirvonen EA, Nuutinen LS, Kauko M. Ventilatory effects, Blood Gas Changes, and oxygen consumption during laparoscopic hysterectomy. Anesth Analg 1995; 80: 961.
24. Fleming RY, Dougherty TB, Feig BW. The safety of helium for abdominal insufflation. Surg Endosc 1997; 11: 230.
25. Neuberger TJ, Andrus CH, Wittgen CM, et al. Prospective comparison of helium versus carbon dioxide pneumoperitoneum. Gartrointest Endosc 1996; 43: 38.
26. Rademaker BM, Odoom JA, Dewit LT, et al. Hemodynamic effects of pneumoperitoneum for laparoscopic surgery: a comparison of CO_2 with N_2O insufflation. Eur J Anaesthesiol 1994; 11: 301.
27. Ciofola MJ, Clergue F, Seebacher J, et al. Ventilatory effects of laparoscopy under epidural anaesthesia. Anesth Analg 1990; 70: 357-61.
28. Sha M, Ohmura A, Yamada M. Diaphragm function and pulmonary complications after laparoscopic cholecystectomy. Anesthesiology 1991; 75 (Suppl): A255.
29. Welkowitz LA, Rapp L, Martinez J, et al. Instructional set and physiologic response to CO_2 inhalation. Am J Psychiatry 1999; 156: 745.
30. Kuntz C, Wunsch A, Bodeker C, et al. Effect of pressure and gas type on intra- abdominal, subcutaneous and Blood pH in laparoscopy. Surg Endosc 2000; 14: 367.
31. Iwasaka H, MiyaKawa H, Yamamoto H, et al. Respiratory mechanics and arterial blood gases during and after laparoscopic cholecystectomy. Can J Anesth 1996; 43: 128.
32. Guyton AC. Text book of Medical Physiology, 8th ed. WB Saunders: 1991.
33. Staszewska-Barczak J, Dusting GJ. Importance of circulating angiotensin II for elevation of arterial pressure during acute hypercarbia in the anaesthetized dogs. Clin Exp Pharmacol Physiol 1981; 8: 189.
34. Rasmussen JP, Daucot PJ, de Aplma RG, et al. Cardiac function and hypercarbia. Arch Surg 1981; 113: 1196.
35. Waxels JC, Mios OD. Effects of carbon dioxide and pH on myocardial function in dogs with acute left ventricular failure. Crit Care Med 1987; 15: 116.
36. Cullen DJ, Eger EL. Cardiovascular effects of carbon dioxide in man. Anesthesiology 1974; 41: 345.
37. Scott DB, Julian DG. Observations on cardiac arrhythmias during laparoscopy. Br Med J 1972; 1: 411-4.
38. Bhavani-Shankar K, Steinbrook RA, Brooks DC. Arterial to end tidal carbon dioxide pressure difference during laparoscopic surgery in pregnancy. Anesthesiology 2000; 93: 370.
39. Cheng KI, Tang CS, Tsai EM, et al. Correlation of arterial and end tidal carbon dioxide in spontaneously breathing patients during ambulatory gynecologic laparoscopy. J Formos Med Assoc 1999; 98: 814.
40. Casati A, Comotti L, Tommasino C, et al. Effects of pneumoperitoneum and reverse Trendelenburg position on cardiopulmonary function in morbidly obese patients receiving laparoscopic gastric banding. Eur J Anaesthesiol 2000; 17: 300.
41. Frei FJ, Konrad R. The arterial end tidal CO_2 partial pressure difference during anesthesia. Anaesthesist 1990; 39:101.
42. Wikox S, Vandem LD. Alas, poor Trendelenburg and his position! A critique of its uses and effectiveness. Anesth Analg 1988; 67: 574-8.
43. Scott DB. Cardiac Arrhythmias during laparoscopy. Br Med J 1972; 2:49-50.

Effect of Carboperitoneum on CNS Physiology

INTRODUCTION

Like other systems alterations in patient position, carboperitoneum raised intra-abdominal (IAP) and intra-thoracic pressure during laparoscopic surgery can modify cerebral haemodynamics as well. Josephs et al[1] first observed that establishment of pneumoperitoneum produces a significant rise in intracranial pressure (ICP).

CO_2 absorption was implicated in the increased cerebral blood flow (CBF) as measured by transcranial doppler ultrasonography.[2] However, De Cosmo and colleagues[3] observed a rise in middle cerebral artery (MCA) blood flow velocity without an increase in $EtCO_2$ concentration. Intracranial pressure (ICP) also rises with abdominal insufflation with or without a rise in $PaCO_2$[4] and carboperitoneum exacerbates the raised ICP following closed head injury.[5] The increase in ICP is proportional to the IAP attained.[6] Rosenthal et al[7] in an experimental model observed that the elevated ICP associated with CO_2 pneumoperitoneum was unresponsive to hyperventilation and hypocapnia; however ICP was higher with hypoventilation and hypercapnia. CBF and ICP therefore rise during pneumoperitoneum regardless of $PaCO_2$, but hypercapnia may aggravate these effects. The haemodynamic changes that appear after an increased IAP, such as increased mean arterial pressure (MAP) can be considered secondary to CNS responses activated to maintain cerebral perfusion pressure after increased ICP.

This increase in ICP during pneumoperitoneum is usually temporary, with the ICP normalising within 10 minutes of desufflation. The increase in ICP during laparoscopy has been attributed mainly to the increase in vena caval pressure during intra-abdominal insufflation and the subsequent engorgement of the cerebral veins within the rigid cranium. Patients subjected to laparoscopy also become mildly hypercapnic due to the absorption of CO_2 through the peritoneum and this causes intracranial arteriolar dilatation and increased cerebral perfusion. Therefore, intraoperative hypercapnia produces cerebral hypertension.

Halverson and colleagues[8] examined the effects of position during laparoscopy on ICP in an experimental model. The Trendelenberg position increased ICP further during abdominal insufflation, whereas the reverse Trendelenberg position did not reduce it sufficiently. The increased ICP during Trendelenberg position was mainly due to decreased venous return. In an animal model, a rise in IAP combined with head-down position produced a 150 per cent rise in ICP.[9] A study by Abe et al[10] in a series of fourteen patients undergoing laparoscopic hysterectomy in head down position demonstrated significant increase in mean CBF-velocity with respect to baseline levels. Other workers like Kirkinen et al[11] stated that there was no significant change in the mean blood-flow velocity in the MCA in a study group of fifteen patients undergoing the same surgery in the head down position. Similar observations were made by Colomina and Godet et al.[12] They observed no significant difference in mean MCA blood flow in healthy ASA I and II patients undergoing lengthy laparoscopic procedures in head down position. However, both the latter studies demonstrated significant changes in the haemodynamic variables studied, resulting in significant changes in the ICP. They concluded that the consequences of increased IAP on cerebral haemostasis and ICP are particularly relevant for patients affected with cranial trauma or other neuropathologies and who might require examination by the laparoscopic technique. They stated that lengthy laparoscopic procedures in the head down position performed in otherwise healthy patients do not significantly affect cerebral circulation. Nevertheless, this technique should be reconsidered in patients with associated neurological pathologies when the means for proper measurement of cerebral haemodynamics are not available.

Cooke and Browne[13] reported that there was a significant increase in reports of postoperative headache and nausea in patients who underwent laparoscopic abdominal surgery as compared to those who underwent open operation. They suggested that this was because of an increase in ICP as a result of carboperitoneum. Colomina and Godet[12] also reported moderately intense headache in eight of seventeen patients undergoing lengthy laparoscopic surgeries in head down position. The headaches occurred in the immediate postoperative period and were similar in all patients-holocranial location and slightly pulsatile. All cases resolved with conservative treatment consisting of bed rest and oxygen therapy and did not delay discharge. They suggested that it may be related to the effect of plasma absorption of CO_2 breakdown products in the closed abdominal cavity after electrocautery. Several other studies have quantified the increase in plasma concentrations of carboxy-haemoglobin and met-haemoglobin.[14-16] Results have shown that the levels reached are not in the range of toxicity and thus no clinical signs of toxicity in the immediate postoperative period would be expected.

In experimental models a significant rise in ICP was observed even at low IAP pressures (8 mmHg) with the animals in Trendelenberg position.[1] Hence, caution is to be advocated in diagnostic laparoscopy in patients of trauma suspected to be suffering from head injury. However, Ahmed and Whelan[17] recommend that diagnostic laparoscopy for penetrating abdominal injuries in a defined set of conditions was safe and accurate, effectively eliminating nontherapeutic laparotomy and shortening hospitalisation. They recommend that it can be used for penetrating injuries of the abdomen with stable vital signs, intact sensorium without evidence of raised intracranial pressure, ability to give informed consent for the procedure and absence of contraindications for pneumoperitoneum. They suggest that in the algorithm for management of penetrating abdominal injuries, laparoscopy should be placed somewhere between CT scan and laparotomy, either instead of or after CT scan. If the deployment is appropriate, it should lead to significant cost reduction for the trauma service.

Until recently, the presence of ventriculoperitoneal shunt (VPS) was considered an absolute contraindication to laparoscopy because intra-abdominal insufflation causes a rapid increase in ICP.[18] Patients with VPS usually have hindbrain abnormalities and, thus, are thought to be more susceptible to hindbrain herniation with such intracranial hypertension. In patients with VPS, increase in ICP during insufflation can potentially be greater and more sustained than in other patients. This has been mainly attributed to increased resistance to shunt outflow by the pneumoperitoneum. However, in the presence of an incompetent shunt valve, retrograde insufflation of cerebrospinal fluid (CSF) may also contribute to the increase in ICP intraoperatively. Furthermore, acute distal catheter obstruction by soft tissue during intra-abdominal insufflation can lead to shunt failure, resulting in an acute increase in the ICP intraoperatively, which may persist postoperatively until the obstruction is relieved.[20]

To minimise changes in ICP and the risk of hindbrain herniation in patients with VPS, studies have reported using lower insufflation pressure during laparoscopy.[19] Another option is intraoperative distal shunt catheter clamping.[12,19] A more extreme alternative is exteriorisation of the shunt by neurosurgeons during surgery and internalisation after laparoscopy.[18] In the presence of high ICP, intraoperative ICP monitoring and ventricular drainage of CSF from the VPS reservoir maybe warranted.[21] However other studies have shown that routine anaesthetic monitoring maybe adequate[22] and retrograde valve failure chances are remote even with IAP as high as 80 mmHg.[23]

Routine anaesthetic monitoring may be safe but patients should be regularly observed over the first postoperative day for signs of increased ICP, and on discharge should be advised to contact the hospital should any neurological symptoms occur. However, ICP measurement may be done when clear indications are present.

To summarise, the effects of carboperitoneum and raised IAP on CNS physiology can be divided into two phases—an early mechanical effect and a secondary late, arterial or chemical effect (Fig. 6.1).

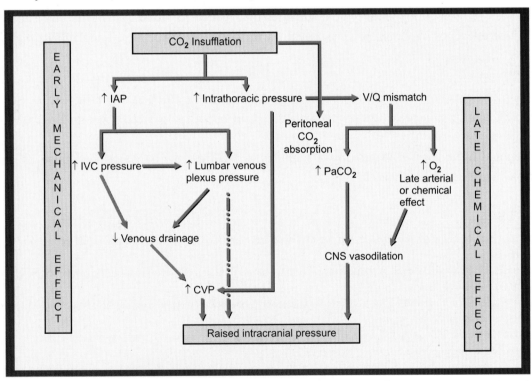

Fig. 6.1: Effects of carboperitoneum on CNS physiology

The rise in ICP during the early phase is due to elevated intrathoracic and intra-abdominal pressures. Elevated IAP compresses the IVC and reduces venous drainage from the CNS and lumbar plexus thereby raising the CSF pressure.[24] Raised IAP also causes cephalad displacement of the diaphragm thus increasing intrathoracic pressure. This leads to increased cardiac filling pressure and CVP in the superior vena cava, which leads to a rise in the ICP. This concomitant increase in ICP and CVP can be explained by the Monroe-Kellie hypothesis that states that if one of the four compartments of the CNS (vascular, parenchymal, osseous or CSF) expands rapidly, there is insufficient time for other compartments to buffer those changes and the ICP rises.

A late chemical effect is observed 10-15 minutes after CO_2 insufflation and is due to reflex vasodilatation caused by the rise in CO_2.[25] Increase in intra-thoracic pressure also leads to ventilation-perfusion (V/Q) mismatch leading to elevated CO_2 level and decreased O_2 levels. In addition there is peritoneal absorption of CO_2. Both hypoxia and hypercapnia are potent cerebral vasodilators leading to a rise in the ICP. Arterial CO_2 tension is the most important single factor controlling CBF.[26] Harper[27] showed that in dogs CBF changes by about 2.5 per cent for every 1 mm change in PCO_2 and this relationship is virtually linear between 30 to 60 mmHg (4-8 KPa). The effect of CO_2 on CBF is almost certainly due to a direct action on the smooth muscles of cerebral arterioles, mediated by local tissue pH changes.[28]

The cerebral circulation does not respond to PaO2 changes around the normal values. When PaO_2 falls below 50 mmHg (6.7 KPa) CBF increases, and is doubled at a PaO2 of about 30 mmHg (4kPa).[26] The cerebral vasodilatation produced by hypoxia may be due to local tissue acidosis caused by a fall in tissue pH and affecting smooth muscle of cerebral arterioles.[29]

CONCLUSIONS

Intracranial pressure rises during laparoscopic surgeries mainly due to raised IAP in the early phase and later due to chemical effects of hypercapnia. This could be further exacerbated in Trendelenberg position.

CLINICAL PEARLS

1. Laparoscopy in patients with cerebral trauma or pathology may produce a rise in ICP.
2. Elevated ICP may not decrease with hyperventilation and hypocapnia, but hypercapnia aggravates this rise and should be avoided.
3. Caution should be advocated in prolonged surgeries in the Trendelenburg position mainly in patients with co-existent neurological pathologies.

REFERENCES

1. Josephs LG, Este Mc Donald JR, Birkett DH, et al. Diagnostic laparoscopy increases intracranial pressure. J Trauma 1993; 36(6): 815-19.
2. Fujii Y, Tanaka H, Tsuruoka S, et al. Middle cerebral arterial blood flow velocity increases during laparoscopic cholecystectomy. Anesth Analg 1994; 78: 80.
3. De Cosmo G, Iannace E, Primeri P, et al. Changes in cerebral haemodynamics during laparoscopic cholecystectomy. Neurol Res 1999; 21: 658.
4. Emelijanov SI, Fedenko VV, Levite EM, et al. Pneumoperitoneum risk prognosis and correction of venous circulation disturbances in laparoscopic surgery. Surg Endosc 1998; 12: 1224.
5. Johannsen G, Andersen M, Juhl B. The effect of general anaesthesia on the haemodynamic events during laparoscopy with CO2 insufflation. Acta Anaesthesiol Scand 1989; 33: 132.
6. Rosenthal RJ, Hiatt JR, Phillips EH, et al. Intracranial pressure: Effects of pneumoperitoneum in a large animal model. Surg Endosc 1997; 11: 367.
7. Rosenthal RJ, Freedman RL, Chidambran A, et al. Effects of hyperventilation and hypoventilation on PaCO2 and intracranial pressure during acute elevation of intra-abdominal pressure with CO_2 pneumoperitoneum: Large animal observations. J Am Coll Surg 1998; 187: 32.
8. Halverson A, Buchanan R, Jaceb L, et al. Evaluation of mechanism of increased intracranial pressure with insufflation. Surg Endosc 1998; 12: 226.
9. Ravaoherisoa J, Meyer P, Afriat R et al. Laparoscopic surgery in a patient with venticuloperitoneal shunt: monitoring of shunt fraction with transcranial Doppler. Br J Anaesth 2004; 92:434-7.

10. Abe K, Hashimoto N, Taniguchi A, et al. Middle cerebral arterial blood flow velocity in during laparoscopy in head-down position. Surg Laparosc Endosc 1998; 8:1-4.

11. Kirkinen P, Hirvonen E, Kauko M, et al. Intracranial blood flow during laparoscopic hysterectomy. Acta Obstet Gynecol Scand 1995; 74:71-4.

12. Colomina MJ, Godet C, Pellise f, et al.Transcranial Doppler monitoring during laparoscopic anterior lumbar interbody fusion. Anesth Analg 2003; 97:1675-9.

13. Cooke SJ, Paterson-Brown S. Association between laparoscopic abdominal surgery and postoperative symptoms of raised intracranial pressure. Surg Endosc 2001; 15:723-5.

14. Beebe DS, Swica H, Carlson N, et al. High levels of carbon monoxide are produced by electrocautrey of tissue during laparoscopic cholecystectomy. Anesth Analg 1993; 77: 338-41.

15. Wu JS, , Luttman DR, Meininger TA, et al. Production and systemic absorption toxic byproducts of tissue combustion during laparoscopic surgery. Surg Endosc 1997; 11: 1075-9.

16. Wu JS, Monk T, Luttman DR, et al. Production and systemic absorption toxic byproducts of tissue combustion during laparoscopic cholecystectomy. J. Gastrointest Surg 1998; 2: 399-405.

17. Ahmed N, Whelan J, Brownlee J, et al. The contribution of laparoscopy in evaluation of penetrating abdominal wounds. J Am Coll Surg 2005; 201: 213-16.

18. Muffarej F, Nolan C, Shastri S, et al.Laparoscopic procedures in adults with ventriculoperitoneal shunts. Surg Laparosc Endosc Percutan Tech 2005; 15: 28-9.

19. Kimura T, Nakajima K, Wasa M, et al. Successful laparoscopic fundoplication in children with ventriculoperitoneal shunts. Surg Endosc. 2002; 16:215.

20. Baskin JJ, Vishteh AG, Wesche DE, et al. Ventriculoperitoneal shunt failure as a complication of laparoscopic surgery. JSLS. 1998; 2:177-80.

21. Uzzo RG, Bilsky M, Mininberg DT, et al. Laparoscopic surgery in children with ventriculoperitoneal shunts: effect of pneumoperitoneum on intracranial pressure-preliminary experience. Urology. 1997; 49: 753-7.

22. Jackman SV, Weingart JD, Kinsman SL, et al. Laparoscopic surgery in patients with ventriculoperitoneal shunts: safety and monitoring. J Urol. 2000; 164: 1352-4.

23. Neale ML, Falk GL. In vitro assessment of back pressure on ventriculoperitoneal shunt valves. Is laparoscopy safe? Surg Endosc. 1999; 13: 512-5.

24. Halverson A, Buchanan R, Jaceb L, et al. Decreased cerebrospinal fluid absorption during abdominal insufflation. Surg Endosc 1999; 13: 797.

25. Hargrearies DM. Hypercapnia and raised cerebrospinal fluid pressure. Anesthesia 1990; 45(12): 7-12.

26. Wylie and Churchill-Davidson's: A Practice of Anaesthesia. 5th Edn.

27. Harper AM. Physiology of the cerebral blood flow. Br J Anaesth 1965; 37: 225.

28. Lassen NA. The luxury perfusion syndrome and its possible relation to acute metabolic acidosis localised within the brain. Lancet 1966; 2: 1113.

29. Kegure K, Scheinberg P, Reinmuth OM, et al. Mechanism of cerebral vasodilatation in hypoxia. J Appl Physiol 1970; 29: 223.

Effect of Carboperitoneum on Renal Physiology

REVIEW OF NORMAL RENAL PHYSIOLOGY

Insufflation of CO_2 to produce carboperitoneum results in an increase in the intra-abdominal pressure. Increase in IAP along with patient positioning are the main trespasses to normal homeostasis in laparoscopic surgery. These trigger off a neurohormonal cascade which ultimately results in decreased renal blood flow and oliguria. However to understand this chain of events it is essential to review the normal renal physiology.

Under normal circumstances the kidneys receive 20-25 per cent (l.25 1/min) of the cardiac output (CO). Most (85%) of the renal blood flow (RBF) perfuses the outer cortex of the kidney. The remaining 15 per cent of RBF perfuses the juxtamedullary nephrons. Blood flow to the kidneys is determined by the cardiac output and renal vascular resistance. RBF is maintained relatively constant, despite significant changes in mean arterial pressure (MAP), by autoregulatory resistance changes in the renal afferent arterioles (Fig. 7.1).

Approximately 20 per cent of the renal plasma (650 ml/min) is filtered as an essentially protein-free plasma through the glomerular capillary into the Bowman's capsule. The glomerular filtration process is governed by Starling's forces and averages 125 ml/min.

EFFECTS OF ELEVATED INTRA-ABDOMINAL PRESSURE (IAP) ON RENAL PHYSIOLOGY

In 1923, Thorington and Schmidt[1] observed that urine output improved following paracentesis in a patient with malignant ascites. They subsequently demonstrated in a canine study that animals become oliguric at an IAP of 15-30 mmHg and anuric when it exceeds 30 mmHg.

The decrease in renal perfusion during pneumoperitoneum produces a reduction in glomerular filtration rate (GFR),[2,3] urinary output,[3,4] sodium excretion[3] and creatinine clearance.[5] These changes are greater at an intra-abdominal pressure (IAP) greater than 15 mmHg,[5] although some deterioration in renal function also occurs at an IAP of 10 mmHg.[6]

The adverse effects of elevated IAP on renal haemodynamics are due to the decline in cardiac output and the direct effect on RBF observed during carboperitoneum. Harman et al[6] observed that the decline in RBF persists despite normal or even supranormal values of cardiac output when IAP is >20 mmHg. At an IAP less

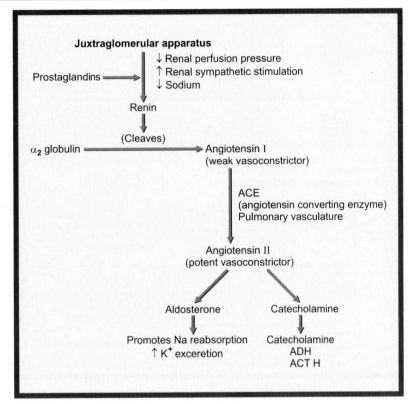

Fig. 7.1: Renin-angiotensin-aldosterone axis

than 15 mmHg the efficacy of maintaining normal or supranormal CO for maintaining renal function is uncertain[6]. Thus, besides changes in renal vascular resistance, the other determinants of RBF appear to be critical in understanding the pathophysiology of elevated IAP on renal function. The main factors affecting renal vascular resistance are mechanical compression and neurohormonal response to the elevated IAP (Fig. 7.2).

Renal venous pressure may rise due to direct mechanical compression and the resultant increase in renal vascular resistance decreases the renal blood flow.[7] Renal vasoconstriction may also occur due to sympathetic stimulation due to elevated IAP[8] or hypercarbia.[9] The primary renal effect of CO_2 insufflation is a decrease in renal blood flow, which may last up to two hours after deflation[5]. The use of different insufflating gases does not alter the decrease in urine output.[7] Renal vasoconstriction also impairs the oxygen balance of renal medulla and is one of the main factors for acute tubular necrosis.[10]

An increase in plasma renin activity, norepinephrine and epinephrine is considered to be a stress response to CO_2 insufflation.[11,12] Opioid analgesia during anesthesia may blunt this response so that the increase may be quite modest and not clinically significant.[10]

Increased endothelin concentration during carboperitoneum in an experimental model can cause a reduction in RBF, GFR and sodium excretion.[13] Antidiuretic hormone (ADH) levels rise during pneumoperitoneum[10,13] and pretreatment with an ADH antagonist improves urine output.[2] This increase in ADH is multifactorial and pneumoperitoneum alone is not responsible for its rise. Surgery itself induces high concentrations of ADH for several days.

Diminished RBF due to various causes is a potent trigger of the renin-angiotensin-aldosterone axis. Angiotensin II causes renal and systemic vasoconstriction and a release of catecholamines. Urinary sodium has been observed

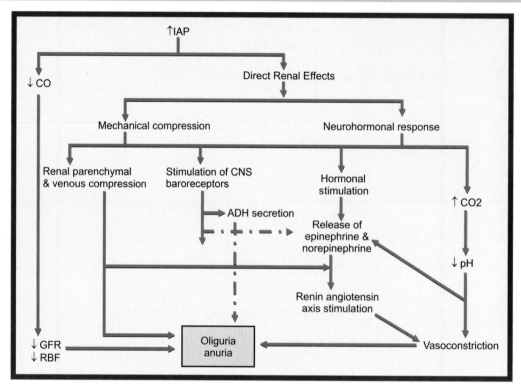

Table 7.2: Effect of carboperitoneum on renal physiology

to decrease and potassium concentration to increase, an effect consistent with elevated aldosterone levels.[14] Insufflation of cool CO_2 into the abdominal cavity may cause renal vasoconstriction.[15] The core temperature decreases approximately 0.2°C/50L of CO_2 flow. Warm CO_2 causes vasodilatation and maintains urine output during laparoscopic surgery lasting up to three hours.[15]

There is no correlation between the systemic haemodynamic response to peritoneal insufflation and renal arterial blood flow.[16]

The recently introduced technique of gasless laparoscopy has a more favourable effect on renal physiology. Higher urine output has been documented as well as no changes in renal oxygenation were seen with this method, when compared with conventional pneumoperitoneum.[4,10] Hence, this method may prove to be beneficial in patients with limited renal function and those with a transplanted kidney.

CONCLUSION

Renal blood flow is greatly compromised during laparoscopic surgery due to a combination of various factors. One must particularly remember this in patients with deranged renal function and in surgeries of long duration. Renal protection strategies may need to be adopted. Restriction of IAP and judicious use of diuretics may be needed to augment RBF in special cases.

CLINICAL PEARLS

• Intra-abdominal pressure is the major determinant of renal blood flow during laparoscopy.
• Monitor urine output in prolonged laparoscopic surgery.

REFERENCES

1. Thorington JM, Schmidt CF. A study of urinary output and blood pressure changes resulting in experimental ascetics. Am J Med Sci 1923; 165: 880-86?

2. Dolgor B, Kitano S, Yoshida T, et al. Vasopressin antagonist improves renal function in a rat model of pneumoperitoneum. J Surg Res 1998; 79: 109.

3. Hamilton BD, Chow GK, Inman SR, et al. Increased intra-abdominal pressure during pneumoperitoneum stimulates endothelin release in a canine model. J Endourol 1998; 12: 193.

4. Koivusato AM, Kellokumpu I, Puskari S, et al. Splanchnic and renal deterioration during and after laparoscopic cholecystectomy. A comparison of the carbon dioxide pneumoperitoneum and the abdominal wall lift method. Anesth Analg 1997; 85: 886.

5. Mc Dougall EM, Bennett HF, Menk TG, et al. Functional MR imaging of the porcine kidney: Physiologic changes of prolonged pneumoperitoneum. J Soc Laparoendosc Surg 1997; 1: 29.

6. Harman PK, Kron I, MC Lochlan HD, et al. Elevated intra-abdominal pressure and renal function. Ann Surg 1982; 196: 594-7.

7. Shuto K, Kitono S, Yeshida T, et al. Haemodynamic and arterial blood gas changes during carbon dioxide and helium pneumoperitoneum in pigs. Surg Endosc 1995; 9: 1173.

8. Julius S, Sanchez R, Malayan S, et al. Sustained blood pressure elevation to lower renal compression in pigs and dogs. Hypertension 1982; 4: 782-8.

9. Price HL. Effects of carbon dioxide on the cardiovascular system. Anesthesiology 1960; 21: 652-7.

10. Koivusalo AM, Kellekumpu I, Scheinin M, et al. A comparison of Gasless Mechanical and conventional carbon dioxide pneumoperitoneum methods for laparoscopic cholecystectomy. Anesth Analg 1998; 86: 153-8.

11. Koivusalo AM, Kellekumpu I, Scheinin M, et al. Randomised comparison of the neuroendocrine response to laparoscopic cholecystectomy using either conventional or abdominal wall lift techniques. Br J Surg 1996; 83: 1532-6.

12. O'Leary, Hubbard, Termey W, Cunninfram A. Laparoscopic cholecystectomy: Haemodynamic and neuro-endocrine response after pneumoperitoneum and changes in position. Br J Anaesth 1996; 76: 640-4.

13. Walder AD, Aitkenhead AR. Role of vasopressin in the haemodynamic response to laparoscopic cholecystectomy. Br J Anaesth 1997; 78: 264.

14. Shenasky JH, Gillinneater JY. The renal haemodynamic and functional effects of external counter pressure. Surg Gynecol Obst 1972; 134: 253-8.

15. Backlund M, Kellekumpu I, Scheinin T, et al. Effect of temperature of insufflated CO_2 during and after prolonged laparoscopic surgery. Surg Endosc 1998; 12: 126.

16. Junghans T, Bohm B, Graudel K, et al. Does pneumoperitoneum with different gases, body positions, and intraperitoneal pressures influence renal and hepatic blood flow? Surg 1997; 121: 206.

Stress Response and Laparoscopy

INTRODUCTION

The normal body responds to injury through a series of complex neural and hormonally mediated changes, termed "the neurohormonal stress response". These changes attempt to restore an injured organism to a normal state of homeostasis and health. The magnitude of systemic stress response is proportional to the degree of operative trauma. Minimal access surgery is definitely associated with less surgical trauma and therefore should lead to decrease in the stress response. Indeed the very term "minimally invasive surgery" suggests the possibility that laparoscopy is accompanied by a diminished physiological stress response, however, this is not yet proven.

NORMAL STRESS RESPONSE[1]

Systemic response to surgery is characterised by:

Sympathetic nervous system activation

Endocrine stress responses:

    Pituitary hormone secretion

    Insulin resistance

Immunological and haematological changes:

    Acute phase reaction

    Neutrophil leucocytosis

    Lymphocyte proliferation

    Cytokine production

HORMONAL RESPONSE TO SURGERY[1]

Tissue surgery: Stimulates afferent sensory limb of CNS

      ↓

      Spinothalamic tract

      ↓

Pons and medulla
↓
Hypothalamus
↓
Hypothalamic releasing factors
↓
Pituitary hormones
↓
Endocrine target hormones
↓
Adrenal gland
↓
End organ hormonal response

The onset of surgery is associated with a rapid secretion of hormones derived from the anterior and posterior pituitary; β-endorphin, ACTH, growth hormone, prolactin, arginine, vasopressin together with activation of sympathetic nervous system and release of adrenaline and noradrenaline. This is closely followed by increases in circulating cortisol, aldosterone and renin. In the presence of a marked increase in catabolic hormone secretion, there is suppression of important anabolic hormones: insulin and testosterone. These hormonal changes result in a measurable neurohormonal stress response that is characterised by substrate mobilisation and ultimately a catabolic state with negative nitrogen balance.

The outstanding feature of catabolic hormonal response to surgery is the failure of normal feedback mechanisms that control secretion. For example, ACTH secretion from the pituitary is rapidly followed by cortisol release from the adrenals, which fail to inhibit the further secretion of trophic hormones.

Table 8.1: Hormonal responses to surgery

Endocrine gland	Hormones	Change in secretion
Anterior pituitary	ACTH	↑
	Growth hormone	↑
	TSH	↑ or/ ↓
	FSH + LH	↑/↓
Posterior pituitary	AVP	↑
Adrenal cortex	Cortisol	↑
Pancreas	Insulin	↓
	Glucagon	↑
Thyroid	Thyroxine, triiodothyronine	↓

ACTIVATION OF STRESS RESPONSE FACTORS

Cytokines[1,2]

Cytokines are a group of low molecular weight glycoproteins which include the interleukins and interferons. These are produced at the site of injury and have a major role in mediating immunity and inflammation. After major surgery, the main cytokines released are interleukin I (IL-1), tumour necrosis factor α (TNF-α) and IL-6.

TNF-α[1,2]

It is one of the earliest appearing mediators after operative injury, and has a half-life of less than 20 minutes. TNF-α is a potent inducer of IL-6 production and is responsible for the systemic manifestations of fever, tachycardia, increased catabolism and hypotension.

Interleukin-6[1,2]

Serum IL-6 concentration is roughly proportional to the severity of surgery. It is a pleiotropic proinflammatory cytokine, which appears to potentiate the biosynthesis of acute phase proteins by hepatocytes as its levels precede the rise of C-reactive proteins (CRP). IL-6 also initiates the activation of hypothalamic pituitary-adrenal axis and induces ACTH synthesis. Within 30 to 60 minutes after the start of surgery, IL-6 concentration increases and becomes significant after two to four hours.

C-Reactive Protein[1,2]

C-reactive protein is the most sensitive acute phase protein and has been used as an objective biochemical marker to reflect the degree of operative injury.

Following tissue injury a number of changes occur, which are stimulated by cytokines, particularly IL-6; this is known as an acute phase response.

FEATURES OF ACUTE PHASE RESPONSE

1. Fever
2. Granulocytosis
3. Production of acute phase proteins in liver:
    CRP
    Fibrinogen
    α_2 macroglobulin
4. Changes in serum concentration of transport proteins like albumin
5. Changes in serum concentration of divalent cations like copper, ceruloplasmin and zinc
6. Actvation of hypothalamic-pituitary-adrenal axis

STRESS RESPONSE IN LAPAROSCOPIC SURGERY

Conventional surgery usually involves a large skin incision, muscular destruction, increased third space losses due to an exposed abdomen, greater manipulation of the bowel and is accompanied by postoperative pain. Trauma implicated in laparoscopic surgery is definitely much less as compared to laparotomy. It involves an iatrogenic carboperitoneum, increased intra-abdominal pressure, altered acid base balance due to CO_2 insufflation and altered circulatory and pulmonary mechanics. [1,2] The contribution of any single parameter to the neurohormonal response is inherently difficult to define and measure.

ENDOSCOPIC SURGERY AND ENDOCRINE METABOLIC RESPONSE

Various studies have been done to compare stress markers in laparotomy and laparoscopy. It appears that most studies have compared open cholecystectomy with laparoscopic cholecystectomy. A summary of the effects of endoscopic, predominantly laparoscopic techniques on various endocrinal metabolic responses compared with similar open operations is presented in Table 8.1.

Table 8.1: Effect of endoscopic surgery on intraoperative and postoperative endocrine metabolic responses [31]

Author	Operation	Duration of study (hours)	Parameter
Joris (1992)	Lap. Vs. open cholecystectomy	48	p-cortisol→ p-catecholamines→ p-glucose↓
Rademaker (1992)	Lap. Vs. open cholecystectomy	6	p-cortisol→ p-glucose→
McMahon (1993)	Lap. Vs. mini cholecystectomy	7 Days	p-cortisol→ u-catecholamines→ u-3-Methylhistidine→ s-albumin, s-transferrin→
Jakeways(1994)	Lap. Vs. open cholecystectomy	12	p-cortisol→ p-lactate, s-albumin→, p-glucose↓
Redmond (1994)	Lap. Vs. open cholecystectomy	3 Days	p-cortisol→
Glaser (1995)	Lap. Vs. open cholecystectomy	48	p-epinephrine, p-norepinephrine→, b-glucose↓, p-ACTH, p-cortisole→
Glerup(1995)	Lap.vs.open herniorrhaphy	24	Functional hepatic nitrogen clearance↓ p-glucagon, p-cortisol↓
Senagore (1995)	Lap.vs.open colectomy	7 Days	Nitrogen balance improved u-3-methylhistidine→
Targarona (1996)	Lap.vs. Open cholecystectomy	80	p- cortisol, p-ACTH, p-GH, p-prolactin, p-glucagun, p-insulin,p-glucose, p-FFA→
Deuss (1994)	Lap.vs.open cholecystectomy	48	p- cortisol, p-ACTH, p-GH, p-prolactin→
Fukushima (1996)	Lap.vs. open sigmoidectomy	5 Days	p-glucagon, u-catecholamines→
Essen (1995)	Lap.vs. open cholecystectomy	24	Protein synthesis rate→ Insulin sensitivity↑
Bellon (1997)	Lap.vs. Open cholecystectomy	7 Days	p-cortisol→
Ortega (1996)	Lap.vs. Open cholecystectomy	24	p-ADH↑; p-cortisol, p-ACTH, p-insulin, p-glucose, p-catecholamines→
Hammarqvist (1996)	Lap.vs. Open cholecystectomy	48	Muscle glutamine, ribosome, nitrogen loss→

→: no difference between endoscopic and open surgery; ↓: reduction of response in endoscopic vs. open surgery; ↑: improvement in response in endoscopic vs. open surgery; lap.: laparoscopic; p: plasma; u: urine; s: serum; b: blood; u-vma: vaniline mandelic acid; ACTH: adrenocorticotrophic hormone; ADH: antidiuretic hormone; GH: growth hormone; FFA: free fatty acids.

The results are relatively uniform in demonstrating no significant differences in classic endocrine catabolic responses (glucose and protein economy), although a few studies have shown reduced responses in favour of laparoscopic surgery.[3] In conclusion, endocrine response to laparoscopic and open cholecystectomy does not differ significantly.[4] Plasma concentration of cortisol and catecholamines, metabolic and anaesthetic requirement are similar after both procedures. However, most data come from cholecystectomy, where morbidity is also low. Further data with repeated sampling for a prolonged period and focusing on protein economy and pituitary sympathetic responses are required from major abdominal operations to allow conclusions on potential clinical applications.

Some[5,6] studied the impact on stress response and the influence of anaesthesia on endocrine and immunological changes by investigating the plasma levels of norepinephrine, cortisol, TNF-α and IL6 in patients scheduled for laparotomy and laparoscopic cholecystectomy. They confirmed that laparoscopic cholecystectomy is associated with less immunoendocrine response and the type of anaesthesia does not interfere with plasma changes of assessed hormones.

Studies[7] have compared objective stress response of laparoscopic and open abdominal rectopexy by measuring urinary catecholamines, interleukin and serum cortisol for acute phase response; and C-reactive proteins and ESR for delayed stress response. It was concluded that there is benefit in terms of the immediate objective stress response in laparoscopic surgery than in open surgery; while the delayed response is equal in both.

Joris et al[8] in 1992 and Mc Mahon in 1993[9] compared metabolic and respiratory changes after laparoscopic and open cholecystectomy. They concluded that metabolic and acute phase responses (glucose, leucocytosis, C-reactive protein) were less after laparoscopy compared to laparotomy. Although plasma cortisol and catecholamine concentrations were not significantly different between the two groups, postoperatively interleukin-6 concentration was less in laparoscopy group.

Gideon P Naude et al[10] in 1996 undertook a study to compare the stress response of patients undergoing laparoscopic cholecystectomy using CO_2 and helium as insufflating gases. They concluded that stress response to laparoscopic cholecystectomy is independent of the insufflating gas used and both groups demonstrated significant increase in epinephrine, norepinephrine and cortisol levels throughout the procedures. Except for a larger increase in epinephrine in the helium group there were no significant differences between the groups.

Taragarona et al[11] undertook a study to investigate the response to injury of two surgical models (laparoscopic versus open cholecystectomy) by evaluating neuroendocrine, acute phase and metabolic components. They concluded that surgical response after laparoscopic cholecystectomy is similar to that after open cholecystectomy but acute phase response component is less intense in laparoscopy group (interleukin-6 / C-reactive protein and prealbumin). This finding may be a consequence of reduced size of operative wound with laparoscopic cholecystectomy.

Karayiannakis[12] et al in 1996 did a randomised clinical trial of 41 patients undergoing laparoscopic cholecystectomy and 42 patients undergoing open cholecystectomy. Neuroendocrine and metabolic stress responses were compared. Plasma levels of cortisol, adrenaline, noradrenaline, glucose, IL-6 and CRP were measured before, during and at 4,8 and 24 hours after operation. They found that plasma levels of cortisol and catecholamines increase during and after both laparoscopic and open cholecystectomy, however, their postoperative responses were significantly higher in open cholecystectomy group. They concluded that systemic stress response is significantly decreased after laparoscopic cholecystectomy.

Pinnonen, Melville et al and Heruzzo et al[13-15] in separate studies documented significant increase in ADH levels in patients undergoing laparoscopy, especially at the end of carboperitoneum insufflation after excluding factors like decrease in blood pressure, changes in serum osmolality and oxygenation. They postulated that the relationship between increased intra-abdominal pressure (IAP) and ADH secretion is mediated by trapping of blood in the lower part of the body and decreased venous return to the heart which is sensed by intrathoracic blood volume receptors located in the right atrium.

Monsour et al[16,17] compared the hormonal stress markers, ACTH, cortisol, insulin and glucagon, in pigs undergoing laparoscopic and open cholecystectomy.[16] Cooper et al studied 22 women undergoing laparoscopy for serum cortisol, prolactin, growth hormone and serum glucose levels. Both groups came to the same conclusion: that laparoscopy is as stressful as laparotomy. Both the groups hypothesised that acute stretch of the peritoneum by CO_2 insufflation may activate receptors that trigger ACTH and cortisol release. It has also been proposed that acute stretch of the peritoneum can trigger vagal responses, which in turn trigger the neural stimulus for hormonal release.

Deuss et al[18] compared laparoscopic cholecystectomy vs open cholecystectomy where they found that ACTH levels become maximally elevated after skin incision and cortisol levels become maximally elevated 2 hours after extubation. The maximum levels of ACTH and cortisol were greater for the laparoscopic group as compared to the open group, however these differences were not statistically significant. They concluded that peritoneal incision itself is the major stimulus for ACTH and cortisol secretion, independent of the size of the skin incision.

Milheiro[19] in a study on 40 humans undergoing open and laparoscopic cholecystectomy found elevation in cortisol and renin levels but the difference in the rise in laparoscopy group vs open group was not statistically significant.

O'Leary[20] studied 16 patients undergoing laparoscopic cholecystectomy and concluded that maximal stimulus to hormone secretion is not pneumoperitoneum but the drugs used for reversal of anaesthesia, return to consciousness, postoperative pain and anxiety.

Nyugen et al[21] have shown elevation of CRP levels at 1 hour postoperatively that peaked at 48-72 hours after both laparoscopic and open gastric bypass. CRP levels were significantly lower after laparoscopic gastric bypass procedure. The lower CRP response reflects a reduced operative trauma after laparoscopic gastric bypass (GBP).

The hypothesis that laparoscopy produces an attenuated hormonal stress response compared to the open surgical approach was finally tested in a prospective and randomised fashion by Ortega et al. [22] In patients with laparoscopic vs open cholecystectomy the classical hormonal stress response was measured including the adrenocortical (serum ACTH, cortisol, urinary free cortisol), adrenomedullary (plasma and urinary epinephrine and norepinephrine) and pituitary (ADH and growth hormone) hormonal axis as well as the components of glucose metabolism (serum glucose, glucagon and insulin). Growth hormone levels were similar in both groups; serum ADH levels were highest in the laparoscopic group. Serum ACTH levels rose intraoperatively and peaked during the first 4 postoperative hours in both groups; however the postoperative deviation from baseline tended to be higher in the open group; cortisol levels were similar in both groups. Plasma epinephrine and norepinephrine levels were similar between the two groups.

All the above studies indicate that a considerable activation of the neuroendocrine axis does occur after laparoscopic surgery, despite the absence of a substantial skin incision and minimal postoperative pain. Probably, apart from the neurogenic afferent stimuli from the wound, other visceral afferent stimuli may also play an important role. Abdominal distension after creation of pneumoperitoneum has been suggested as a possible stimulus for sympathetic stress response.[21]

ENDOSCOPIC SURGERY AND INFLAMMATORY RESPONSE AND IMMUNE FUNCTION

There is an increasing body of data that suggests that acute-phase-response, as measured by C-reactive protein (CRP), interleukin-6 and total lymphocyte count, is attenuated after laparoscopic surgical procedures. It is perhaps those studies that demonstrate an attenuated acute phase response after laparoscopic cholecystectomy that best support the concept that the laparosocpic procedure is less traumatic. With herniorrhaphy, studies show no difference in inflammatory responses whether the operation is performed open or endoscopically. With colonic operations, studies suggest a larger increase in IL-6 and CRP with endoscopic operations. This finding is difficult to explain except that longer duration of endoscopic surgery is often related to a larger increase in these parameters postoperatively.[23, 24]

The effect of endoscopic techniques on postoperative immune function and inflammatory responses has been studied in several clinical studies (Table 8.2).

Table 8.2: Effect of endoscopic surgery on postoperative immune function (clinical studies) [31]

Author	Operation	Duration of study (hours)	Parameter	Comments
Joris (1992)	Lap. Vs. open cholecystectomy	48	CRP↓, IL↓, leucocytosis↓	
Mealy (1992)	Lap. Vs. open cholecystectomy	48	CRP↓, complement C-3→	
Roumen (1992)	Lap. Vs. open cholecystectomy	24	CRP or IL-6↓	
McMahon (1993)	Lap. Vs. mini cholecystectomy	148	IL-6, CRP, PMN elastase→	Minilap vs.lap. cholecystectomy: less difference in trauma size
Cho(1994)	Lap. Vs. open cholecystectomy	48	IL-6, CRP↓	If ERCP preceded operation, higher IL-6 responses occurred
Jakeways(1994)	Lap. Vs. open cholecystectomy	48	IL-6, CRP↓	
Berggren(1994)	Lap. Vs. open cholecystectomy	24	CRP, IL-6→	
Redmond (1994)	Lap. Vs. open cholecystectomy	3 days	CRP→;monocyte release of O_2^- and TNF↓; PMN release of O_2^- and chemotaxis ↓; WBC count↓	Sample only on preoperative and postoperative days 1 and 3; difference mostly on postoperative day 1
Stage (1997)	Lap. Vs. open colonic resection	10 Days	IL-6, CRP↑	
Hill (1995)	Lap.vs.open herniorraphy	24	IL-6, CRP→	
Thorell (1996)	Lap.vs. Open cholecystectomy	24	IL-6→	
Schrenk (1996)	Lap.vs.open herniorraphy	5 Days	IL-6, TNF, CRP→	
Targarona (1996)	Lap.vs. Open cholecystectomy	80	IL-6, CRP↓	
Wright (1996)	Lap.vs.open herniorrhaphy	24	IL-6, CRP→	
Fukushima (1996)	Lap.vs. open sigmoidectomy	5 Days	IL-6↑, CRP→	
Gebhard (1996)	Lap.vs. open pneumothorax surgery	3 Days	CRP, thromboxane, prostacyclin↓	
Bellon (1997)	Lap.vs. Open cholecystectomy	7 Days	IL-6v; IL-1α, TNF α, IL-10→	
Klava (1997)	Different open vs. lap.procedures	8	Monocyte HLA-DR expression→	

→: no difference between endoscopic and open surgery; ↓: reduction of response in endoscopic vs. open surgery; ↑: improvement in response in endoscopic vs. open surgery; CRP: C-reactive protein; PMN: polymorphonuclear leucocytes; WBC: White blood cells; TNF: Tumour necrosis factor; IL: Interleukin; HLA-DR: class II human leucocyte antigen; ERCP: endoscopic retrograde cholangiopancreaticography; C-3: Complement 3 fraction.

In experimental studies, laparoscopy has been demonstrated to reduce impairment in the delayed hypersensitivity response, release of O_2 radicals, tumour necrosis factor and the impairment of candida ingestion by peritoneal macrophages.

In summary, the data on inflammatory and immunological parameters suggest a slight reduction in inflammatory responses (CRP, IL-6), following endoscopic versus open cholecystectomy. The studies on other immunological parameters are inadequate to allow further conclusions.[11]

EFFECT OF ENDOSCOPIC SURGERY ON PULMONARY FUNCTION AND HYPOXAEMIA

The differences in pulmonary function parameters and hypoxaemia between endoscopic and open procedures have also been studied extensively (Table 8.3).

Table 8.3: Effect of endoscopic surgery on postoperative pulmonary function and hypoxaemia[31]

Author	Operation	Duration of study (hours)	Pulmonary function	Hypoxaemia	Other findings
Frazee (1991)	Lap. Vs. open cholecystectomy	24	FVC, FEV1↑		
Joris (1992)	Lap. Vs. open cholecystectomy	48	FVC, FEV1, VT↑	PaO$_2$↑	
Mealy (1992)	Lap. Vs. open cholecystectomy	24	VC, FEV↑	Pa O$_2$→	
Putensen-Himmer (1992)	Lap. Vs. open cholecystectomy	72	FVC, FEV1, FRC↑	Pa O$_2$↑	
Rademaker (1992)	Lap. Vs. open cholecystectomy	24	FVC, peak flow, FEV1↑		No additional approvement with epidural bupivacaine
Schauer (1993)	Lap. Vs. open cholecystectomy	12 Days	FVC, FEV1, peak flow↑	O$_2$ satutation↑	Less atelectasis in laparoscopic group
Mc Mahon (1994)	Lap. Vs. mini cholecystectomy	48	FVC, FEV1, peak flow↑	O$_2$ satutation↑	Insignificant reduction in chest infection in lap. Froup (1% vs. minilap 8%), n=132
Redmond (1994)	Lap. Vs. open cholecystectomy (8 cm)	24		Pa O$_2$↑	Insignificantly fewer respiratory
infections					
					in open (6/22) vs. lap. Cholecystectomy (0/22)
Stage (1997)	Lap.vs.open colonic resection	30 Days	FEV1, PF, FVC→		
Karayiannakis (1996)	Lap. Vs. open cholecystectomy	48	FEV1, FVC, FRC↑	PaO$_2$↑	Less atelectasis in lap. Group
Olsen (1997)	Lap. Vs. open fundoplication	3 Days	FVC, peak flow↑	O2 satutation↑	

→: no difference between endoscopic vs. open surgery; ↑: improved function in endoscopic vs. open surgery; FVC: forced vital capacity; FEV1: forced expiratory volume in 1 second; VT: tidal volume; VC: vital capacity; FRC: functional residual capacity; PaO2: arterial oxygen tension; PF: peak flow.

In contrast to the results from endocrine, metabolic, inflammatory and immunological parameters, the results for pulmonary function and hypoxaemia generally favour endoscopic surgery, although most studies have demonstrated impairment of all types of pulmonary functions.[8, 25]

There is less postoperative hypoxaemia in endoscopic versus open procedures.[8, 25] There is also a trend towards less atelectasis and respiratory infections in the endoscopic versus open surgery groups. Most of the above studies are based on cholecystectomy and there is an inadequate number of studies to allow conclusions about other abdominal operations.[8, 24, 25] However, postoperative pulmonary dysfunction is most prominent after upper abdominal procedures, a finding that also applies to endoscopic procedures when performed in the upper versus lower part of the abdomen.[31]

POSTOPERATIVE GASTROINTESTINAL PARALYSIS AND OTHER PHYSIOLOGICAL RESPONSES TO SURGERY

Any abdominal operation is followed by an obligatory neurally mediated paralytic response in the gastrointestinal tract. Experimental studies comparing laparoscopic versus open laparotomy clearly suggest a shortened gastrointestinal paralysis with endoscopy procedure. The clinical implication of the above findings may be of major importance as they allow early oral nutrition which in turn reduces catabolism and septic complications.[17, 21, 31]

SPLANCHNIC TISSUE OXYGENATION

There seems to be no difference in splanchnic tissue oxygenation whether cholecystectomy is performed laparoscopically or as an open procedure. Postoperative sleep disturbances may be reduced by laparoscopic cholecystectomy, but the role of concomitant reduced requirement of opioids has not been established.[17, 21]

CLINICAL IMPLICATIONS

It appears from the data comparing endoscopic and open surgery in a variety of operations, that only small, if any, differences exist in various endocrine, metabolic, inflammatory responses and changes in immune function except for the reduced CRP and IL-6 responses in laparosocopic cholecystectomy. This applies to relatively minor operations such as herniorrhaphy; major abdominal operations such as colectomy are less well studied and need further evaluation. Various factors (like intraoperative hypothermia, postoperative immobilisation, semistarvation and pain) that may contribute to morbidity must be considered. In addition, the exact role of endoscopic procedure to improve outcome after a variety of abdominal operations such as fundoplication, colectomy and appendicectomy remains to be established.[12, 15, 20, 26, 27]

The important question remains as to why the advantageous outcome results are not more obvious. In this context, it is important again to take into consideration other factors that may limit early recovery and even contribute to morbidity. Such factors include traditional regimens with unnecessary drains, gastrointestinal tubes inadequate pain relief and inadequate oral nutrition, which limit mobilisation and rehabilitation, and all of which may contribute to a cascade of events leading to postoperative dependence. Immobilisation may amplify catabolism, contribute to thromboembolic complications, impaired pulmonary function and oxygenation.[12, 15, 20, 26, 27]

CONCLUSION

More number of studies and more frequent assessments of various neurological and endocrine parameters and immune markers are required to evaluate the true and potential advantages of endoscopic versus open surgical techniques.

CLINICAL PEARLS

1. Endoscopic surgery is almost as stressful as open surgery.
2. Acute Phase response (C-reactive protein, IL-6 and TLC) is attenuated after laparoscopic surgical procedure.
3. Less postoperative hypoxia and shortened GI paralysis after endoscopic procedures.

REFERENCES

1. Sanjib DA, Korula M. The stress response and its implications in surgery and anaesthesia. The Indian Anaesthetists forum – online journal, April 2004; 1: 1-11.
2. Desborough JP. The stress response to trauma and surgery. Br J Anesth 2000; 85(1): 109-17.
3. Ortega AE, Peters JH, Incarbone R, Estrada L, et al. A prospective randomised comparison of the metabolic and stress hormonal responses of laparoscopic and open cholecystectomy: J Am Coll Surg 1996; 183: 249.
4. Redmond HP, Watson WG, Houghton T, Condron C, et al. Immune functions in patients undergoing open vs.laparoscopic cholecystectomy: Arch Surg 1994; 129: 1240.
5. Glering H, Heindorff H, Fluyvbferg A, Jension SL, et al. Elective laparoscopic cholecystectomy nearly abolishes the postoperative hepatic catabolic stress response: Ann Surg.1995; 221: 214.
6. Glaser F, Sanwald GA, Buhr HJ, Kuntz C, et al. General stress response to conventional and laparoscopic cholecystectomy: Ann Surg 1995; 221: 372.
7. Mealy K, Gallagher H, Barry M, Lennon F, et al. Physiological and metabolic response to open and laparoscopic cholecystectomy: Br J Surg 1992; 709: 1061.
8. Joris J, Cigarini I, Legrand M, Jacquet N, et al. Metabolic and respiratory changes in cholecystectomy performed via laparotomy or laparoscopy. Br J Anesth 1992; 69: 341.
9. McMahon AJ, D'Dwyer PJ, Cruikshank AM, McMillan D, et al. Comparison of metabolic response to laparoscopic and minilaparotomy cholecystectomy: Br J Surg 1993; 80: 1255.

10. Gideon PN, Marianna K, Ryan MD, Nana A, et al. Comparative stress hormone changes during helium versus CO_2 laparoscopic cholecystectomy: Journal of Laparoendoscopic Surgery 1996; Vol.6, Number 2.

11. Targarona EM, Pons MJ, Balague C, Erpert JJ, et al. Acute phase is the only significantly reduced component in the injury response after laparoscopic cholecystectomy: World J Surg 1996; 20: 528.

12. Karayiannakis AJ, Makri GG, Mantzioka A, Karatzas G. Postoperative pulmonary function after laprosocopic and open cholecystectomy: Br J Anesth 1996; 77: 448.

13. Pinnonen R, Vunamaki O. Vasopressin release during laparoscopy: role of increased intra-abdominal pressure. Lancet 1982; 1: 175-6.

14. Melville RJ, Friziz HI, Forsling ML, Le Quescne LP. The stimulus for vasopressin release during laparoscopy. Surg Lobstet Gynecol 1985; 161: 253-6.

15. Herruzo JA, Catellano G, Larrodira L, Morillas JD, et al. Plasma argentine vasopressin concentration during laparoscopy: Hepatogastroendtrology 1989; 36: 499-503.

16. Mansour MA, Stiegmann GV, Yamamota M, Berguer R. Neuroendocrine stress response after minimally invasive surgery in pigs. Surg Endos Nov-Dec 1992; 6(6): 294-7.

17. Cooper GM, Scoggins AM, Ward ID, Murph D. Laparoscopy - a stressful procedure, Anaesthesia 1982; 37: 266-9.

18. Deuss U, Dietrich D, Kaulen K, Frey W, et al. The stress response to laparoscopic cholecystectomy: Investigations of endocrine parameters: Endoscopy 1994; 26: 235.

19. Milheiro A, Sousa FC, Manso EC, Leitao F. Metabolic responses to cholecystectomy: Open vs. laparoscopic approach. J Laparo Endo Sc.Surg 1994; 4: 311-7.

20. O'Leary E, Hubbard K, Tormey W, Cunningham AJ. Laparoscopic cholecystectomy: Hemodynamic and neuroendocrine responses after pneumoperitoneum and changes in position: Br Janesth 1996; 76: 640-4.

21. Nguyen NT, HO HS, Fleming NW, et al. Cardiac function during laparoscopic vs open gastric bypass; a randomized comparison. Surg Endos 2002; 16: 78-83.

22. Ortega AE, Peters JH, Incarbone R, Estrada L, et al. A prospective randomized comparison of the metabolic and stress hormonal responses of laparoscopic and open cholecystectomy. J Am Coll Surg Sept1996; 183(3): 249-56.

23. Jakeway MSR, Mitchell V, Hashim LA, Chadwick SJO, et al. Metabolic and inflammatory responses after open or laparoscopic cholecystectomy. Br J Surg 1994; 81: 127.

24. Berggrin U, Gordh T, Grama D, Haglund U, et al. Laparosocpic versus open cholecystectomy: hospitalization, sick leave, analgesia and trauma responses: Br J Surg 1994; 81: 1362.

25. Rademaker B, Ringers J, Odoom JA, Dehlat LT, et al. Pulmonary cholecystectomy: comparison with subcosial incision and influence of thoracic epidural analgesia: Aneasth. Analg 1992; 75: 381.

26. Hannargvest F, Westman B, Leifonmarck EE, Anderson K, et al. Decreases in muscle glucamine, ribosomes and the nitrogen losses are similar after laparoscopic compared with open cholecystectomy during immediate postoperative period: Surgery 1996; 119: 417.

27. Thorel A, Nygren J, Essn P, Gutniak M, et al. The metabolic response to cholecystectomy: insulin resistance after open compared with laparoscopic operation: Eur J Surg 1995; 162: 187.

28. Harmon GD, Senagore AJ, Kilride MJ, Warzynski MJ. Interleukin-6 response to laparoscopic and open colectomy: L DIS.Colon Rectum1994; 37: 754.

29. Senagore AJ, Kilbride MJ, Luchtefeld MA. Superior nitrogen balance after laparoscopic assisted colectomy: Ann Surg 1995; 221: 171.

30. Essen P, Thorell A, McNurlan MA, Anderson S, et al. Laparoscopic cholecystectomy does not prevent the postoperative protein catabolic responses in muscle: Ann Surg 1995; 222: 36.

31. Henrik Kehlet; Surgical stress response. Does endoscopic surgery confer an advantage: World J of Surgery 23, 801-7, 1999.

CHAPTER 9

General Anaesthesia for Laparoscopic Surgery

INTRODUCTION

Laparoscopic surgery may be minimally invasive anatomically but physiologically it is otherwise. It is not a benign procedure and often leads to major physiological perturbations, which if not rectified could progress to untoward effects. Although these changes are described elsewhere in this book, a brief description is given in this chapter. Until the late 1960s morbidity and mortality were accepted as unavoidable aspects of therapeutic process. The current realization that less invasive method of treatment may reduce the risk of death and morbidity has given rise to concept of "minimally invasive therapy" with the general aim to minimize trauma of the interventional process whilst still achieving satisfactory therapeutic result.[1] A UK report Commissioned by the Department of Health,[2] did not favour the term "minimal invasive surgery" with its connotation of increased safety and minor procedure," preferring instead the term "minimal access surgery."

Laparoscopic approach for treatment of various abdominal ailments is increasingly applied and also tends to be readily proposed for ill patients. This approach is also being used for new surgical procedures. Many surgeons beginning laparoscopy for gastrointestinal surgery are still inexperienced and a learning curve increases the risk of morbidity and mortality.[3] Laparoscopy with carboperitoneum is a standard procedure in gynaecological and gastrointestinal surgery. In gynaecological practice, Cognat et al[4] estimated the incidence of acute cardiovascular collapse during this procedure[5] to be 1:2000, while in 1:10,000 it was impossible to resuscitate the patient. There are other reports of fatal complications like cardiac failure, pulmonary oedema and myocardial infarction during these procedures.[5-7]

Therefore, it is imperative that anaesthesiologists and surgeons thoroughly understand pathophysiology of pneumoperitoneum for safer conduct of anaesthesia and prevent potential complications.

PATHOPHYSIOLOGY OF PNEUMOPERITONEUM

RESPIRATORY SYSTEM

Detailed elsewhere.

Ventilation is impaired by abdominal distension[8-11] and position[2,12,13] of the patient. The elevation of the diaphragm results in mismatching of ventilation and pulmonary perfusion.[8,11] An increase in arteriolo alveolar CO_2 difference [$D(a-A)CO_2$], reflecting an increase in the physiologic dead space has been reported.[9,10] However, other authors failed to demonstrate any significant change in $D(a-A)CO_2$ due to pneumoperitoneum.[14-15]

Induction of general anaesthesia decrease functional residual capacity (FRC) and lung compliance.[16] Insufflation of intraperitoneal CO_2 may further exacerbate these changes. Kandall[17] et al in a recent study of 20 patients undergoing laparoscopic cholecystectomy documented a 49 per cent and a 39 per cent decrease in thoracic and lung compliance, respectively, with insufflation of CO_2 to an intra-abdominal pressure (IAP) of 15 mmHg. Increased IAP decreases diaphragmatic excursion and increases the pressure forced on the lower lung lobes, resulting in decreased alveolar ventilation. An increase in less ventilated alveoli results in an increased ventilation perfusion mismatch causing elevated dead space and shunt volume.[18] This may produce hypoxemia in these patients. Intraoperative hypoxemia is however uncommon in healthy patients.[19,20] Joris et al found insignificant increased intrapulmonary shunt despite reductions in cardiac output and oxygen delivery in 20 healthy patients during laparoscopic cholecystectomy. Cunningham et al[21] reported a case of intraoperative hypoxemia complicating laparoscopy in an obese patient with sickle hemoglobinopathy. Hypoxemia may be also caused by regurgitation and aspiration of gastric contents.

INCREASE IN $PaCO_2$

During intraperitoneal insufflation of CO_2, an increase in $PaCO_2$ was observed both in animals[22] and humans[8,12,23-25] when ventilation was controlled at a constant minute volume. With patients in head up position as for laparoscopic cholecystectomy, similar results were observed.[14,20,27] During laparoscopy with local anaesthesia[9,20,26] $PaCO_2$ remained unchanged but minute ventilation significantly increased. Because of decreased total respiratory compliance during pneumoperitoneum,[19,18,28] hyperventilation was achieved by increasing respiratory rate rather than tidal volume, thus minimizing the increase in ventilatory work.[8,19,26] $PaCO_2$ increases in patients breathing spontaneously under general anaesthesia.[9,11,29] The hyperventilation was insufficient probably because of anaesthetic induced ventilatory depression.[10,24] Duration of pneumoperitoneum influences the extent of the increase in $PaCO_2$. It takes 15-25 minutes for $PaCO_2$ to plateau.[14,24,30] The increase in $PaCO_2$ also depends on intra-abdominal pressure.[22] Patients with preoperative cardiopulmonary disease demonstrate significantly larger increase in $PaCO_2$ than those without underlying diseases.[18]

The causes of increased $PaCO_2$ during laparoscopy are several, and the contribution of each factor varies from patient to patient.
1. Absorption of CO_2 from the peritoneal cavity.
2. $\dot{V}A/\dot{V}Q$ mismatch – increased physiologic dead space.
    Abdominal distension.
    Position of patient.
    Controlled mechanical ventilation.
    Reduced cardiac output.
3. Increased metabolism
4. Depression of ventilation by anesthetics (spontaneous breathing)
5. Accidental events
    CO_2 embolism.
    Pneumothorax.
    CO_2 emphysema (subcutaneous or body cavity).
    Selective bronchial intubation.

The observation of an increase in $PaCO_2$, when CO_2, but not nitrous oxide, was used as peritoneal insufflating gas, suggests absorption of CO_2 from the peritoneal cavity as a potential mechanism for the rise in $PaCO_2$.[22,25,30] This hypothesis was further supported by the increased production of CO_2 (VCO_2) reported when CO_2 but not nitrous oxide was the inflating gas.[20] Amount of CO_2 absorbed was also influenced by patient physical status.

Wittgen et al[18] compared 20 healthy patients undergoing laparoscopic cholecystectomy with 10 ASA II-III patients. Sick patients had significant decrease in pH and increase in $PaCO_2$ during pneumoperitoneum. ASA III or IV patients may have rise in $PaCO_2$ which is incorrectable by increasing minute ventilation.[31] Hall et al[32] reported a case of acute profound hypercarbia occurring late in the procedure caused by CO_2 insufflation and was first detected by capnography. Large increases in $PaCO_2$, as high as 70 mmHg, have been reported for spontaneously breathing patients under general anaesthesia during insufflation, or in case of CO_2 embolism.

POSTOPERATIVE CHANGES

Laparoscopic surgery may reduce postoperative pulmonary complications by avoiding division of abdominal musculature and hence restrictive pattern of breathing. Schauer et al[33] observed that the laparoscopic procedure was associated with 30-38 per cent less impairment of pulmonary function including FRC, forced expiratory volume in 1 second, maximum forced expiratory flow and total lung capacity. However respiratory abnormalities similar to those observed after open cholecystectomy may occur.[34] This respiratory impairment may be due to visceral afferents from gallbladder area or somatic afferents arising from the abdominal wall, which exert an inhibitory action on phrenic nerve discharge and thus lead to diaphragmatic dysfunction. Erice et al[35] concluded that the internal site of surgical intervention is the crucial variable determining diaphragmatic inhibition after they observed a decrease in maximum transdiaphragmatic pressure with laparoscopic cholecystectomy and not laparoscopic hernia repair.

HAEMODYNAMIC CHANGES

Raising IAP by insufflating gas intraperitoneally, induces significant alterations of haemodynamics.[4,11,12,27,36] Magnitude of IAP, nature of insufflating gas, patient position, depth and nature of anaesthesia and patient's physical condition are some factors which influence these haemodynamic alterations. These disturbances are characterized by decrease of cardiac output, elevation of arterial pressure, and increase of systemic and pulmonary vascular resistance[15,22] (Fig. 9.1). The decrease in cardiac output is proportional to the increase in intra-abdominal pressure. Many authors have used invasive monitoring[31,37-39] and others non-invasive means to demonstrate depression of cardiac output.[40,41] While majority report depression of cardiac output by raised intra-abdominal pressure, there are few authors who have showed no change in cardiac output.[42-48] Cardiac output has also been reported to increase or remain unchanged[27,45-47] during pneumoperitoneum. These discrepancies might be due to differing rates of CO_2 insufflation, IAP, steepness of the tilt, depth of anaesthesia and techniques to assess haemodynamics. However all recent studies showed a decrease of cardiac output (25 to 35%) during peritoneal insufflation regardless of whether the patient was placed in the head down[28] or head-up position.[15,36] The combined effect of anaesthesia, patient position (10 degrees head up) and increased IAP (14 mmHg) can reduce the cardiac output to as much as 50 per cent of preoperative values.[36] The usual intraoperative cardiovascular monitoring; blood pressure, pulse rate and clinical assessment of peripheral circulation, give no information on changes in SVR or reduction in stroke index (cardiac output).[48]

Most authors have studied effects of CO_2 pneumoperitoneum on haemodynamic on young and healthy humans (ASA I & II). Only a few studies have focused on patients with a higher ASA classification. Stuttmann and coworkers monitored 20 ASA III and IV patients during laparoscopic cholecystectomy. They concluded that the laparoscopic procedure may lead to temporary myocardial insufficiency due to haemodynamic changes, but it seems to be safe provided sufficient recognition and treatment of pathologic changes are guaranteed.[49] During laparoscopy, cardiac output remains significantly lower (30–35%) than prior to induction of anaesthesia despite surgical stimulation.[36]

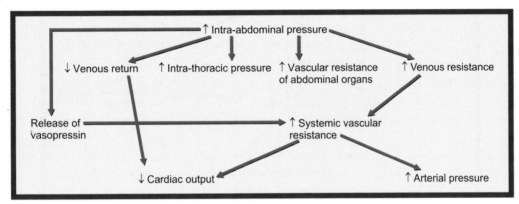

Fig. 9.1: Haemodynamic changes during laparoscopy

Whether these haemodynamic changes are well tolerated is poorly documented. In ASA I, II patients the fall in cardiac output is well tolerated. Venous oxygen saturation (SvO_2) and plasma concentration of lactate remained within normal values during pneumoperitoneum suggesting satisfactory tolerance in healthy patients.[50] The decrease in preload and the increase in afterload resulting from peritoneal insufflation might induce deleterious effects in patients with impaired cardiac function, anaemia or hypovolemia. Indirect data suggest more pronounced alterations of haemodynamics in patients with cardiac disease.[18] $PaCO_2$ rises more in these patients than in healthy patients, and the $D(a-A)CO_2$ also increases much more in cardiac patients reflecting a greater enlargement of the physiologic dead space (increase of pulmonary units with high $\dot{V}A/\dot{V}Q$).

Haemodynamic embarrassment during laparoscopy can be minimised by reducing the insufflation pressure. This is particularly important in patients with cardiac disorders or hypovolemia. If pneumoperitoneum causes an excessive fall in cardiac output and blood pressure the insufflation pressure should be reduced to the lowest possible level

INTRA-ABDOMINAL ORGANS

Increase in IAP can impair renal, hepatic and mesenteric blood flow.

An increase in IAP raises renal vascular resistance, decreases cardiac output, which may result in decrease renal blood flow. Correcting cardiac output to normal or supra-normal values when IAP is > 20 mmHg does not restore renal function to normal. The effectiveness of maintaining cardiac output at normal or higher levels on renal function when IAP < 15 mmHg is uncertain. Increase in renal vascular resistance account for the direct effects of increased IAP on renal blood flow (RBF) and function. Increase in renal vascular resistance with increase IAP may in part be due to neural, hormonal or intrinsic influence.

Mesenteric (splanchnic) perfusion is also affected by rise in IAP (Fig. 9.2). Superior mesenteric blood flow, intestinal mucosal microcirculation and intramucosal pH are all reduced. The perfusion of abdominal organs such as liver, kidney or the gastrointestinal tract can be measured by indirect methods (e.g. tonometry) or direct measurements (e.g. laser Doppler flowmetry). There are reports of fatal intestinal ischaemia following laparoscopic cholecystectomy.[51,52] Under conditions with pre-existing intestinal vascular disease a high pressure pneumoperitoneum might aggravate ischaemic changes and be followed by a disastrous outcome for the patient. The other concern is of bacterial translocation following splanchnic ischaemia and ischaemic reperfusion injury.

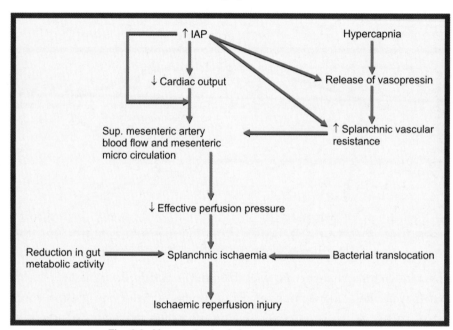

Fig. 9.2: Mesenteric circulation during laparoscopy

Increase in IAP significantly decreases organ blood flow (OBF) in all abdominal organs except the adrenal gland. These changes in OBF are more marked than changes in cardiac output, which suggest a contribution of local control mechanisms.[53] Hepatic blood flow is also affected by rise in IAP.

EFFECT ON PERIPHERAL VASCULAR SYSTEM

Effect on peripheral vascular system or circulatory changes in lower extremities –the main concern is thromboembolic events. Patients undergoing a laparoscopic procedure are often operated in reverse Trendelenburg position with an IAP of 12-15 mmHg. These factors can lead to venous stasis, which may favour the occurrence of deep vein thrombosis. A number of reports of deep vein thrombosis,[54-59] nonfatal pulmonary embolism or even fatal pulmonary embolism[54] have been published. Influence of IAP on the haemodynamics of the lower extremities may explain how this complication may occur and how it can be avoided.

INTRA CRANIAL PRESSURE CHANGES

Laparoscopic inspection of the abdominal cavity during trauma emergencies, may jeopardize safety of the patient, as these patients may have associated head injury. Some investigators have, by clinical and experimental observations, shown that increased IAP causes an elevation in intracranial pressure and decrease in cerebral perfusion pressure. This data was obtained with and without pre-existing brain injury.[60-62] The precise mechanism of the effects of increased abdominal pressure on intra-cromal pressure (ICP) is yet not clear, but interference with venous drainage from cerebral veins and decreased effective cerebral perfusion pressure seem to play a role. Peritoneal insufflation with helium or nitrous oxide as potentially alternative gases increase the mean ICP, but is significantly less than with CO_2.[63] It appears that the rise in ICP during early phase is due to elevated intra thoracic pressure and IAP while the late phase is due to an arterial or chemical effect. ICP also rises with abdominal insufflation with or without a rise in $PaCO_2$.[64] Pneumoperitoneum exacerbates the raised ICP following closed head injury. Rosenthal et al[65] in an experimental model observed that the elevated ICP associated with CO_2 pneumoperitoneum was unresponsive to hyperventilation and hypocapnia; however ICP was higher with hypoventilation and hypercapnia. Cerebral blood flow CBF and ICP therefore rise during pneumoperitoneum regardless of $PaCO_2$, but hypercapnia, may aggravate this.

PATIENT POSITION

During laparoscopic surgery the patient is positioned to produce gravitational displacement of the abdominal viscera away from the surgical site. Head-down tilt is used for pelvic and submesocolic surgery. The head-up position is preferred for supramesocolic surgery. In addition, patient is often placed in the lithotomy position. Gravity has profound effects on the cardiovascular and pulmonary system. Overall effect will depend on degree of tilt, whether change in position is before or after pneumoperitoneum, suppression or modification of compensatory reflexes by anesthesia and cardiovascular drugs. Compensatory reflexes like baroreceptors – which respond to increased hydrostatic pressure with systemic vasodilation and bradycardia, maintain cardiovascular status.[66,67] Although these reflexes may be impaired during general anaesthesia, the haemodynamic changes induced by this position during laparoscopy remain insignificant.[46,48,68] However, central blood volume and blood pressure changes are greater in patients with coronary artery disease, particularly in cases of compromised ejection fraction, leading to a potentially deleterious increased myocardial demand.[13] The Trendelenburg position may also affect the cerebral circulation, particularly in case of high intra-cranial pressure, and results in elevation of the intraocular venous pressure, which can worsen acute glaucoma. The head-down position decreases transmural pressure in the pelvic viscera, reducing blood loss but increasing the risk of gas embolism.[13]

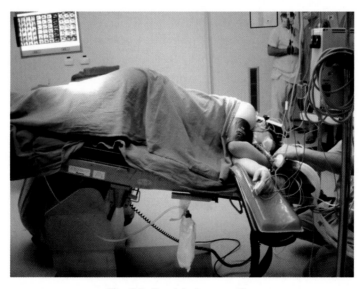

Fig. 9.3: Trendelenburg position

Head up position decreases venous return and thus decreases cardiac output.[36,67] This decrease in cardiac output compounds the hemodynamic changes induced by pneumoperitoneum. The steeper tilt, accentuates the decrease in cardiac output.[15] When head up tilt is obtained after creation of pneumoperitoneum, haemodynamic effects are minimal.

The head down position (Fig. 9.3) facilitates the development of atelectasis. Steep head down tilt results in decreased FRC, total lung volume and pulmonary compliance. These changes are more marked in obese, elderly or debilitated patients, who may not tolerate these changes. The head up position is usually considered to be more favorable to respiration.[13,69,70] Brachial plexus palsy, regurgitation of gastric contents and inadvertent endobronchial intubation[71] are other problems of Trendelenburg position.

ANAESTHESIA FOR LAPAROSCOPY

PREOPERATIVE EVALUATION OF THE PATIENT AND PREMEDICATION

Preoperative evaluation is essentially same as for other surgical patients. Pneumoperitoneum stresses cardiovascular and respiratory system more than other systems. In patients with heart disease, cardiac function should be evaluated in the light of haemodynamic changes induced by pneumoperitoneum and patient position. Patients with CHF are certainly more prone to develop cardiac complications than patients with ischaemic cardiac disease during laparoscopy. The patient's cardiac status should be assessed and quantified. Goldman index and Lee score can be used for quantification of cardiac risk factors. For these patients, the postoperative benefits of laparoscopy must be balanced against the intraoperative risks when the choice of laparoscopy versus laparotomy is discussed.

Although a history of chronic obstructive pulmonary disease (COPD) and cancer was strongly associated with the development of acidosis, only an elevated acute physiological score (APS) (≥ 10) was predictive of this complication in a study.[72] The ABG values did not predict the complication of respiratory acidosis. Formal PFTs do identify patients with diffusion deficits as being more likely to experience hypercarbia and acidosis. In patients with a poor state of health preoperatively, as reflected by the APS, individuals with known COPD or cancer, more extensive preoperative evaluation that include preoperative PFT is advisable. However diffusion defects less than 80 per cent of predicted values do not eliminate laparoscopic cholecystectomy as an operative choice. In patients with respiratory disease, laparoscopy appears preferable to laparotomy because of reduced postoperative respiratory dysfunction. These positive effects counterbalance the risk of pneumothorax during pneumoperitoneum and the risk of inadequate gas exchange secondary to $\dot{V}A/\dot{V}Q$ mismatching.

Because of venous stasis in the legs during laparoscopy,[73] prophylaxis of deep vein thrombosis should be initiated prior to surgery, as for laparotomy.

Premedication should be adapted to the patient's physical status and to the requirements of the procedure. Because of the potential risk of regurgitation and aspiration, antacids, H_2-receptor antagonists and gastroprokinetic drugs are recommended.[74,75] Preoperative administration of NSAIDs may be helpful in reducing postoperative pain and opiate requirements.

ANAESTHETIC TECHNIQUES

Principle concerns are
- Haemodynamic instability
- Cardiac arrhythymias

- Respiratory embarrassment—hypercapnia and hypoxia
- Gastric regurgitation and aspiration
- Outpatient nature of surgical treatment
- Postoperative nausea and vomiting (PONV)
- Deep vein thrombosis
- Complications of laparoscopy.

GENERAL ANAESTHESIA

General anaesthesia with endotracheal intubation and controlled ventilation is recommended for these procedures. The advantages of the endotracheal tube and adequate muscle relaxation are protection from aspiration of gastric contents and a quite operative field.[76] During pneumoperitoneum, controlled ventilation must be adjusted to maintain EtCO$_2$ at about 35 mmHg. This may require 20-25 per cent increase in minute ventilation. Increase in rate rather than of tidal volume might be preferable, to minimize rise in peak airway pressure and barotrauma.

These patients require management of haemodynamic perturbations caused by pneumoperitoneum. Most patients responds to pneumoperitoneum by fall in cardiac output, rise in blood pressure and bradycardia. The anesthetic agents should not depress myocardium, should preferably decrease peripheral vascular resistance and not potentiate bradycardia. Anesthesia technique should not decrease hepatic blood flow, which is already compromised by raised IAP during pneumoperitoneum. There are important considerations in use of analgesics and muscle relaxants in these patients which are mentioned below.

For the choice of volatile anesthetic the factors to be considered are—

Myocardial depression, increase in SVR, arrhythmogenic propensity in presence of increased PaCo$_2$, recovery pattern, and PONV.

Anaesthetics that directly depress the myocardium should be avoided in favour of anesthetics with vasodilating properties such as isoflurane.

VOLATILE ANAESTHETICS (FIG. 9.4)

All modern volatile anesthetics cause concentration related decrease in arterial pressure.[77,78] Decrease in arterial pressure produced by halothane and enflurane can be primarily attributed to reduction in myocardial contractility and cardiac output. In contrast decrease in arterial pressure associated with isoflurane, desflurane and sevoflurane anesthesia occur as a result of reduction in LV afterload.[79] Isoflurane, desflurane and sevoflurane maintain cardiac output because these agents produce less pronounced reduction in myocardial contractility and greater decrease in SVR than does halothane or enflurane in humans. Isoflurane and desflurane may also preserve autonomic nervous system regulation of the circulation to a greater degree than other volatile anesthetics. Decline in arterial pressure produced by volatile anaesthetics may be attenuated by surgical stimulation or concomitant administration of nitrous oxide.[80,81] The vasodilating effects of isoflurane, desflurane and sevoflurane cause less pronounced increase in right atrial pressure than those observed during halothane or enflurane anaesthesia.

All modern volatile anesthetics including desflurane and sevoflurane depress the contractile function in normal myocardium in vitro and in vivo. Enflurane and isoflurane produce direct negative inotropic effects, as indicated by decreases in maximal velocity of shortening, peak developed force and maximal rate of force development

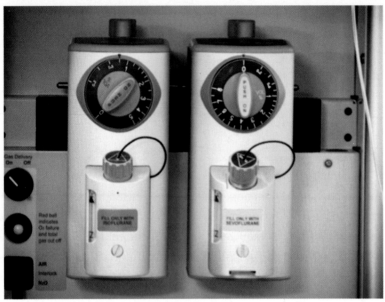

Fig. 9.4: Vaporizers

during isotonic contraction in isolated feline papillary muscles. This reduction in intrinsic myocardial contractility by enflurane and isoflurane contribute to the cardiovascular depression observed with these agents in humans. Simultaneous alteration in systemic and pulmonary haemodynamics and autonomic nervous system activity often complicate assessment of left ventricular (LV) systolic function. Halothane produced a larger reduction in the rate of increase of LV positive pressure (dp/dt) than did isoflurane when equianesthetic concentrations were directly compared in the presence and absence of autonomic nervous system function,[82] suggesting that difference in myocardial depression caused by these anaesthetics occurred independent of autonomic nervous system activity.[83]

Desflurane produces systemic and coronary haemodynamic effects which are similar to those produced by isoflurane.[84] Desflurane and isoflurane have been shown to depress myocardial function to equivalent degrees using isovolumic and ejection phase measures of contractility in dogs,[85] pigs[86] and humans.[80] However, the unique cardiovascular stimulation associated with rapid increases in inspired desflurane concentration in humans may lead to transient increases in myocardial contractility resulting from augmentation of sympathetic nervous system tone.

The effects of sevoflurane on myocardial contractility are virtually indistinguishable from those produced by isoflurane in dogs.[87] Sevoflurane produces less myocardial depression than does enflurane in volunteers. As assessed by the heart rate corrected velocity of circumferential fiber shortening versus the LV end-systolic wall stress relationship derived from echocardiograph, volatile anesthetics appear to depress the contractile state in normal ventricular myocardium in the following order: halothane > enflurane > isoflurane = desflurane = sevoflurane.

Halothane produces more pronounced myocardial depression in ischaemic than in normal myocardium. Isoflurane and halothane produced greater negative inotropic effects in ventricular myocardium obtained from cardiomyopathic hamsters than from normal hamsters. These findings suggested that myocardial depression caused by volatile anaesthetics in failing myocardium was accentuated and they provided indirect evidence that patients with underlying contractile dysfunction might be more sensitive to the negative inotropic effects of volatile agents. Halothane and isoflurane also produced beneficial decrease in LV preload and afterload in patients with heart failure and coronary artery disease respectively.

Prolong duration of anaesthesia alters the cardiovascular effects of volatile anaesthetics. Heart rate may also increase during prolong halothane or enflurane anaesthesia but arterial pressure remains constant. Recovery from circulatory depression is greatest during halothane anaesthesia and less pronounced during prolonged administration of isoflurane and desflurane. The time dependent improvement in haemodynamics observed with volatile anaesthetics is antagonised by propranolol and may result from enhanced sympathetic nervous system activity.

Halothane and to a lesser extent other volatile anaesthetics have been shown to sensitize myocardium to the arrhythmogenic effects of epinephrine.[88] The doses of epinephrine required to produce ventricular arrhythmia during desflurane or sevoflurane anaesthesia are similar to but significantly more than those observed during administration of isoflurane and halothane. Halothane catecholamine sensitization also promotes abnormal automaticity of dominant and latent atrial pacemaker. These effects may produce premature ventricular contractions and arrhythmia originating from the bundle of His.

Volatile anaesthetics produce direct negative chrontropic actions *in vitro* by depressing sinoatrial node activity. However alterations in heart rate *in vivo* are determined primarily by the interaction of volatile agents and baroreceptor reflex responses.[89,90] Heart rate increases to various degrees with enflurane but these increases may be insufficient to preserve cardiac output.[91] Isoflurane increases heart rate in response to simultaneous decreases in arterial pressure. These findings occur with this volatile agent because baroreceptor reflexes are relatively preserved compared with equi MAC of halothane and enflurane. Desflurane and isoflurane induced tachycardia may be more pronounced in paediatric patients or in the presence of vagolytic agents and conversely may be attenuated in neonates[92] and geriatric patients or by concomitant administration of opioids.[93] Rapid increases in the inspired desflurane concentration at greater than 1.0 MAC may be associated with further transient increase in heart rate and arterial pressure resulting from sympathetic nervous system activation.[94] Similar increases in heart rate are observed when the inspired isoflurane concentration is rapidly increased.[95] The cardiovascular stimulation induced by rapid increases in desflurane or isoflurane concentrations in humans results from activation of tracheopulmonary and systemic receptors and is attenuated by pretreatment with β-adreno receptor antagonists, α_2-adrenoreceptor agonists or opioids. Sevoflurane neither alters heart rate[96] nor causes cardiovascular stimulation during rapid increases in anaesthetic concentration in humans.[97]

Few clinical investigations have focused on the effect of superficial general anaesthesia on the haemodynamic events provoked by increased IAP. During "fairly light anaesthesia" (as with balanced anesthesia) and controlled ventilation the circulation is stimulated by the surgical procedure and CO_2 absorption. Blood pressure may rise abruptly and patient might have bradycardia or tachycardia. Narcotics based techniques have the same fate. Marshall et al[98] used deeper anaesthesia with 1 per cent halothane and spontaneous respiration and found that CO_2 – insufflation upto 2 kpa provoked increased HR and mean arterial pressure (MAP), whereas cardiac output was unchanged. This indicated a SV reduction and an increased TPR. Lenz et al[48] used balanced anaesthesia and showed that SV and CO decreased during increased IAP. Deeper plane of anesthesia with sevoflurane and isoflurane results in blunting of rise in arterial pressure and better intraoperative haemodynamic adjustment. Infusion of vasodilating drugs such as nicardipine (a calcium channel blocker), reduces the haemodynamic repercussions of a pneumoperitoneum. Feig BW[31] et al have shown that use of intravenous nitroglycerine resulted in rapid return of the SVR, MAP, pulmonary capillary wedge pressure and cardiac index to baseline levels. Isoflurane, sevoflurane are also compatible with hypercarbia and raised catecholamine in view of arrhythmogenicity. We believe that maintaining deep level of anaesthesia with short acting, nonflammable agents like isoflurane, sevoflurane or desflurane blunt the haemodynamic response to pneumoperitoneum. The contribution of nitrous oxide to nausea and vomiting is still controversial,[100,101] but it may distend the bowel, which generally has no clinical significant effect on surgical conditions during laparoscopy except in patients of intestinal obstruction.

CONSIDERATION IN CHOOSING INTRA-VENOUS ANAESTHETIC AGENTS

The concerns are:
- Myocardial depression action of agent
- Action on peripheral vascular system
- Recovery profile
- PONV

Thiopentone, propofol, etomidate or midazolam, may be used for induction of anaesthesia, propofol and etomidate are suitable for total intravenous anaesthesia. Their relevant features are described here.

PROPOFOL

Propofol is one of a group of alkylphenols that have hypnotic properties.

Propofol is used for induction and maintenance of anaesthesia. The most prominent effect of propofol is a decrease in arterial blood pressure during induction of anaesthesia.

An induction dose of 2 to 2.5 mg/kg produces 25 to 40 per cent reduction in systolic blood pressure.[102-108] Similar changes are seen in mean and diastolic blood pressure. The decrease in arterial pressure is associated with a decrease in cardiac output / cardiac index (15%), stroke volume index (~ 20%) and systemic vascular resistance (15% to 25%). The left ventricular stroke work index is also decreased (by ~ 30%). The decrease in systemic pressure after an induction dose of propofol appears to be due to vasodilation and possibly myocardial depression. The direct myocardial depression action of propofol is controversial. These haemodynamic properties, early recovery profile and low PONV make this agent suitable for laparoscopic surgery.

The heart rate may increase, decrease or remain unchanged when anesthesia is maintained with propofol. An infusion of propofol results in a significant reduction in both myocardial blood flow and myocardial oxygen consumption, a finding that suggest preservation of the global myocardial oxygen supply-demand ratio.

BARBITURATES

Thiopentone may be used as an induction agent for laparoscopic surgery. The cardiovascular depression from barbiturates is a result of both central and peripheral (direct vascular and cardiac) effects.[109-114] The primary cardiovascular effects of barbiturate induction is peripheral vasodilation resulting in pooling of blood in the venous system. Decrease in contractility leading to fall in cardiac output may be due to direct negative inotropic action, decreased ventricular filling because of increased capacitance and transiently decreased sympathetic outflow from the CNS. The increase in heart rate (10 to 30%) that accompanies thiopentone administration probably from baroreceptor – mediated sympathetic reflex stimulation of heart in responses to the drop in cardiac output and pressure. The cardiac index is unchanged or reduced and mean arterial pressure is maintained or slightly reduced. Thiopentone infusions and lower doses tend to be accompanied by smaller haemodynamic changes than those noted with rapid bolus injections. Pneumoperitoneum produces fall in cardiac output, so use of thiopentone for anaesthesia calls for caution, as it also reduces cardiac output.

Benzodiazepines

Benzodiazepines, especially midazolam can be used for anaesthesia in these surgeries. Benzodiazepines have modest haemodynamic effects. The predominant haemodynamic change is a slight reduction in arterial blood pressure which results from a decrease in systemic vascular resistance. The mechanism by which benzodiazepines maintain relatively stable haemodynamics involves the preservation of homeostatic reflex mechanisms[112] but some evidence indicates that baroreflex is impaired by, both midazolam and diazepam.[115] Midazolam causes a slightly greater decrease in arterial blood pressure than the other benzodiazepines, but the hypotensive effect,[116] is minimal and about the same as seen with thiopentone.

Despite the hypotension, midazolam, even in doses as high as 0.2 mg/kg is safe and effective for induction of anaesthesia even in patients with severe aortic stenosis. The haemodynamic effects of midazolam and diazepam are dose related, higher the plasma level, the greater the decrease in systemic blood pressure. Delayed recovery is the only problem when midazolam is used for anaesthesia in laparoscopic surgery.

ETOMIDATE

It is a cardiostable anaesthetic agent. An induction dose of 0.3 mg/kg given to cardiac patients for non-cardiac surgery results in almost no change in heart rate, mean arterial pressure, mean pulmonary artery pressure, pulmonary capillary wedge pressure, central venous pressure, stroke volume, cardiac index and pulmonary and systemic vascular resistance.[117] In patients with ischaemic heart disease or valvular disease,[18] etomidate (0.3 mg/kg) produces minimal alterations in cardiovascular parameters. A relatively larger dose of etomidate, 0.45 mg/kg also produces minimal change in cardiovascular parameters in patient with ischaemic heart disease or valvular disease. In patients with mitral or aortic valve disease, etomidate may produce greater change in mean arterial pressure than in patients without cardiac valvular disease.[117,119] Therefore it is a good choice for laparoscopic procedures in cardiac patients.

TOTAL INTRAVENOUS ANAESTHESIA (TIVA) (FIG. 9.5)

Propofol introduction in anaesthesia practice has spurred the use of total intravenous anaesthesia (TIVA). Propofol has a good recovery profile because of short context sensitive half-life. Propofol with short acting analgesics like alfentanyl, fentanyl or sufentanil (our practice) gives good operating conditions and recovery profile.

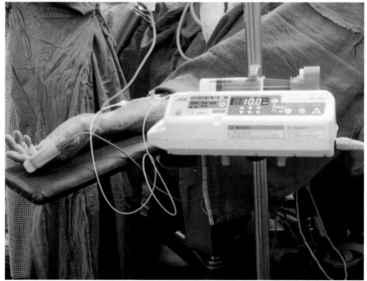

Fig. 9.5: Propofol TIVA

A combination of midazolam infusion, fentanyl and norcuron as TIVA give good operative and haemodynamic conditions but delayed recovery profile and may be used in laparoscopic procedures.

MUSCLE RELAXANTS

The administration of muscle relaxants is necessary to prevent high intra-abdominal and intrathoracic pressures induced by carboperitoneum during laparoscopy, and to improve intraoperative surgical conditions.[120,121] Use of muscle relaxants decreases peak airway inspiratory pressure (PIP), thereby minimizing effects on haemodynamics, risk of pneumothorax and respiratory dead space.[24,46,121]

During laparoscopy, a decrease in total pulmonary compliance and an increase in peak airway pressure are well known,[19,122] whereas increase in PIP is variable. These discrepancies could be attributed to differences in IAP (volume insufflated), compliance of abdomen and method of measurement. Previous studies using paralysed and nonparalysed patients have attempted to evaluate the effect of the respiratory muscles on the pressure-volume relationship of the respiratory system. Putensen et al[123] found that neuromuscular block did not alter elastic properties of the lungs in eight pigs anaesthetized with pentobarbital. Several human clinical studies support the view that muscle relaxants have no effect on pressure-volume relationship or PIP.[124,125] Chassard et al[126] showed that increase in PIP is not affected by muscle relaxants at the level of IAP recommended for carboperitoneum in humans. Some clinical studies have suggested that excessive IAP during insufflation can be overcome by adequate muscle relaxation,[120] but this is not so, as has been proven by many authors. Moreover the action of muscle relaxants is potentiated by volatile anaesthetic agents, so one can use no or minimal muscle relaxant for laparoscopic surgery. Chassard et al[126] has shown that same volume injected in the abdominal cavity produced similar IAP whether or not muscle relaxants were used, and elastance was not affected by relaxation. Many authors[127-131] have reported anaesthetic management without the need for neuromuscular blocking drugs during carboperitoneum.

Clinical use of muscle relaxants is governed by two philosophies. One end of the scale has been popularized by Gray and coworkers in Liverpool, England. In this approach nitrous oxide, oxygen, and large doses of muscle relaxants constitute the sole anaesthetic. Often this practice is advocated in a patient who has an unstable circulatory system. Awareness is the main problem of this philosophy.[132,133] The other end of the scale are workers who advocate use of muscle relaxants as adjunct to anesthesia and not as a substitute for it. By giving them only in an anaesthetized patient (e.g. no movement, hypertension, tachycardia, tearing, grimacing) and monitoring neuromuscular function, large doses of muscle relaxants can be avoided.

Narcotic medication may be used to supplement analgesia. The propensity to induce postoperative nausea vomiting, intraoperative spasm of sphincter of Oddi and cardiovascular stability are the main concerns for selection of these agents. Use of parenteral perioperative NSAIDs and the tendency for less postoperative pain associated with laparoscopic approach may reduce or obviate perioperative narcotic administration.

The laryngeal mask airway results in less sore throat and might be proposed as an alternative to endotracheal intubation.[134] It allows controlled ventilation and accurate monitoring of end-tidal CO_2 ($EtCO_2$). Use of LMA, PLMA, their efficacy, advantages and disadvantages are detailed elsewhere in this book.

IAP should be monitored, kept as low as possible to reduce hemodynamic and respiratory changes, and not be allowed to exceed 15 mmHg. Increase in IAP can be avoided by ensuring a deep plane of anaesthesia and paralysis. In poor risk patients IAP should be kept as minimum as possible; usually at 10 mmHg.

Some authors have used spontaneous ventilation, avoiding tracheal intubation and muscle relaxants.[127,128] However, Peterson et al[135] revealed that almost one third of the deaths associated with laparoscopic procedures were related to anesthetic complications during general anaesthesia without intubation. In these cases the laryngeal mask airway might improve the safety of anaesthesia for laparoscopy in patient breathing spontaneously[129] and is therefore recommended.

Postoperative nausea and vomiting are among the most common and distressing symptoms after laparoscopic surgery.[136] A highly potent and selective 5-HT$_3$ receptor antagonist, ondansetron, has proved to be an effective oral and parenteral prophylaxis against postoperative emesis.[137]

LOCAL AND REGIONAL ANAESTHESIA

Local anaesthesia has been employed quite frequently for laparoscopic gynaecologic procedures – most commonly tubal ligation. It offers several advantages like reduced anaesthesia time, quicker recovery, decreased postoperative nausea and vomiting, early awareness of complications and less haemodynamic changes.[138-140] Sequelae of general anaesthesia, such as airway trauma, sore throat, fatigue and nausea and vomiting can be avoided. However, this anaesthetic approach requires a precise and gentle surgical technique. This also requires supplementation with intravenous sedation, to allay patient's anxiety, discomfort and pain. The combined effect of carboperitoneum and sedation can lead to hypoventilation and arterial oxygen desaturation.[141] With local anaesthesia, IAP should be as low as possible to reduce pain and ventilatory disturbances. A laparoscopic procedure that requires multiple puncture sites, considerable organ manipulation, steep tilt, and a large carboperitoneum makes spontaneous breathing difficult for the patient, results in discomfort and must not be conducted under local anaesthesia.[76]

Regional anaesthesia reduces the metabolic response.[142] Regional anaesthesia, such as an epidural technique, combined with the head-down position, can be used for gynaecologic laparoscopy without major impairment of ventilation.[9,143] It reduces the need for sedatives and narcotics, produces better muscle relaxation and can be proposed for other laparoscopic procedures. Shoulder pain, however, is difficult to control and makes the patient restless, during epidural anaesthesia for a laparoscopic procedure.[144] An extensive sensory block (T_4 to L_5) is therefore necessary for surgical laparoscopy, leading to some discomfort. The epidural administration of opiate or/and clonidine might help to provide adequate analgesia. Patient cooperation, an experienced and skilled laparoscopist, reduced IAP and tilt are necessary to guarantee the success of epidural anesthesia, which should be avoided for long procedures. The assumed advantage of less physiologic stress has not been demonstrated[142] and comparable levels of circulating stress hormones can be measured when compared to general anaesthesia. No increase in gastrointestinal reflux has been documented during laparoscopies under local or epidural anaesthesia. This may be explained partially by the concomitant increase in lower esophageal sphincter pressure, which also occurs with the pneumoperitoneum.[145]

MONITORING (FIG. 9.6)

Patients undergoing laparoscopic surgery are prone for haemodynamic disturbances, arrhythmias, hypercapnia, hypoxia and air embolism. Non-invasive blood pressure, heart rate, ECG, pulse oximetry and capnometry should be used to detect arrhythmias, embolism and other effects of haemodynamic perturbation. These monitors however only poorly reflect the haemodynamic changes induced by the pneumoperitoneum. SVR, CI, PCWP, left ventricular stroke work index (LVSWI), oxygen consumption and oxygen delivery ($\dot{D}O_2$) are not routinely monitored. Invasive haemodynamic monitoring may be required in ASA III-IV patients, but the increased intrathoracic pressure may complicate the interpretation of the measured central venous and pulmonary artery pressures. Use of transoesophageal echocardiography might be more helpful in patients with severe cardiac disease.

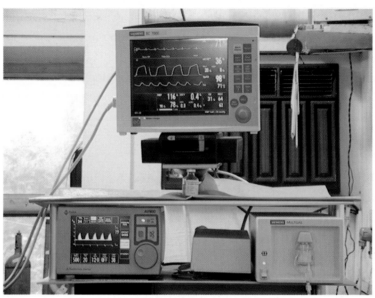

Fig. 9.6: Monitor

Bradycardia is the most frequent arrhythmia observed during laparoscopic procedures. It occurs early during the insertion of Veress needle or initiation of pneumoperitoneum and occurs due to stretching of the peritoneum leading to vagus nerve stimulation. Modern anaesthetics like propofol, fentanyl, vecuronium are all vagomimetic and potentiate bradycardia. Nodal rhythm and ventricular premature beats are other arrhythmias often observed.

End-tidal CO_2 (EtCO$_2$) is commonly used as a noninvasive substitute for PaCO$_2$ in evaluating the adequacy of ventilation during laparoscopic procedures. Wahba and Mamazza[146] studied 28 healthy patients undergoing elective laparoscopic cholecystectomy to determine the increase in minute ventilation required to maintain the preinsufflation arterial CO_2 tension and whether end-tidal CO_2 could safely be used as an index of PaCO$_2$ and, therefore of the adequacy of ventilation during pneumoperitoneum. End-tidal CO_2 (EtCO$_2$) was not a satisfactory noninvasive index of PaCO$_2$ if it exceeded 41 mm of Hg and if large volumes of CO_2 were insufflated. End-tidal CO_2 proved to be a reasonable approximation of PaCO$_2$ in patients with no cardiopulmonary disease. In contrast, patients with preoperative cardiopulmonary disease demonstrated significant increases in PaCO$_2$ not reflected by comparable increase in end-tidal CO_2 during insufflation.[18] PaCO$_2$ may be underestimated by end-tidal CO_2 if there is a reduction in cardiac output or an increase in V/Q mismatch, and occasionally end-tidal CO_2 may overestimate PaCO$_2$.[147] In patients with significant cardiopulmonary disease it would seem prudent to monitor PaCO$_2$ levels during the procedure to avoid problems with hypercarbia and acidosis.

Monitoring of intra-abdominal pressure (IAP)- IAP should be kept below 15 mmHg. In sick and cardiac patients low IAP should be aimed. A sudden rise in IAP may indicate requirement of more muscle relaxants.

Monitoring of muscle relaxation and body temperature are useful during long surgical laparoscopy. Precordial doppler ultrasound allows early recognition of gas embolism and is recommended by some authors.[148,149] Urine output should be monitored in long laparoscopic procedures.

POSTOPERATIVE CARE AND PAIN RELIEF

Monitoring should be continued in the postanaesthesia care unit. Haemodynamic changes produced by carboperitoneum outlast its release. Hypertension of short duration is not uncommon after recovery from anaesthesia. Joris and Lamy[50] reported an increase in cardiac output in ASA I patients, accompanied by significant decrease in venous oxygen saturation (SvO_2) and an increase in plasma concentration of lactate. This increase in oxygen extraction may be due to a high incidence of shivering in these patients. A fall in PaO_2 after laparoscopic cholecystectomy has been reported.[150,151] Although laparoscopy tends to be considered a minor surgical procedure, oxygen should be administered postoperatively even in healthy patients.[152] Hypercapnia can also develop immediately after release of carboperitoneum.[153] Indeed improvement of cardiac output may increase absorption of CO_2. We mobilize our patients fairly early. After 2 hours in the postoperative period they are made to ambulate with the help of an assistant. Early mobilization decreases pain, reduces muscle spasm and increases confidence of patients. Patients are also encouraged to have liquids after 3 hours. The IV fluids are stopped after 3 to 4 hours postoperatively and oral fluids like apple juice, tea, decarbonated cold drinks and water are allowed.

Although pain reported after laparoscopic cholecystectomy is not always less than after laparotomy[150,151,154-156] analgesic consumption is significantly reduced. The nature of pain varies according to the surgical technique; after laparotomy, patients complain more of parietal (abdominal wall) pain, whereas after laparoscopic cholecystectomy patients report visceral pain similar to that of biliary colic and shoulder-tip pain resulting from diaphragmatic irritation.[150] Neck and shoulder pain are reported by 80 per cent of patients at 24 hours and by as many as 50 per cent at 48 hours.[157] CO_2 as insufflating gas induces more discomfort than does nitrous oxide.[158] Different treatment options have been proposed to provide pain relief. Topical anaesthesia[159,160] or infiltration of the fallopian tubes decrease postoperative pain and analgesic consumption after laparoscopic sterilization.[161] Intraperitoneal administration of local anaesthetic (0.25% or 0.125% bupivacaine) reduces shoulder–tip pain and analgesic requirement.[162,163] Preoperative administration of nonsteroidal anti-inflammatory drugs[164-172] (NSAIDs) may decrease pain and analgesic consumption, though some investigators failed to demonstrate significant effect of preoperative NSAIDs.[173-177]

For pain relief we mostly depend upon a multimodal approach. Combination of local anaesthetics, nonsteroidal analgesics and narcotics are administered. Around 20 ml of 0.25 per cent bupivacaine is instilled subdiaphragmatically and all port sites are infiltrated with 0.25 per cent bupivacaine. Intramuscular or IV diclofenac sodium 75 mg is administered after induction of anaesthesia. Postoperatively diclofenac sodium is given 12 hourly intramuscularly. Injection tramadol 50 mg is administered as required. Whereas inj. fentanyl or morphine supplementation is given for rescue analgesia.

POSTOPERATIVE BENEFITS OF LAPAROSCOPY

Laparoscopy produces fast recovery and a heightened feeling of well being. Postoperative fasting, duration of intravenous infusion and the hospital stay are significantly reduced after laparoscopy.[150,154,178,179] Surgical trauma is seemingly less, therefore pain and pulmonary dysfunction should also be less. Pulmonary function derangement is less after laparoscopic surgery and recovery is quicker.[150,151,154,156,179,180] Thoracic epidural analgesia does not improve lung function after laparoscopic cholecystectomy.[156] Although a laparoscopic approach might decrease the risk for patients with chronic obstructive pulmonary disease, diaphragmatic function is still significantly impaired.[11]

CARBOPERITONEUM RELATED COMPLICATIONS

CARBON DIOXIDE GAS EMBOLISM

Gas embolism is a rare but potentially fatal complication of carboperitoneum.[149,181] During insufflation, gas may enter the circulation directly if a needle or a trocar accidentally punctures a blood vessel or indirectly if gas is trapped in the portal circulation.[99,182-185] When CO_2 is used for insufflation during laparoscopy, fatal gas embolism rarely occurs since CO_2 easily dissolves or is carried in blood as carboxyhemoglobin and bicarbonate. The lethal dose of CO_2 is five times greater than that of air.[186]

Early recognition and treatment of gas embolism improves outcome.[183,186] The initial flow rate of the insufflation gas should not exceed 1 litre/min. If gas embolism is suspected, insufflation should be immediately discontinued, the abdomen deflated, the patient turned on to the left (right side up) in a steep head down position (Durant position). This reduces the amount of gas reaching the right heart.[187] 100 per cent oxygen is administered and all inhalation anaesthetic agents are discontinued.

PULMONARY ASPIRATION

Patients undergoing laparoscopy are usually considered at risk of developing the acid aspiration syndrome.[74,75] Fortunately, the intra-abdominal pressure also increases the competence of the gastro-esophageal sphincter, and thus contains the risk of gastric regurgitation.[76,77] Despite tracheal intubation with a cuffed tube, seeping of gastric contents around the cuff and pulmonary aspiration is still possible during laparoscopy.[188] The regurgitation may be "silent" and totally missed by the anaesthesiologist. Only later, as chemical pneumonitis sets in, would clinical signs of pulmonary aspiration become obvious.

Patients scheduled for laparoscopic surgery are usually premedicated with H_2 blockers and metoclopramide.

PNEUMOTHORAX, SUBCUTANEOUS EMPHYSEMA AND PNEUMOMEDIASTINUM

Increased intraperitoneal pressure during laparoscopy can open embryonic channels to the mediastinum, pleural cavity and pericardium[189] leading to the formation of pneumothorax.

Subcutaneous emphysema is not an uncommon complication in laparoscopic surgery for hernias, reflux oesophagitis and obesity. Rise in end-tidal CO_2 ($EtCO_2$) and hypoxia are the usual presentation. The patient should be ventilated after deflation of pneumoperitoneum till end-tidal CO_2 ($EtCO_2$) is normalized.

THROMBOEMBOLISM

Pneumoperitoneum causes slowing of blood flow in the peripheral vascular system, which may favour deep vein thrombosis (DVT).[102-107] Patients may require protection from DVT and hence pulmonary embolism. The following patients are predisposed to DVT:
- Morbid obese
- Cancer
- Congestive heart failure
- History of previous DVT
- Prolonged laparoscopic procedure.

These patients should be given antithrombotic prophylaxis with low molecular weight heparin and/or intermittent pneumatic compression perioperatively.

CARDIOVASCULAR

Bradyarrhythmia is very common during laparoscopy. Arrhythimas, venticular and supraventicular occur not infrequently during this surgery. These may be due to carboperitonium, hypoxia or reduced cardiac output.

Haemodynamic perturbations include hypertension, hypotension and occasionally cardiovascular collapse.

POSTOPERATIVE NAUSEA AND VOMITING (PONV)

PONV is common following laparoscopic surgery. It may delay discharge from day care facility. It can be prevented by the use of appropriate anti-emetics.

REFERENCES

1. Wickham JEA: Minimally invasive surgery: Future developments. Br med. J 15; 1994; 308(6922): 198-6.
2. Working Group of department of heart and the Scottish department of home health: Minimal access surgery: Implications for the NHS: Edinburgh. HM Stationary office 1994.
3. Mintz M: Le risqué et al. La prophylaxis des accidents en coelioscopic gynecologique: enquete portant Sue 100,000 case. J. Gynecol obstet Biol Reprod (Paris) 1976; 5: 691.
4. Cognat M, Gerald D, Vigneaud A le risqué d'reece cardiaque au cours de la coclioscopic. J Gynecol obstet Bio' Reprod (Paris) 1976; (7):925-40.
5. Brantly JC, Riley PM; Cardiovascular collapse during laparoscopy: A report of two cases. Am J obstet Gynecol 1998; 159: 735-7.
6. Holohan TV. Laparoscopic cholecystectomy. Lancet 1991; 28; 338(8770): 801-3.
7. Schirmer BD, Edge SB, Dix I et al (1990). Laparoscopic cholecystectomy. Treatment of choice for symptomatic cholelithiasis. Am Surg 1990; 213(6) 665-77.
8. Alexander GD, Noe FE, Brown EM. Anesthesia for pelvic laparoscopy. Anesth Analg 1969; 48(1):14-8.
9. Ciofolo MJ, Clergue F, Seebacher J et al. Ventilatory effects of laparoscopy under epidural anesthesia. Anesth Analg 1990; 70(4): 357-61.
10. Lewis DG, Ryder W, Burn N, et al. Laparoscopy an investigation during spontaneous ventilation with halothane. Br. J Anesth 1972; 44(7):685-91.
11. Sha M, Ohmura A, Yamada M. Diaphragm and pulmonary complication after laparoscopic cholecystectomy. Anesthesiology 1991; 75: Suppl 3A, A 255.
12. Schaeffler P, Heberer JP, Manhes H, et al. Repercussion a circulatoires at ventilatoires de la coelioscopic ches l'obese: Ann Fr Anesth Reanim 1984; 3:10.
13. Wilcox S, Vandam LD. Alas, poor trendelenburg and his position! Anesth Analg 1988; 67(6):574-8.
14. Joris J, Ledoux D, Honore P, Lamy M. Ventilatory effects of CO_2 insuffation during laparoscopic cholecystectomy. Anesthesiology 75 Suppl. 1991; 3A: A121.
15. Nyarwaya JB, Samii K, Mazost JX, deWalteville JC. Are pulse oximetric and capnographic monitoring reliable during laparoscopic surgery for cholecystectomy? Anesthesiology 1991; 75: Suppl 3A: A453.
16. Wahba RWM: Perioperative functional residual capacity. Can J Anesth 1991; 38: 384.
17. Kendall AP, Bhatt S, Oh TE: Pulmonary consequences of carbon dioxide insufflation for laparoscopic cholecystectomy. Anaesthesia 1995; 50(4):286-9.
18. Wittgen CM, Andrus CH, Fitzgerald SD, et al. Analysis of the hemodynamic and ventilatory effects of laparoscopic cholecystectomy Arch Surg 1991; 126(8):997-1001.
19. Puri GD, Singh H: Ventilatory effects of laparoscopy under general anaesthesia. Br J Anaesth 1992; 68(2):211-3.
20. Brown DR, Fishburne JI. Roberson VO: Ventilatory and blood gas changes during laparoscopy with local anesthesia. Am J obstet Gynecol 1976; 124(7):741-5.
21. Cunningham AJ, Schlanger M: Intraoperative hypoxemia complicating laparoscopic cholecystectomy in a patient with sickle hemoglobinopathy. Anesth Analg 1992; 75(5):838-43.
22. Ivankovich AD, Milctich DJ, Albrecht RF, et al. Cardiovascular effects of intraperitoneal insufflation with carbon dioxide and nitrous oxide in the dog. Anesthesiology 1975; 42(3):281-7.
23. Seed RF, Shakespeare TF, Muldron MJ. Carbon dioxide homeostasis during anaesthesia for laparoscopy. Anaesthesia 1970; 25(2): 223-31.
24. Hodgson C, McChelland RMA, Newton JR. Some effects of the peritoneal insufflation of carbon dioxide at laparoscopy. Anesthesia 1970; 25:382.
25. Magno R, Medegard A, Bengtason R, Tronstad SE. Acid base balance during laparoscopy. Acta obstet Gynecol Scand 1979; 58(1): 81-5.

26. Diamant M, Benumof JL, Saidman IJ et al. Laparoscopic sterilization with local anaesthesia. Complication and blood gas changes. Anesth Analg 1977; 56:335.

27. Verschelen L, Serreyn R, Rolly G et al. Physiological changes during anaesthesia administration for gynecologic laparoscopic. J Reprod Med 1984; 29(10): 697-700.

28. Johnson C, Anderson M, Juhl B. The effects of general anaesthesia on hemodynamic event during laparoscopy with CO_2 insufflation. Acta Anesthesiol Scand 33-132, 1989. Social

29. Kenefick JP, Leader A, Maltby JR, et al. Laparoscopy blood-gas values and minor sequelae associated with three techniques based on isoflurane. Br J Anaesth 1987; 59:189.

30. Sagaard P, Viale Jp, Annat G, et al. Diffusion du gas carbonique dana l'organisme au. a cours de la cholecystectomie par voie coelioscopique. Ann Fr Anesth Reanim Suppl 1991; 10 R 50.

31. Feig BW, Berger DH, Dougherty TB, et al. Pharmacological intervention can reestablish baseline hemodynamic parameters during laparoscopy. Surgery 1994; 116(4):733-41.

32. Hall D, Goldstein A, Tynan E, Braunstein L. Profound hypercarbia late in the course of laparoscopic cholecystectomy: Detection by continuous capnometry. Anesthesiology 1993; 79(1):173-4.

33. Schauer PR, Luma J, Ghiatas AA et al. Pulmonary function after laparoscopic cholecystectomy. Surgery 1993; 114:389.

34. Frazee RC, Roberts JW, Okeson GC et al. Open versus laparoscopic cholecystectomy. A comparison of postoperative pulmonary function. Arch Surg 1991; 213:631.

35. Erice F, Fox Gs, Salib YM et al. Diaphragmatic function before and after laparoscopic cholecystectomy. Anesthesiology 1993; 79:966.

36. Joris JL, Noirot DP, Legrand MJ et al. Hemodynamic changes during laparoscopic cholecystectomy. Anesth Analg 1993; 76(5): 1067-71.

37. Safran D, Sagambati S, Orlando R. Laparoscopy in high-risk cardiac patients. Surg Gynecol obstet 1993; 176:548-54.

38. Zollinger A, Krayer S, Singer T, et al. Haemodynamic effects of pneumoperitoneum in elderly patients with an increased cardiac risk. Euro J Anaesthesiol 1997; 14(3): 266-75.

39. Hirvonen BA, Nuufinen LS, Kauko M. Haemodynamic changes due to trendelenburg positioning and pneumoperitoneum during laparoscopy surgery 1994; 166:733.

40. Elliott S, Savill P, Eckersall S. Cardiovascular changes during laparoscopic cholecystectomy: A study using transoesophageal Doppler monitoring. Eur J Anaesthesiol 1998; 15(1):50-5.

41. Haxby EJ, Gray MR, Rodriguez C, et al. Assessment of cardiovascular changes during laparoscopic hernia repair using oesophageal Doppler. Br J Anesth 1997; 78(5): 515-9S.

42. Westerband A, VanDc Water, Amzallag M, Lebowitz PW. Cardiovascular changes during laparoscopic cholecystectomy. Surg Gynecol obstet 1992; 175(6):535-8.

43. Richardson JD, Trinkli EK. Haemodynamic and respiratory alterations with increased intra-abdominal pressure J Surg Res 1976; 20(5): 401-4.

44. Kelman GR, Swapp GH, Smith I, et al. Cardiac output and arterial blood gas tension during laparoscopy. Br J Anesth 1972; 44(11):1155-65.

45. Marshall RL, Jebson PJR, Davie IT, Scott DB. Circulatory effects of carbon dioxide insufflation of the peritoneal cavity for laparoscopy. Br J Anesth 1972; 44(7):680-12.

46. Motew M, Ivankovich A, Bieniarz J, et al: Cardiovascular effects and acid-base and blood gas changes during laparoscopy. Am J obstet Gynecol 1973; 1; 115(7):1002-12.

47. Ekman LG, Abrahamsson J, Biber J, et al. Haemodynamic changes during laparoscopy with positive end-expiratory pressure ventilation. Acta Anesthesiol Scand 198; 32(6):447-53.

48. Lenz RJ, Thomas TA, Wilkens DG, Cardiovascular changes during laparoscopy. Anesthesia 1976; (1): 31: 4-12.

49. Stuttmann R, Vogi C, Eypasch, Doehn M. Haemodynamic changes during laparoscopic cholecystectomy in the high risk patients. Endosc Surg 1995; 3:174.

50. Joris J, Lamy M. Changes in oxygen transport and ventilation during pneumoperitoneum for laparoscopic cholecystectomy. Anesthesiology 1992; 77: Suppl –3A, A 149.

51. Paul A, Troidl H, Peters S, Stuttmann R. Fatal intestinal ischaemia following laparoscopic cholecystectomy. Br J Surg 1994; 81(12): 1207-8.

52. Dwerryhouse SJ, Melson DS, Burton PA, Thompson MH. Acute intestinal ischaemia after laparoscopic cholecystectomy. Br J Surg 1995; 82(10):1413.

53. Caldwell CB, Ricotta JJ. Changes in visceral blood flow with elevated intra-abdominal pressure. J Surg Res 1987; 43(1): 14-20.

54. Jorgensen JO, Hanel K, Lalak NJ, et al. Thromboembolic complications of laparoscopic cholecystectomy. BMJ 1993; 300: 318-19.

55. Deziel DJ, Millikan KW, Economou SG, et al. Complication of laparoscopic cholecystectomy a national survey of 4292 hospitals and an analysis of 77604 cases. Am J Surg 1993; 165(1): 9-14.

56. Airan M, Appel M, Berci G, Coburg AJ, et al. Retrospective and prospective multi-institutional laparoscopic cholecystectomy study organized by the society of American Gastrointestinal endoscopic surgeons. Surg Endosc 1992; 6(4):169-76.

57. Dubois F. Berthelot G, Levard H. Laparoscopic cholecystectomy: Historic perspective and personal experience. Surg Laparosc Endosc 1991; 1(1):52-7.

58. Jorgensen JO, Lalak NJ, North I, et al. Venous stasis during laparoscopic cholecystectomy. Surg Laparosc Endosc 1994; 4(2): 128-33.

59. Scott TR, Zucker KA, Bailey RW. Laparoscopic cholecystectomy: a review of 12397 patients. Surg Laparsc Endosc 1992; 2(3):191-8.

60. Josephs LG, Esto-McDonald JR, Birkett DH, et al. Diagnostic laparoscopy increases intracranial pressure. J Trauma 1994; 30(6):815-8.

61. Mijangos JI, Thwin N, Hinchey EJ, Oung EM. Change in intracranial pressure during carbon dioxide pneumoperitoneum in normovolemic and hypovolemia animals. Surg Forum 1994; 45:583.

62. Bloomfield GL, Dalton JM, Sugerman HJ, et al. Treatment of increasing intracranial pressure secondary to the acute abdominal compartment syndrome in a patient with combined abdominal and head trauma. J Trauma 1995; 39(6):1168.

63. Schob OM, Allen DC, Benzel E, et al. A comparison of the pathophysiologic effects of carbon dioxide, nitrous oxide and helium pneumoperitoneum on intracranial pressure. Am J Surg 1996; 172(3):248-53.

64. Emelijanov SI, Fedenko VV, Levite EM, et al. Pneumoperitoneum risk prognosis and correction of venous circulation disturbances in laparoscopic surgery. Surg Endosc 1998; 12:1224.

65. Rosenthal RJ, Freedman RL, Chidambran A, et al. Effects of hyperventilation and hypoventilation on $PaCO_2$ and intracranial pressure during acute elevation of intra abdominal pressure with CO_2 pneumoperitoneum. Large animal observations. J Am Coll Surg 1998; 187:32.

66. Sibbald WJ, Paterson NAM, Holliday RL, Baskerville J. The Trendelenburg position: haemodynamic effects in hypotensive and normotensive patients. Crit Care Med 1979; 7(5):218-24.

67. Anzai Y, Nishikawa T. Heart rate responses to body tilt during spinal anesthesia. Anesth Analg 1991; 73(4):385-90.

68. Torrielli R, Cesarini M Winnock S, et al. Modifications hemodynamique durant la coeliscopie: 'Etudemene'e - bioimpedance electricque thoracique. Can J Anesth 1990; 37(1):46-51.

69. Lumb AB, Nunn JF. Respiratory function and ribcage contribution to ventilation in body positions commonly used during anesthesia. Anesth Analg 1991; 73(4):422-6.

70. Marco AP, Yeo CJ, Rock P. Anesthesia for a patients undergoing laparoscopic cholecystectomy. Anesthesiology 1990; 73(6): 1268-70.

71. Heinonen J, Tarri S, Tammisto T. Effect of the trendelenburg tilt and other procedures on the position of endotracheal tubes. Lancet I: 1969; 26; 1(7600):850-3.

72. Wittgen CM, Naunheim KS, Andrus CH, et al. Preoperative pulmonary function evaluation for laparoscopic cholecystectomy. Arch Surg 1993; 128:880-86.

73. Beebe DS, McNevin MP, Belani KG, et al. Evidence of venous stasis after abdominal insufflation for laparoscopic cholecystectomy. Anesthesiology 1992; 77: Suppl 3A: A148.

74. Tay HS, Chiu HH. Acid aspiration during laparoscopy. Anesth Intensive care 1989; 6(2):134-7.

75. Duffy BL. Regurgitation during pelvic laparoscopy. Br J Anesth 1979; 51(11):1089-90.

76. Spielman FJ. Laparoscopic surgery P 151. IN Hood DD, Kirby RR, Brown DL (eds). Problems in anaesthesia: Anesthesia in obstetrics and Gynaecology. Vol. 3 JB Lippincott. Philadelphia 1989.

77. Eger IJ IInd, Smith NT, Stoelting RK. Cardiovascular effects of halothane in man. Anesthesiology 1970; 32(5):396-409.

78. Calverley RK, Smith NT, Prys Roberts C et al. Cardiovascular effects of enflurane anesthesia during controlled ventilation in man. Anesth Analg 1978; 57:619-28.

79. Lowe D, Hettrick DA, Pagel PS, Waltier DC. Influence of volatile anesthesia on left ventricular afterload in vivo. Difference between desflurane and sevoflurane. Anesthesiology 1996; 85:112-20.

80. Cahalan MK, Weiskopf RB, Eger EI II. Hemodynamic effects of desflurane/nitrous oxide anesthesia in volunteers. Anesth Analg. 1991; 73(2):157-64.
81. Eger IJ II. Nitrous oxide: N_2O New York, Elsevier, 1985.
82. Pagel PS, Kampine JP, Schmeling WT, Waltier DC. Comparison of the systemic and coronary hemodynamic actions of desflurane, isoflurane, halothane, and enflurane in the chronically instrumented dog. Anesthesiology 1991; 74(3):539-51.
83. Martin BC. Are the myocardial and metabolic effect of isoflurane really different from those of halothane and enflurane? Anesthesiology 1981; 55:398-408.
84. Eger EJ II. New inhaled anesthetics. Anesthesiology 1994; 80(4):906-22.
85. Martin BG, Bernard JM, Douisout ME, et al. Comparison of the effects of isoflurane and desflurane on cardiovascular dynamics and regional blood flow in the chronically instrumented dog. Anesthesiology. 1991; 74(3):568-74.
86. Weiskopf RB, Homes MA, Eger IJ IInd. Cardiovascular effects of I653 in swine. Anesthesiology 1988; 69(3):303-9.
87. Berhard JM; Wouters PE; Kersten JR et al. Direct inotropic and lusitropic effects of sevoflurane. Anesthesiology 1994; 81(1): 156-67.
88. Sumikawa K, Ishizaka N, Suzaki M. Arrhythmogenic plasmas levels of epinephrine during halothane, enflurane and pentobarbital anesthesia in dogs. Anesthesiology 1983; 58:322-25.
89. Bristow JD, Prys-Roberts C, Fisher A. Effects of anesthesia on baroreflex control of heart rate in man. Anesthesiology 1969; 31(5):422-8.
90. Kotrly KJ, Ebert TJ, Vucins E et al. Baroreceptor reflex control of heart rate during isoflurane anesthesia in humans. Anesthesiology 1984; (3):173-9.
91. Calverley RK, Smith NT, Jones CW et al. Ventilatory and cardiovascular effects of enflurane anesthesia during spontaneous ventilation in man. Anesth Analg 1978; 57:610-18.
92. Murat I, Lapeyre G, Saint-Maurice C. Isoflurane attenuates baroreflex control of heart rate in human neonates. Anesthesiology 1989; 70(3):395-400.
93. Cahalan MK, Lurz FW, Eger EJ IInd. Narcotics decrease heart rate during inhalational anesthesia. Anesth Analg 1987; 66(2): 166-70.
94. Ebert TJ, Muzi M. Sympathetic hyperactivity during desflurane anesthesia in healthy volunteers. A comparison with isoflurane. Anesthesiology 1993; 79(3):444-53.
95. Weiskopf RB, Moore MA, Eger EJ II, et al. Rapid increase in desflurane concentration is associated with greater transient cardiovascular stimulation than with rapid increase in isoflurane concentration in humans. Anesthesiology 1994; 80(5):1035-45.
96. Ebert TJ, Harkin CP, Muzi M. Cardiovascular responses to sevoflurane A review. Anesth Analg 1995; 81:811-22.
97. Ebert TJ, Muzi M, Lopatka CW. Neurocirculatory responses to sevoflurane in humans. A comparison to desflurane. Anesthesiology 1995; 83:88-95.
98. Marshall RL, Japson PJR, Danie JT, Scott DB. Circulatory effects or carbon dioxide insufflation of the peritoneal cavity. Br J Anesth 1972; 44:1155-61.
99. Landercasper J, Miller GJ, Strutt PJ et al. Carbon dioxide embolization and laparoscopic cholecystectomy. Surg Laparosc Endosc 1993; 3:407-10.
100. Hovorka J, Korttila K, Erkola O. Nitrous oxide dose not increase nausea and vomiting following gynecological laparoscopy. Can J Anesth 1989; 36(2):145-8.
101. Sengupta P, Plantevin OM. Nitrous Oxide and day-case laparoscopy, effect on nausea vomiting and return to normal activity. Br J Anesth 1988; 60(5):570-3.
102. Aun C, Major E. The cardiorespiratory effect of ICI 35 868 in-patients with valvular heart disease. Anesthesia 1984; 39:1096-1100.
103. Grounds RM, Twighy AJ, Carli F et al. The hemodynamic effects of intravenous induction. Comparison of the effects of thiopentone and propofol. Anesthesia 1985; 40:735-40.
104. Coates DP, Monk CR, Prys-Roberts C, Turtle M: Hemodynamic effect of infusions of the emulsion formulation of propofol during nitrous oxide anesthesia in humans. Anesth Analg 1987; 66:64-70
105. Larsen R, Rathgeber J, Bagdahn A, et al. Effects of propofol on cardiovascular dynamic and coronary blood flow in geriatric patients. A comparison with etomidate. Anesthesia 1988; 43 suppl. 25-31.
106. Patrick MR, Blair U, Feneck RO, Sebel PS. A caparison of the haemodynamic effect of propofol and thiopentone in patients with coronary artery disease. Post Grad Med J 1985; 61 suppl. 23-27.

107. Coates D, Prys-Roberts C, Spelina K. Propofol by intravenous infusion with nitrous oxide: Dose requirements and haemodynamic effect. Post Grad Med J 1985; (suppl 3): 76-79.

108. Claeys MA, Gepts E, Camu F. Haemodynamic changes during anesthesia induced and maintained with propofol. Br J Anesth 1983; 60:3-9.

109. Todd MM, Drummond JC, UHS. The hemodynamic consequences of high-dose thiopental anesthesia. Anesth Analg 1985; 64: 681-7

110. Rodriguez E, Jorden R: Contemporary trends in paediatric sedation and analgesia. Med Clin North Am 2002; 20:199-222.

111. Dundee J Wyant G. Intra venous Anesthesia. 2nd ed. Edinburgh. Churchill Livingstone 1998.

112. Reves JA, Gelman S. cardiovascular effect of intravenous anesthetic drugs. In Covino B, Fozzard H, Rehdevs K (eds). Effect of anesthesia. American physiological society 1995 pp 179.

113. Tarabadkar S, Kopriva D, Srinivasan N et al. Hemodynamic impact of induction in patient with decreased cardiac reserve. Anesthesiology 1980; 53:543.

114. Seltzer JL, Gerson JI, Allen FB. Comparison of the cardiovascular effects of bolus vs. incremental administration of thiopentone. Br J Anaesth 1980; 52(5):527-30.

115. Marty J, Gauzit R, Lefevre P et al. Effect of diazepam and midazolam on baroreflex control of heart rate & on sympathetic activity in humans. Anesth Analg 1986; 65:113-9.

116. Lebowitz DW, Cote ME, Daniel AL. Comparative cardiovascular effects of midazolam and thiopentone in healthy patients. Anesth Analg 1982; 61(9):771-5.

117. Gooding JM, Weng JT, Smith RA, et al. Effect of etomidate on the cardiovascular system. Anesth Analg 1977; 56(5): 717-9.

118. Calvin MP, Savage TM, Newland PE, et al. Cardiorespiratory changes following induction of anaesthesia with etomidate in patients with cardiac disease. Br J Anaesth 1979; 51(6):551-6.

119. Haessler R, Madler C, Klasing S. Propofol/fentanyl versus etomidate/fentanyl for the induction of anesthesia in patients with aortic insufficiency and coronary artery disease. J Cardiothorac Vasc Anesth. 1992; 6(2):173-80.

120. Hanley ES. Anesthesia for laparoscopic surgery. Surg Clin North Am 1992; 72(5):1013-9.

121. Gabbott DA, Dunkley AB, Roberts FL. Carbon dioxide pneumothorax occurring during laparoscopic cholecystectomy. Anesthesia 1992; 47(7):587-8.

122. Barodczky GI, Engelmar E, Levarlet M, Simon P. Ventilatory effects of pneumoperitoneum monitored with continuous Spirometry. Anesthesia 1993; 48(4):309-11.

123. Putensen C, Leon MA, Putensen-Himmer G. Effects of neuromuscular blockade on the elastic properties of the lung, thorax and total respiratory system in anesthetized pigs. Crit Care Med 1994; 22(12):1976-80.

124. Westernbrook PR, Stubbs SE, Sessler AD et al. Effects of anesthesia and muscle paralysis on respiratory mechanics in normal man. J Suppl Physiol 1973; 34(1):81-6.

125. Norlander O, Herzog P, Norden I. Compliance and airway resistance during anaesthesia with controlled ventilation. Acta Anesthesiol Scand 1968; 12(3):132-52.

126. Chassard D, Berrada K, Tournadre J and Bouletreau P: The effects of neuromuscular block on peak airway pressure and abdominal elastance during pneumoperitoneum. Anesth Analg 1996; 82(3):525-7.

127. Kurer FL, Welch DB. Gynaecological laparoscopy: Clinical experiences of two anesthetic techniques. Br J Anesth 1984; 56(11): 1207-12.

128. Myatt JK, Smith M, Plantevin OM, Crowther A. Anesthesia for day-stay laparoscopy. Br J Anesth 1986; 58(10):1200-1.

129. Goodurn APL, Rowe WL, Ogg TW. Day care laparoscopy. A comparison of two anesthetic techniques using laryngeal mask during spontaneous breathing. Anesthesia 1992; 47(10):892-5.

130. Skacel M, Sengupta P, Plantevin OM. Morbidity after day-care laparoscopy. A comparison of two techniques of tracheal intubation. Anaesthesia 1986; 41(5):537-41.

131. Poindexter AN, Abdul Malak M, Fast JE. Laparoscopic tubal sterilization under local anesthesia. Obstet Gynecol 1990; 75(1): 5-8.

132. Bogetz MS, Katz JA. Recall of surgery for major trauma. Anesthesiology 1984; 61(1):6-9.

133. Editorial: On being aware. Br J Anaesth 1979; 51(8):711-2.

134. Barker P, Langton JA, Murphy PJ, Rowbotham DJ. Regurgitation of gastric contents during general anesthesia using the laryngeal mask airway. Br J Anaesth 1992; 69(3):314-15.

135. Peterson HB, DeStefano F, Rubin GL, et al. Deaths attributable to tubal sterilization in the United State 1977-1981. Am J Obstet Gynecol 1983; 15;146(2):131-6.

136. Malins AF, Field JM, Nesling FM, Cooper GM. Nausea and vomiting after gynecological laparoscopy: complication of premedication with oral ondansetron, metoclopramide and placebo. Br J Anesth 1994; 72(2):231-3.

137. Raphael JH, Norton AC. Antiemetic efficacy of prophylactic ondansetron in laparoscopic surgery: randomized double blind comparison with metoclopramide. Br J Anesth 1993; 71(6):845-8.

138. Fishburne JI: Anesthesia for laparoscopy: considerations, complications and technique. J Reprod Med. 1978; 21(1):37-40.

139. Mackenzie IZ, Turner E, O'sullivan GM et al. Two hundred-outpatient laparoscopic clip sterilisations using local anesthesia. Br J obstet Gynaecol 1987; 94(5):449-53.

140. Paterson HB, Hulka J, Spielman FJ,et al. local versus general anesthesia for laparoscopic serialization: A randomised study . Obstet Gynecol 1987; 70(6):903.

141. Brady CE, Harkleroad LE, Pierson WP. Alterations in oxygen saturation and ventilation after intravenous sedation for peritoneoscopy. Arch Intern Med 1989; 149(5):1029-32.

142. Lehtinen AM, Laatikainen T, Koskimies AI, Hovorka J. Modifying effects of epidural anesthesia or general anesthesia on stress hormone response to laparoscopy for in vitro fertilization. J Invitro Fert Enbryo Transf 1987; 4(1): 23-9.

143. Bridenbaugh LD, Soderstrom RM. Lumbar epidural block anesthesia for outpatient laparoscopy. J Reprod Med 1979; 23(2): 85-6.

144. Lefebvre G, Vauthier-Brouzes D, Darbois Y et al. La oscilloscopie sons anesthesie peridural: technique. Indications resultats a´ propos de 220 cases. J Gynecol Obstet Biol Reprod (Paris) 1991; 20(3):355-60.

145. Jones MJ, Mitchell RW, Hindocha N. Effect of increased intra-abdominal pressure during laparoscopy on the lower esophageal sphincter. Anesth Analg 1989; 68(1):63-5.

146. Wahba RWM, Mamazza J. Ventilatory requirements during laparoscopic cholecystectomy. Can J Anaesth 1993; 40(3):206-10.

147. Bhavani Shankar R, Moseley H, Kumar AV et al. Capnometory and anesthesia. Can J Anaesth 1991; 39(6):617-32.

148. Yacoub OF, Cadona I, Coveler, Dodson MG. Carbon dioxide embolism during laparoscopy. Anesthesiology 1982; 57(6): 533-5.

149. Gomar C, Fernandez C, Villalonga A, Nalda MA. Carbon dioxide embolism during laparoscopy and hysteroscopy. Ann Fr Anesth Reanim 195; 4(4):380-2.

150. Joris J, Cigarini I, Legrand M et al. Metabolic and respiratory changes after cholecystectomy performed via laparotomy or laparoscopy. Br J Anesth 1992; 69(4):341-5.

151. Putensen- Himmer G, Putensen C, Lammer H et al. Comparison of postoperative respiratory function after laparoscopy or open laparotomy for cholecystectomy. Anesthesiology 1992; 77(4):675-80.

152. Vegfors M, Cederholm I, Lennmarken C et al: Should oxygen be administered after laparoscopy in healthy patients? Acta Anaesthesiol Scand 1988; 32(4):350-2.

153. Blobner M, Felber AR, Gogler et al. caroban dioxide uptake from pneumoperitoneum during laparoscopic cholecystectomy. Anesthesiology 1992; 77: Suppl 3A: A37.

154. Mealy K, Gallagher H, Barry M et al. Physiological and metabolic responses to open and laparoscopic cholecystectomy. Br J Surg 1992; 79(10): 1061-4.

155. Rademaker BM, Ringers J, Odoom JA et al. Pulmonary function and stress response after laparoscopic cholecystectomy: comparison with subcostal incision and influence of thoracic epidural analgesia. Anesth Anlag 1992; 75(3):381-5.

156. Reed AP, Han D, Sampson IH. Does laparoscopic cholecystectomy prevent postoperative pulmonary function deterioration? Anesthesiology 1991; 75 Suppl 3A: A127.

157. Colline KM, Docherty PW, Plantevin OM. Postoperative morbidity following gynaecological outpatient laparoscopy. A reappraisal of the service. Anesthesia 1984; 39(8):819-22.

158. Sharp JR, Pierson WP, Brady CE. Comparison of CO_2 and N_2O induced discomfort during peritoneoscopy under local anaesthesia. Gastroenterology 1982; 82:453.

159. Koetsawang S, Srisupandit S, Apimas SJ, Champion CB. A Comparative study of topical anesthesia for laparoscopic sterilization with the use of tubal ring. Am J Obstet Gynecol 1984; 150(8):931-3.

160. Mckenzie R, Phitayakorn P, Uy NTL et al. Topical etidocaine during laparoscopic tubal occlusion for postoperative pain relief. Obstet Gynecol 1986; 67(3):447-9.

161. Alexander CD, Wetchler VB, Thompson RE. Bupivacaine infiltration of the mesosalpinx in ambulatory surgical laparoscopic tubal sterilization. Can J Anesth 197; 34(4):362-5.

162. Narchi P, Benhamou D, Fernandez H. Intraperitoneal local anesthesia for shoulder pain after day-case laparoscopy. Lancet 1991; 338(8782-8783):1569-71.

163. Narchi P, Benhamou D, Aubrum F et al. Analgesia using mesosalpinx infiltration combined with intraperitoneal lidocaine for yoon ring laparoscopy. Anesthesiology 1992; 77:3A, A17.

164. Delucia JA, White PF. Effect of intraoperative ketorolac on recovery after outpatient laparoscopy. Anesthesiology 1991; 75: Suppl. 3A:A14.

165. Gillberg LE, Harsten AS, Stahl LB. Preoperative diclofenac sodium reduces post-laparoscopy pain. Can J Anaesth 1993; 40(5):406-8.

166. Bellamy CD, Chovan J, Brose EL, Gunzen Hauser L. Ketorolac superior to sufentanil, giving longer pain relief with less nausea and less recovery time after laparoscopy. Anesthesiology 1991; 75: Suppl. 3A: A29.

167. Ding Y, White PF. Comparative effects of ketorolac, dezocine and fentanyl as adjuvants during outpatient anesthesia. Anesth Analg 1992; 75(4):566-71.

168. Greenberg CP, Levine MI, Brown AR. Ketorolac is an effective analgesic for outpatient laparoscopy & shoulder arthroscopy. Anesthesiology 1992; 77: Suppl. 3A: A21

169. Shenton O, Fabrick J, Pagulayan G. Evaluation of toradol for pain control after laparoscopic cholecystectomy. Anesthesiology 1992; 77: Suppl 3A: A440.

170. Liu J, Ding Y, White PJ et al: Effect of ketorolac on postoperative analgesia and ventilatory function after laparoscopic cholecystectomy. Anesth Analg 1993; 776:1061.

171. Comfort VK, Code WE, Rooney ME, Yip RW: Naproxen Premedication reduces postoperative tubal ligation pain. Can J Anesth 1992; 39(4):349-52.

172. Rosenblum M, Wellar RS, Conard PL, et al. Ibuprofen provide longer lasting anesthesia than fentanyl after laparoscopic surgery. Anesth Analg 1991; 73:275.

173. Crocker S, Paech M. Preoperative rectal indomethacin for anesthesia after laparoscopic sterilization. Anaesth Intensive Care 1992; 20(3):337-40.

174. Edwards ND, Berclay K, Catling SJ et al. Day care laparoscopy surgery of postoperative pain and an assessment of the value of diclofenac. Anesthesia 1991; 46:1077.

175. Pandit SK, Kothary SP, Lebenbom-Mansour M et al: Failure of ketorolac to pervent severe postoperative pain following outpatient laparoscopy. Anesthesiology 1991; 75: Suppl. 3A: A33.

176. Green CR, Pandit SK, Kothary SP et al. No fentanyl sparing effect of intraoperative iv ketorolac after laparoscopic tubal ligation. Anesthesiology 1992; 77: Suppl. 3A: A7.

177. Calhoun B, Viani B, LaRue D. The effect of ketorolac on patients undergoing outpatient laparoscopy. Anesthesiology 1992; 77 Suppl. 3A: A48.

178. Grace PA, Quereshi A, Coleman et al. Reduced postoperative hospitalization after laparoscopic cholecystectomy. Br J Surg 1991; 78(2):160-2.

179. Mc Anema OJ, Austin O, Hiderman WP et al. laparoscopic versus open appendicectomy. Lancet 1991; 338(8768):693.

180. Frazee R, Roberts J, Okeson G et al. Open versus laparoscopic cholecystectomy a comparison of postoperative pulmonary function. Ann Surg 1991; 213:651.

181. Philips JM, Keith D, Hulka J et al. Gynecological laparoscopy in 1975. J Reprod Med 1976; 16:105-17.

182. Root B, Levy MN, Pollack S et al. Gas embolism death after laparoscopy delayed by "trapping in portal circulation. Anesth Analg 1978; 57:232-7.

183. Clark CC, Weeks DB, Gurden JP. Venous carbon dioxide embolism during laparoscopy. Anesth Analg 1977; 56:650-52.

184. Morison DH (1974). Cardiovascular collapse in laparoscopy. Can Med Assoc J 1974; 111:433-7.

185. Derouin M, Boudreault D, Couture P et al. Detection of CO_2 venous embolization during laparoscopic surgery. Anesthesiology 1994; 81:A560.

186. Mellies CJ. Pneumoperitoneum with an unusual complication. J Missouri Med Assoc 1939; 36:430-35.

187. Shulman S, Chuter T, Weisman C. Dynamic respiratory patterns after laparoscopic cholecystectomy. Chest 1993; 103:1173.

188. Bernhard WN, Cotrell JE, Silvakumaran C et al, Adjustment of intra cuff pressure to pervent aspiration. Anesthesiology 1979; 50:363-6.

189. Batra MS, Driscoll JJ, Coburn WA et al. Evanescent nitrous oxide pneumothorax after laparoscopy. Anesth Analg 1983; 62:1121-3.

CHAPTER 10

Regional Anaesthesia in Laparoscopic Surgery

INTRODUCTION

Laparoscopic procedures are becoming increasingly popular, even in high risk patients. It may possibly be because pulmonary functions are better preserved following laparoscopic surgery. While the forced vital capacity is reduced by 48 per cent after open surgery it is reduced by 27 per cent after laparoscopic surgery.[1,2]

Although most patients desire general anaesthesia, it can be a significant disadvantage in morbid cases. General anaesthesia may be associated with haemodynamic disturbances nausea, vomiting and throat discomfort. The use of epidural / spinal anaesthesia for certain laparoscopic procedures can obviate the side effects and complications of general anaesthesia and muscle relaxation.[1]

PHYSIOLOGY DURING LAPAROSCOPY

RESPIRATORY SYSTEM

Carboperitoneum results in an increased intra-abdominal pressure which leads to a decrease in total lung compliance and functional residual capacity. This results in basal atelectasis and increased airway pressure. The result is impairment in ventilation / perfusion (V/Q) in many lung units. Under general anaesthesia there is increase in CO_2 elimination after insufflation that continues until 10 minutes postdeflation of the abdomen. There is a corresponding rise in arterial CO_2 ($PaCO_2$) concentration which declines in the recovery period; due to decrease in CO_2 production and increase in the ability of a spontaneously breathing patient to eliminate CO_2.[3] Carboperitoneum in patients breathing spontaneously under epidural anaesthesia without sedation results in an increase in minute ventilation with unchanged $EtCO_2$.[4] Arterial blood gases during laparoscopy under regional anaesthesia were maintained within normal limits.[5] The same ventilatory responsiveness does not occur under inhalation anaesthesia. Respiratory depression, combined with mechanical impairment of ventilation explain the high incidence of hypercapnia during laparoscopy in spontaneously breathing patient under inhalational anaesthesia. One hour after CO_2 exsufflation, $PaCO_2$ was unchanged when compared with baseline values. Trendelenburg tilt did not induce any significant change in ventilatory parameters. A mean difference between arterial and end tidal CO_2 ($EtCO_2$) tension of 0.44 KPa has been reported with general and epidural anaesthesia.[6] Causes of increased minute ventilation under regional anaesthesia after carboperitoneum could be due to:[4,7,8]

i. Increased number of lung units with high ventilation perfusion ratios as shown by decrease end tidal PCO_2
ii. Increased alveolo-arterial CO_2 difference
iii. Increase in VD/VT ratio.
iv. Epidurally administered lidocaine increases the slope of ventilatory response to CO_2
v. Persistence of painful stimuli and abdominal distension lead to increased minute ventilation

Thus epidural anaesthesia may be a safe alternative to general anaesthesia for outpatient laparoscopy, as it is not associated with ventilatory depression. It provides excellent postoperative analgesia and lower incidence of postoperative nausea and vomiting.[4]

CARDIOVASCULAR SYSTEM

Mean arterial pressure and heart rate do not change during Trendelenburg positioning or insufflation in patients undergoing epidural anaesthesia. In hyperbaric spinal anaesthesia the level of block can migrate in the cephalad direction during the Trendelenburg position, and predispose to hypotension and bradycardia. However, low dose hypobaric solution does not migrate cephalad in the Trendelenburg position and the risk of hypotension is reduced.[9]

However, laparoscopic procedures conducted under regional anaesthesia require expertise.

DISADVANTAGES OF REGIONAL ANAESTHESIA

Despite the overall safety of epidural anaesthesia, it can be associated with:

a. Insufficient abdominal wall relaxation.
b. Risk of aspiration from Trendelenburg position.
c. Need to convert to general anaesthesia due to patient discomfort.
d. Shoulder tip pain secondary to diaphragmatic irritation which is mediated by phrenic nerve.
e. Difficulty to provide complete analgesia by a regional block. Manipulation of upper gastrointestinal structures require an extensive sensory block (T_4-L_5).
f. Sympathetic block which may exaggerate the development of vagal reflexes.
g. Adequate intraoperative sedation is essential with midazolam, fentanyl or propofol infusion to allay anxiety. Sedation given in conjunction with a regional block however decreases sensitivity of respiratory centre. This can lead to hypoventilation and arterial oxygen desaturation.[8]

Success with local/regional anaesthesia requires a relaxed and cooperative patient, a supportive staff and a skilled surgeon. Low intra-abdominal pressure and a reduced tilt to reduce pain and ventilatory disturbances.[10]

In this chapter we determine the safety and efficacy of epidural / spinal anaesthesia (regional anaesthesia) for various laparoscopic procedures like laparoscopic cholecystectomy, inguinal hernia repair by laparoscopic total extraperitoneal (TEP) approach, laparoscopic segmental colectomy, laparoscopic intraperitoneal onlay poly tetrafluoroethylene mesh repair (IPOM) for umbilical hernia or incisional hernia, short duration outpatient gynaecological laparoscopy, laparoscopic rectopexy, etc. General anaesthesia, however, remains the procedure of choice for all laparoscopic procedures.

ANAESTHETIC MANAGEMENT

PREMEDICATION

Anxiolytics such as benzodiazepines are prescribed. An antiemetic and H_2-receptor antagonist reduce the volume and pH of gastric secretions and thus reduce the incidence of postoperative nausea and vomiting.

LAPAROSCOPIC CHOLECYSTECTOMY

The choice of anaesthetic technique for upper abdominal laparoscopic surgery is general anaesthesia with muscle paralysis and tracheal intubation.[11] Popularity of general anaesthesia over regional anaesthesia in laparoscopic cholecystectomy remains unchallenged despite a few studies showing safety of epidural / combined spinal epidural anaesthesia (Fig. 10.1). Luchetti M et al studied the effectiveness and safety of combined epidural and general anaesthesia for laparoscopic cholecystectomy. They found that the technique provided excellent intra and postoperative analgesia. Recovery time was short because intravenous opioids were not used.[12] In this study combined epidural / general anaesthesia was compared with total intravenous anaesthesia for laparoscopic cholecystectomy and both the techniques were found to be equally safe. If conducted under regional anaesthesia a high epidural block (T_2-T_4 levels) is required to abolish the discomfort of surgical stimulation of the upper gastrointestinal structures. The high block may produce myocardial depression and reduction in venous return, aggravating the haemodynamic effects of carboperitoneum.[11] Combined thoracic epidural and general anaesthesia with laryngeal mask airway has been used in a patient of laparoscopic cholecystectomy with myasthenia gravis. The authors used pre-emptive anti-emetic therapy, a nasogastric tube, reduced intra-abdominal pressure (9-10 mmHg) and proper positioning of the patient which made the use of LMA safe, by reducing the risk of regurgitation and aspiration.[13] However the use of LMA in laparoscopic cholecystectomy is still debatable.

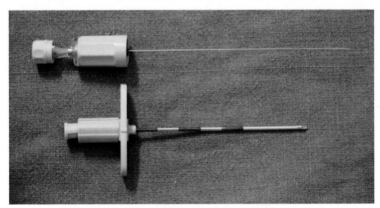

Fig. 10.1: Epidural and spinal needles

There are two studies where laparoscopic cholecystectomy was done under epidural anaesthesia in patients with COPD.[14] In this study authors concluded that laparoscopic cholecystectomy can be safely performed under epidural anaesthesia (Fig. 10.2). The abdominal wall relaxation was adequate contrary to the finding of some other authors. There is a risk of CO_2 partial pressure increasing during surgery which can cause acidosis and arrhythmias. However adequate oxygenation of the patient can prevent this complication. There is a suggestion to use N_2O instead of CO_2 to overcome this problem. N_2O can also help prevent pain because it does not irritate the peritoneum.[15] Other factors which affect the outcome are use of low intra-abdominal pressure combined with intermittent release of pneumoperitoneum, an experienced surgical team and short operative

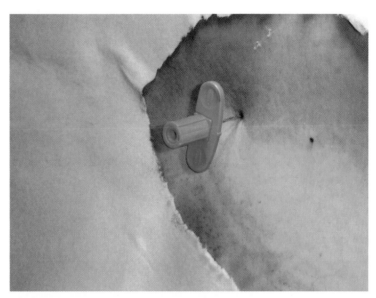

Fig. 10.2: Epidural anaesthesia

time. The patient selection was based on patient's ability to co-operate during the procedure and a non-complicated biliary pathology.

GYNAECOLOGICAL LAPAROSCOPIC PROCEDURES

Conventional dose hyperbaric spinal anaesthesia is not suitable for ambulatory laparoscopic procedures. It is associated with a longer recovery time compared with propofol anaesthesia. Selective spinal anaesthesia (SSA) (Fig. 10.3) competes with newer anaesthetics such as propofol / desflurane in terms of recovery and discharge time. This technique uses minimal doses of 1 per cent lignocaine 10 mg mixed with sufentanil 10 mcg[16] upto a total volume of 3 ml injected with needle orifice in cephalad direction. It allows preservation of motor function and maintains the integrity of the dorsal columns while providing selective pinprick anaesthesia. Patients receiving SSA had satisfactory surgical conditions for laparoscopic gynaecological procedures, were awake postoperatively with less pain and were ambulatory earlier than general anaesthesia patients.[17]

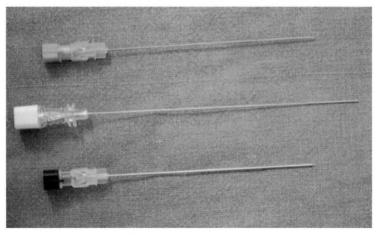

Fig. 10.3: Spinal needles

Vaghadia et al evaluated small dose hypobaric lidocaine (25 mg) in combination with fentanyl (25 µg)[18] for spinal anaesthesia. The patients were seated upright, and spinal anaesthesia was performed at the L_2-L_3 or L_3-L_4 interspace with a 27G Quincke needle. Sensory level upto T6 was obtained. There was no hypotension and the motor and sensory recovery was faster than the group receiving the conventional dose of local anaesthetics. Patient satisfaction was 93 per cent with 90 per cent of patients requesting spinal anaesthesia for laparoscopy in the future.[9] The patients who received selective spinal anaesthesia for outpatient laparoscopy for gynaecological procedures satisfied 'fit to ambulate' criteria at the end of surgery. There was no postural hypotension in these patients because sympathetic recovery occurred before the other modalities.[19]

Lumbar epidural block and small dose selective spinal anaesthesia is a satisfactory anaesthetic technique for outpatient laparoscopic tubal sterilization (Fig. 10.4). Oxygenation during the period of pneumoperitoneum is adequate. The technique results in a shortened postanaesthesia recovery period and fewer postanaesthesia complications compared to general anaesthesia in selected patients.[20,2]

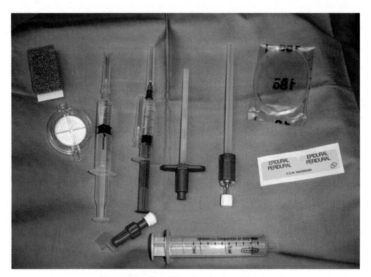

Fig. 10.4: Combined spinal epidural set

Procedures like ovum retrieval for *in vitro* fertilisation (IVF) and gamete intrafallopian transfer are performed under spinal anaesthesia.[21,22] Gynaecological procedures under regional anaesthesia have a high patient and surgeon acceptance with surgical conditions good to excellent.

Topel HC et al performed gasless laparoscopic assisted hysterectomy with epidural anaesthesia. Careful patient selection and attention to technique makes regional anaesthesia safe and viable alternative to general anaesthesia.[23]

Spinal anaesthesia for gynaecological laparoscopy cost the same as general anaesthesia.[24,25]

There are reports in the literature about laparoscopic gynaecological procedures during pregnancy being performed under combined spinal – epidural anaesthesia.[26] More work needs to be done in this field to establish it as a standard procedure.

LAPAROSCOPIC HERNIORRHAPHY

Lower abdominal surgery like endoscopic preperitoneal herniorrhaphy for inguinal hernia can be effectively performed in the supine position under epidural anaesthesia upto a T4 sensory level.[27]

Total extraperitoneal hernia repair (TEP), another approach to inguinal hernia repair which requires extraperitoneal insufflation of gas can be done under regional anaesthesia and sedation.[28,29]

Laparoscopic procedures under regional anaesthesia are safe for patients with severe pulmonary disease. Schmidt et al reported a laparoscopic intraperitoneal onlay polytetrafluoroethylene mesh repair (IPOM) for inguinal hernia under spinal anaesthesia. All patients had severe medical conditions contraindicating general anaesthesia. Hyperbaric bupivacaine (3-3.5 ml) 0.5% was injected at L_2-L_3 interspace with 25 G spinal needle. Segmental level of analgesia upto T_4-T_6 was achieved.[30]

However, Fierro G et al investigated whether laparoscopy was really an advance in the repair of inguinal hernia under regional anaesthesia. In a group of 15 patients; all of them complained of shoulder pain and discomfort which required an intraoperative administration of analgesics in seven patients. Conversion to open repair was needed in one patient. They concluded that although laparoscopy is feasible in repairing inguinal hernia, it is not indicated in high risk patients. Open repair under local anaesthesia is a better option for these patients.[31]

In our experience endoscopic extraperitoneal repair of inguinal hernia can be performed under epidural anaesthesia with sedation. It is safe, has excellent recovery in selected ASA III-IV patients. The procedure has high degree of patient satisfaction.[32]

LAPAROSCOPIC GASTROINTESTINAL SURGERIES

There are very few instances in the literature to show laparoscopic gastrointestinal surgeries being done under neuraxial block. This is probably due to long duration of the procedure and a high thoracic block needed for effective analgesia.

Laparoscopic gastrostomies and jejunostomies can be performed as safely under local anaesthesia with intravenous conscious sedation as under general anaesthesia, and for similar cost. This was seen in a prospective randomized study by Quan-Yang Duh et al. They did not choose regional anaesthesia as an option because it has the disadvantage of not completely relaxing abdominal wall, without the advantage of local anaesthesia with sedation.[33]

Thoracic epidural anaesthesia—analgesia has a significant and favourable impact on dietary tolerance and length of stay after laparoscopic segmental colectomy. Anthony J Senagore et al demonstrated that there is preservation of nutritional status and physical stamina after laparoscopy as compared to open colectomy. Stress reduction through thoracic epidural anaesthesia and analgesia has a favourable impact on the fast-track care plan.[34] There is reduction in the release of catabolic hormones, cortisol and catecholamines and the inflammatory mediators cytokines and arachidonic acid metabolites. Early ambulation maintains muscle strength, limits disruption of orthostatic reflexes, reduces ileus and pulmonary complications. Another benefit of thoracic epidural analgesia is the sparing of lumbar and sacral nerve roots. Absence of lower extremity motor or sensory deficit allows earlier ambulation. There is reduction in the incidence of urinary retention and prolonged catheterisation. There is reduced dosage of local anaesthetic requirement as compared to lumbar administration and hence less hypotension.[35]

A thoracic epidural improves postoperative pulmonary function by reversing diaphragmatic dysfunction after laparotomy and improves forced vital capacity and forced expiratory volumes at 1 second.[36]

A thoracic epidural also reduces myocardial oxygen consumption, pulmonary capillary wedge pressure, pulmonary artery pressure and improves coronory artery perfusion.[37]

LOCAL ANAESTHESIA

Some gynaecological procedures can be performed under local anaesthesia without the disadvantage of general anaesthesia. Peterson et al performed a randomised study to compare laparoscopic tubal ligation with the patient under either general or local anaesthesia. 7.6 per cent patients in the local anaesthetic group required general anaesthesia because of obesity. Hemodynamic stability was greater in the local anaesthetic group. Satisfaction was equal among patients in each group (80%).[38] Local anaesthesia can be used to reduce morbidity in patients under general anaesthesia. The preoperative administration of ketoprofen 100 mg, mesosalpinx infiltration with 5 ml bupivacaine 0.5 per cent peroperatively results in shorter time to discharge, a decrease in parenteral analgesic requirement and a lower incidence of postoperative nausea and vomiting.[39]

Laparoscopic sterilisation can be performed under local anaesthesia with shorter operating time, less discomfort and lower cost.[40] Laparoscopic hernia repair has also been performed under local anaesthesia.[41]

The procedure is technically more challenging when performed under local anaesthesia. Some patients were unable to relax the abdominal muscles because of discomfort from carboperitoneum and some would only tolerate a lower IAP (4-6 mmHg).[33] They require deeper sedation and rarely may be converted to general anaesthesia or open procedure. Clinical conditions and surgeon preference determine whether local anaesthesia can be used since there is no difference in success rate or complications, when compared with general anaesthesia.[40,41]

CONCLUSIONS

While general anaesthesia is recommended for laparoscopic procedures, epidural anaesthesia may be more advantageous because it decreases anaesthesia related respiratory complications, like pneumonia, atelectasis and hypoxaemia in patients at risk for pulmonary complications. There is quicker recovery and less postoperative pain and better cost benefit ratio.

CLINICAL PEARLS

1. Traditional general anaesthesia with controlled ventilation is still the safest technique for certain laparoscopic procedures like laparoscopic fundoplication, and laparoscopic bariatric surgery.
2. Patient co-operation, a skilled laparoscopist, supportive staff, a reduced level of intra-abdominal pressure and low degrees of patient tilt are paramount for the success of laparoscopy under regional anaesthesia.
3. In the future, regional anaesthesia may have an important role to play in laparoscopic surgeries. It would be possible to provide walk in/ walk out regional anaesthesia through the recovery process after ambulatory surgery.[42]
4. Clinical conditions and surgeon preference determine whether local or regional anaesthesia can be used.
5. Epidural anaesthesia – analgesia is an important component of the perioperative care plan in many fast-track programmes.[43]

REFERENCES

1. Frazee RC et al. Open versus laparoscopic cholecystectomy. A comparison of postoperative pulmonary function. Annals of Surgery 1991; 213:651-3.
2. Stewart AVG, Vaghadia H., Collins L. et al. Small-dose selective spinal anaesthesia for short-duration outpatient gynaecological laparoscopy: recovery characteristics compared with propofol anaesthesia. Br J Anaesth 2001; 86(4):570-2.

3. Puri GD, Singh H. Ventilatory effects of laparoscopy under general anaesthesia. Br J Anesth 1992; 68:211.

4. Ciofolo MJ, Clergue F, Seebachea J, et al. Ventilatory effects of laparoscopy under epidural anaesthesia. Anesth Analg 1990; 70(4):357-61.

5. Diamant M, Benumof JL, Saidman LJ, et al: Laparoscopic sterilization with local anaesthesia: Complications and blood gas changes. Anesth Analg 1977; 56:335.

6. Brampton WJ, Watson RJ. Arterial to end tidal carbon dioxide tension difference during laparoscopy: Magnitude and effect of anaesthetic technique. Anaesthesia 1990; 45:210.

7. Sood J, Kumra VP. Anaesthesia for laparoscopic surgery- A review. Indian J Surg 2003; 65(3):232-40.

8. Brady CE 3rd, Harkleroad LE, Pierson WP. Alteration in oxygen saturation and ventilation after intravenous sedation for peritoneoscopy. Arch Intern Med 1989; 149:1029-32.

9. Vaghadia H, Mcleod DH, Mitchell GW. Small-dose hypobaric lidocaine – fentanyl spinal anaesthesia for short duration outpatient laparoscopy, I. A randomized comparison with conventional dose hyperbaric lidocaine. Anesth Analg 1997;84:59.

10. Joris JL. Anaesthesia for laparoscopic surgery. R.D. Miller (ed) In: Text Book of Anaesthesia. 6th edn. Churchill Livingstone. 2005 Chapter 57, pp 2298, Vol 2.

11. Marco AP, Yeo CJ, Rock P. Anaesthesia for a patient undergoing laparoscopic cholecystectomy. Anaesthesiology 1990; 73: 1268-70.

12. Luchetti M, Palonba R, Sica G, Massa G, et al. Effectiveness and safety of combined epidural and general anaesthesia for laparoscopic cholecystectomy. Reg Anesth 1996; 21(5):465-9.

13. Georgiou L, Bousoula M, Spetsaki M. Combined thoracic epidural laryngeal mask airway for laparoscopic cholecystectomy in a patient with myasthenia gravis. Anaesthesia. 2000; 55:821-2.

14. Gramatica L Jr, Brasesio OE, Luna AM, et al. Laparoscopic cholecystectomy performed under regional anaesthesia in patients with chronic obstructive pulmonary disease. Surg Endosc 2002; 16:472-5.

15. Menes T, Spivak H. Searching for the proper insufflation gas. Surg Endosc 2000; 14:1050-6.

16. Viskari D, Berrill A, Vaghadia H: Walkin / Walk-out spinal anaesthesia for outpatient laparoscopy: Evaluation of three hypobaric solutions. Can J Anaesth 1997; 44:A26-B.

17. Lennox PH, Vaghadia H, Martin L. Small dose selective spinal anaesthesia for short duration outpatient laparoscopy: Recovery characteristics compared with desflurane anaesthesia. Anesth Analg 2002; 94:346-50.

18. Chilvers CR, Vaghadia H, Mitchell GW, et al: Small-dose hypobaric lidocaine –fentanyl spinal anaesthesia for short duration outpatient laparoscopy, II. Optinal fentanyl dose. Anesth Analg 1997; 84:65.

19. Vaghadia H, Solylo MA, Henderson CL et al. Selective spinal anaesthesia for outpatient laparoscopy. II: Epinephrine and spinal cord function. Can J Anesth 2001; 48:3, 261-6.

20. Bridenbaugh LD, Soderstrom RM. Lumbar epidural block anaesthesia for outpatient laparoscopy. J Reprod Med 1979; 23(2): 85-6.

21. Silva PD, Kang SB, Sloane KA. Gamete intrafallopian transfer with spinal anaesthesia. Fertil Steril 1993; 59(4): 841-3. (abstract)

22. Endler G, Magyar DM, Hayes MF, et al. Use of spinal anaesthesia in laparoscopy for *in vitro* fertilization. Fertil Steril 1985; 43(5): 809-10. (abstract)

23. Topel HC. Gasless laparoscopic assisted hysterectomy with epidural anaesthesia. J Am Assoc Gynecol Laparosc 1994; 1(4, Part 2): S36.

24. Chilvers CR, Goodwin Alison, Vaghadia Himat et al. Selective spinal anaesthesia for outpatient laproscopy. V: Pharmacoeconomic comparison vs general anaesthesia. Can J Anesth 2001; 48(3):279-83.

25. Hubler M, Litz RJ, Albrecht OM. Combination of balanced and regional anaesthesia for minimally invasive surgery in a patient with myasthenia gravis. Eur J Anaesthesiol 2000; 17:325-8.

26. Pelosi MA. Gasless laparoscopy under epidural anaesthesia during pregnancy. J Am Assoc Gynecol Laparosc 1995; 2(4, suppl): 575. (abstract)

27. Azurin DJ, Leslie SG, Jason C.Cwik et al. The efficacy of epidural anaesthesia for endoscopic preperitoneal herniorrhaphy: A perspective study. Journal of Laparoendoscopic Surgery 1996; 6(6):369-73.

28. Spivak H, Nodelman I, FucoV. Laparoscopic extraperitoneal inguinal hernia repair with spinal anaesthesia and nitrous oxide insufflation. Surg Endosc 1999; 10:1026.

29. Sood J. Anaesthesia for Endohernia Repair. Book of Endoscopic Repair of Abdominal Wall Hernias. Pradeep Chowbey (ed). 2004; Chapter 8, pp. 66-75.

30. Schmidt J, Carbajo MA, Lampert R, Zirngibl H, et al. Laparoscopic intraperitoneal onlay polytetrafluoroethylene mesh repair (IPOM) for inguinal hernia during spinal anaesthesia in patients with severe medical conditions. Surgical laparoscopy Endoscopy and Percutaneous techniques 2001;11(1):34-7.

31. Fierro G, Sanfilippo M, D'Andrea V, Biancari F, Zema M, Vilardi V. Transabdominal preperitoneal laparoscopic inguinal herniorrhaphy (TPLIH) under regional anaesthesia. Int Surg 1997; 82(2):205-7.

32. Chowbey PK, Sood J, Vashistha A, et al. Extraperitoneal endoscopic groin hernia repair under epidural anaesthesia. Surgical laparoscopy, endoscopy and percutaneous techniques 2003; 13(3):185-90.

33. Quan-Yang Duh, Andrea L, Senokoz L, et al. Laparoscopic Gastrostomy and jejunostomy safety and cost with local vs general anaesthesia. Arch Surg. 1999; 134:151-6.

34. Senagore AJ, Whalley D, Delancy CP, et al. Epidural anaesthesia – analgesia shortens length of stay after laparoscopic segmental colectomy for benign pathology. Surgery 129(6): 672-6.

35. Senagore AJ, Delaney CP, Mekhail N, et al. Randomized clinical trial comparing epidural anaesthesia and patient – controlled analgesia after laparoscopic segmental colectomy. Br J Surg 2003; 90:1195-9.

36. Benhamaov D, Sanni K, Noviant Y. Effect of analgesia on respiratory function after upper abdominal surgery. Acta Anaesthesiol Scand 1983; 27:22-5.

37. Neudeiker J, Schwenk W, Junghans T, Pietsch S et al. Randomized controlled trial to examine the influence of thoracic epidural analgesia as postoperative ileus after laparoscopic sigmoid resection. Br J Surg 1999; 86:1292-5.

38. Peterson HB, Hulka JF, Spielman FJ. Local versus general anaesthesia for laparoscopic sterilization: A randomized study. Obstet Gynecol 1987; 70:903.

39. Van EE R, Hemrika DJ, De Blok S. Effect of Ketoprofen and mesosalpinx infiltration on postoperative pain after laproscopic sterilization. Obstet Gynecol 1996; 88:568.

40. Bordahl PE, Raeder JC, Nordentoft J et al. Laparoscopic sterilization under local or general anaesthesia? A randomized study. Obstet Gynecol 1993; 81:137-41.

41. Pendurthi TK, De Moria EJ, Kellum JM. Laparoscopic bilateral inguinal hernia repair under local anaesthesia. Surg Endosc 1995; 9:197-99.

42. Vaghadia H. Spinal anaesthesia for outpatients: controversies and new techniques. Can J Anesth 1998; 45:64.

43. Bardram L, Funch-Jeusen D, Jevsen P, Crawford ME, et al. Recovery after laparoscopic colonic surgery with epidural analgesia, and early oral nutrition and mobilization. Lancet 1995; 345:763-4.

Use of LMA and PLMA in Laparoscopic and Extraperitoneal Endoscopic Surgery

CHAPTER 11

INTRODUCTION

Laparoscopic surgery is a sophisticated technique requiring a highly skilled and experienced anaesthesiologist and surgeon as it introduces some trespasses on the respiratory and cardiovascular system of the patient. The laparoscopic procedures have become increasingly popular over the last decade because of small incisions, reduced postoperative pain, early ambulation, and shortened hospital stay. They are often being performed on an outpatient basis or require only an overnight admission thus demanding extreme caution in the anaesthetic technique. Paradoxically, the popularity of laparoscopic and endoscopic procedures has been matched by the increasing use of the LMA as an airway device since its commercial introduction in 1988.[1]

PHYSIOLOGIC CHANGES DURING LAPAROSCOPIC AND EXTRAPERITONEAL ENDOSCOPIC SURGERY

The physiological changes seen during laparoscopic procedures are due to:
a. Carbon-dioxide insufflation, intraperitoneal or extraperitoneal, with resultant raised intra-abdominal pressure following intraperitoneal insufflation of carbon-dioxide
b. Alteration in patient position

The raised intra-abdominal pressure especially with head down position may be accompanied with the potential danger of regurgitation and pulmonary aspiration. Therefore, it is of utmost importance for the anaesthesiologist to ensure a patent airway which allows adequate ventilation and provides protection against pulmonary aspiration.

PULMONARY MECHANICS IN LAPAROSCOPIC SURGERY

The creation of carboperitoneum results in primary changes in pulmonary physiology. These are mostly mechanical and to a lesser extent arise due to changes in patient position. Peritoneal insufflation produces an increase in intra-abdominal volume and pressure, both of which impede diaphragmatic excursion. Therefore, due to increase of both elastance and resistance of the respiratory system,[2] abdominal insufflation with carbon dioxide raises the peak airway pressure. The decrease in functional residual capacity and the increase in elastic and resistive loads of the respiratory system were described both during abdominal insufflation with carbon dioxide and in obesity.

As a result, peak airway pressures increased [3] whereas pulmonary compliance[4,5] and vital capacity decreased.[6] Use of Trendelenburg position seemed to have little added effect and did not appear to exacerbate the rise in airway pressures.[7]

The increase in intraperitoneal volume can displace the abdominal contents into the thoracic cavity, compressing basilar segments. Physiologically, this is manifested as reduction in functional residual capacity, alveolar dead space and resultant V/Q mismatch.[4] This probably accounts for the relative hypoxemia seen in patients allowed to breathe spontaneously during laparoscopic procedures. The increase in intra-abdominal pressure is also translated across the diaphragm, causing a smaller, but proportionate rise in intrathoracic pressure [3,7] which may be worsened by the use of the Trendelenburg position. [7] The increase in intra-abdominal pressure may exacerbate gastro-oesophageal reflux in predisposed patients, placing them at risk of aspiration if the airway is left unprotected.

Carboperitoneum results in the absorption of carbon dioxide across the peritoneum, and therefore the anaesthetic technique should include controlled hyperventilation. It is desirable to use an automatic lung ventilator capable of compensating for the fall in compliance which occurs following the production of the carboperitoneum. It is essential to monitor the intra-abdominal pressure throughout the procedure which should not exceed 20 mm Hg. Thus although laparoscopy offers advantages to both the patient and the surgeon, it involves considerable alteration in respiratory and cardiovascular homeostasis, and should not be considered a minor procedure.[8]

AIRWAY MANAGEMENT FOR LAPAROSCOPIC SURGERY (FIG. 11.1)

General anaesthesia with tracheal intubation and controlled ventilation is recommended for laparoscopic procedures as it takes care of the raised intra-abdominal pressure as well as it prevents pulmonary aspiration of regurgitated gastric contents.

Although in modern anaesthetic practice, tracheal intubation is an essential component and has become synonymous with safety, it can have serious consequences in the event of unrecognized oesophageal intubation.[9]

There are certain disadvantages of a tracheal tube (TT):

1. Increased pressor response to insertion
2. Increased pharyngolaryngeal morbidity

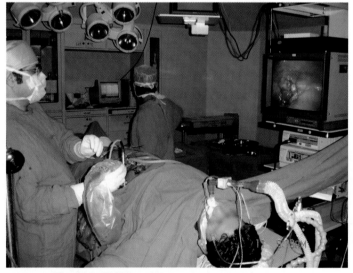

Fig. 11.1: PLMA and laparoscopic appendecectomy

3. Failed intubation in difficult airway
4. Increased anaesthetic and analgesia requirement
5. Endobronchial intubation due to carboperitoneum during laparoscopic surgery.[10]

LMA-FAMILY (FIG. 11.2)

It has been more than 20 years since Dr. Archie Brain in the United Kingdom introduced the first supraglottic airway device the laryngeal mask airway (LMA).[1] Dr Archie Brain designed the LMA as "an alternative to either the endotracheal tube (ETT) or the face mask for use with either spontaneous or positive pressure ventilation."[1] Subsequently the LMA has challenged the assumption that tracheal intubation is the only acceptable way to maintain a clear airway and provide positive pressure ventilation.

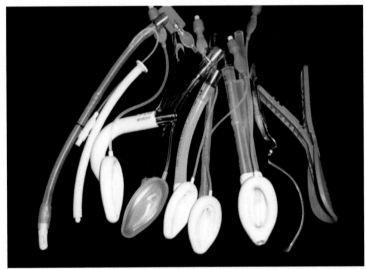

Fig. 11.2: LMA family

Many new supraglottic airway devices have been introduced and include airways with and without sealing characteristics. Presently there are about 17 sealing supraglottic airways that can be classified depending on their main sealing mechanisms: cuffed perilaryngeal sealers, cuffed pharyngeal sealers, and cuffless anatomically preshaped sealers. These can be further subdivided into two main groups:

a. Single-use versus reusable
b. Ability to protect from aspiration of gastric contents.[11]

The LMA family of airway devices includes classic LMA (cLMA), flexible LMA, the intubating LMA (ILMA), the disposable LMA (LMA Unique), the ProSeal LMA and finally the LMA C Trach. Successful use of the LMA does not require the constellation of factors required for direct laryngoscopy and tracheal intubation. Consequently, it can provide an airway in both the "cannot intubate – can ventilate" and the "cannot intubate – cannot ventilate" situations if the problem is supraglottic in nature.[12-14] The *ILMA* is available in adult sizes only (3, 4, 5) and is especially designed for blind tracheal intubation. The disposable *LMA (Unique)* is made of clear medical grade polyvinyl chloride and is supplied sterile. It is used for single use in field or out of box situations. It is available in sizes similar to the classic LMA. The ProSeal Laryngeal Mask Airway *(PLMA)* is a modified version of LMA. Its cuff forms a more effective seal around the glottis than the LMA. The drain tube provides a bypass channel for regurgitated gastric contents and helps in detecting malpositions of the mask. LMA C Trach is a modified ILMA with integrated fibreoptics. The LMA has several advantages and disadvantages over a tracheal tube.

Advantages over ETT

The placement is easier and quicker than tracheal intubation. There is less cardiovascular stimulation, less change in intraocular pressure during insertion and emergence. There is lower frequency of cough and higher oxygen saturation during emergence.[15] Spontaneous ventilation is easier due to a reduced work of breathing. [16,17] Positive pressure ventilation can be performed without muscle relaxation due to better tolerance.[18] The risk of pulmonary infection may be reduced due to non-interference with pulmonary airway resistance[19] and ciliary motility.[20] There is also decreased pharyngolaryngeal morbidity. Incidence of voice abnormalities may be reduced as the vocal cords are not penetrated and mucosal pressures are lower.[21]

Disadvantages

Air leak is likely at airway pressure exceeding 15 to 20 cm H_2O therefore gastric insufflation and gastric reflux are more likely to occur with the result that airway is less effectively protected from pulmonary aspiration. Incidence of aspiration with the LMA in fasted patients is 0.012 per cent.[22]

CLASSIC LMA, FLEXIBLE LMA, LMA UNIQUE (FIG. 11.3)

The LMA provides "hands- free" anaesthesia. The safety record is good for elective surgery. The cLMA represents the salient features of this group. In all these variants of the LMA, the glottic seal is usually lost at peak airway pressures above 20 cm H_2O. Positive pressure ventilation is readily accomplished with the cLMA[15] and the correctly positioned cLMA offers some protection against aspiration.[23]

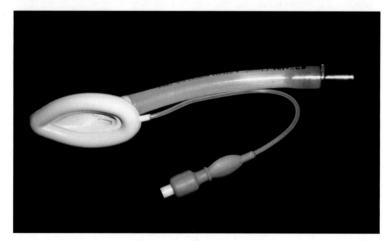

Fig. 11.3: Classic LMA

THE INTUBATING LMA AND LMA CTRACH

The intubating LMA (ILMA) is used as a guide to tracheal intubation and is unsuitable for prolonged procedures because of high pressures exerted against the mucosa.[24] The ILMA has been used for routine intubation, rescue intubation, and intubation of the difficult airway patient after the induction of anesthesia or in the awake state.[25] The ILMA is uniquely suited to the unanticipated "cannot intubate or cannot intubate/cannot ventilate" scenario because of its anatomic shape.[25] LMA C Trach is a modified ILMA with integrated fibreoptics to allow real time visualization of cord structures at time of intubation of the trachea.

THE PROSEAL LMA (PLMA) (FIGS 11.4 TO 11.6)

The ProSeal LMA (PLMA), a new airway device has been in use since 2000 only. It is made from medical grade silicone and has the following new or modified features. The cuff of PLMA has a flat dorsal component designed to press the ventral elliptical cuff more firmly into the periglottic tissues and a wedge shaped proximal component designed to plug gaps in the proximal pharynx. The laryngeal cuff of the PLMA is made of softer silicone than that of the cLMA. It covers the posterior aspect of the bowl of the mask and presses the bowl forwards when inflated. Increased depth of the bowl is designed to improve the seal with the larynx. The ability of the PLMA to protect the airway during regurgitation depends on:
- Correct alignment of the drain tube with the oesophageal sphincter.
- Efficacy of the seal of the distal cuff with the hypopharynx.
- Pressure of regurgitated fluid.

The ProSeal LMA extends the range of surgical procedures for which LMA devices can be used, further encroaching into the domain of the endotracheal tube. It has been used for laparoscopic surgery.[26-33]

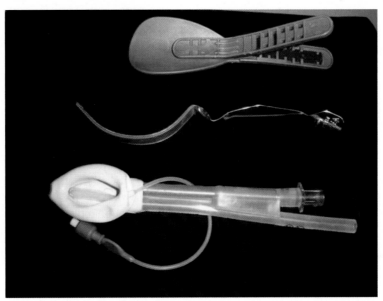

Fig. 11.4: ProSeal LMA

Advantages of PLMA over cLMA

The PLMA offers several advantages over the cLMA:
1. It forms a more effective seal with the respiratory tract (10 cm H_2O higher) and is therefore a better ventilatory device.[34]
2. It forms a more effective seal with the gastrointestinal tract (30 cm H_2O higher) and therefore provides better protection against aspiration and gastric insufflation.[35]
3. It provides easy access to the gastrointestinal tract allowing the passage of a gastric tube, which further reduces the risk of aspiration and gastric insufflation. The passage of a temperature probe through the drain tube facilitates core temperature measurement.[36]

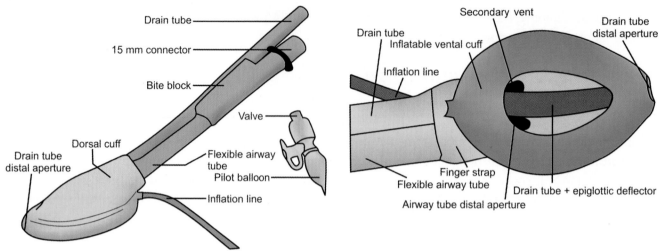

Fig. 11.5: PLMA dorsal view   **Fig. 11.6:** PLMA ventral view

4. It exerts lower pressures against the surrounding mucosa for a given seal pressure, which reduces the risk of mucosal ischemic injury.[37]

5. It provides information about its position in the pharynx, making malpositions with all of its accompanying problems less likely.

6. If a gastric tube is left in situ it can be used to reinsert the PLMA in case of its displacement. [38]

Disadvantages of the PLMA Over the cLMA

The two main disadvantages of the PLMA over the cLMA are that the first time insertion rate is less than cLMA and the airway tube has a narrower bore, making it less suitable for prolonged anaesthesia and less useful as an airway intubator.

ROLE OF LMA AND PLMA IN LAPAROSCOPIC SURGERY

Laparoscopic surgery is evolving and is not only limited to minor gynaecologic surgery or cholecystectomy but has extended to procedures such as appendecectomy, hernia repairs (inguinal, epigastric and incisional), advanced gastrointestinal, urologic and major gynaecologic procedures. The LMA and its variants have been used for laparoscopic surgery in the following situations:

A. Sole airway device.
B. Difficult airway.
C. Failed intubation.
D. Coexisting disease.

SOLE AIRWAY DEVICE[39-46, 26-33]

These extraglottic devices are being used as sole airway devices, for adult as well as paediatric patients [39-43] in varying positions including supine, lateral, lithotomy, extended lithotomy, Trendelenburg, reverse Trendelenburg and prone. They were used initially for short, diagnostic gynaecologic procedures, but now are being used in areas previously thought unheard of. It has been used in children for laparoscopic investigations.[43] Two studies involving the use of PLMA in adults [26,27] showed that the mean (range) success rate was 98 per cent (93-100) and the mean (range) incidence of oropharyngeal and gastric leaks was 4 per cent (0-20) and 1 per cent (0-7), respectively. The peak airway pressures (PIP) increase by 50-100 per cent during carboperitoneum using the classic LMA.[40, 44] The PLMA has been reported superior to the classic LMA in terms of ventilation and gastric insufflation [26] and the ProSeal LMA similar to the TT in terms of ventilation and gastric insufflation in non-obese patients, but has a 12 per cent failure rate in obese patients (>30 kg/m^2).[27]

Patients undergoing laparoscopy might be considered to be at risk of developing the acid aspiration syndrome.[45,46] However, the increased intra-abdominal pressure results in increase in the tone of the lower oesophageal sphincter, which allows maintenance of the pressure gradient across the gastro- oesophageal junction, and which might therefore reduce the risk of regurgitation.[47] These devices have successfully been used for the following laparoscopic procedures by providing adequate ventilation and controlling hypercarbia:

1. Gynaecologic laparoscopy.[28,31-33]
2. General surgical
   a. Laparoscopic cholecystectomy[28-30]
   b. Laparoscopic appendecectomy [28]
   c. Abdominal wall herniorraphy [28]
   d. Colectomy.
3. Others:
   a. Urologic e.g. laparoscopic pyelolithotomy and nephrectomy
   b. Antireflux
   c. Paediatric.

The most common procedures being performed are:

Gynaecologic Laparoscopy

The use of the LMA for gynaecologic laparoscopy was first reported by Brain in 1983.[1] The cLMA, though popular in short gynaecologic laparoscopic procedures, does not offer protection to the trachea against aspiration of regurgitated material.[12] Akhtar et al in 1994, found that up to 40 per cent of UK consultants used the LMA for gynaecologic laparoscopy.[48] Dingley and Asai, in 1996, reported that 23 per cent of consultants and 34 per cent of non-consultants in the UK used the LMA during laparoscopic clip sterilization.[49] Crilly and McLeod, in 2000, found that 20 per cent of Australian anaesthesiologists would use the LMA for laparoscopic sterilization.[50]

Maltby JR et al in a study of 209 females for gynaecologic laparoscopy, found that the ProSeal LMA, cLMA and the endotracheal tube provided equally effective ventilation without clinically important gastric insufflation in non-obese and obese patients. [31] Sharma et al reported the use of PLMA for advanced laparoscopic procedures such as total laparoscopic hysterectomy, laparoscopic assisted vaginal hysterectomy, and ovarian cystectomies.[28] Roth H et al compared the ProSeal laryngeal mask airway and the laryngeal tube suction (LTS) for ventilation in gynaecologic patients undergoing laparoscopic surgery in a study of 25 patients in each group. Both devices were found to provide a secure airway even under conditions of elevated intra-abdominal pressure. In this pilot study, no differences concerning handling or quality of airway seal were detected between PLMA and LTS.[33]

In another prospective, randomized study by Piper et al[32] comprising 104 patients, allocated randomly to two groups: the ProSeal-laryngeal mask versus endotracheal tube, the patients underwent gynaecologic laparoscopic surgery. The use of PLMA was reported as a convenient and practicable approach for anaesthesia in patients undergoing laparoscopic surgery.[32]

Laparoscopic Cholecystectomy

Laparoscopic cholecystectomy is one of the most commonly performed general surgical procedures.[51] Lu et al in a study of 80 adults, found that the ProSeal and cLMA provided adequate ventilation before carboperitoneum, but ventilation was inadequate or failed after carboperitoneum in 20 per cent with classic LMA but none with the ProSeal LMA.[26] Maltby et al in a study of 109 adults, found that the ProSeal LMA and tracheal tube provided equally effective ventilation without clinically important gastric insufflation in non-obese patients, but the ProSeal LMA failed in 12 per cent of obese patients (>30 Kg/m^2) because of respiratory obstruction or air leak.[27] These data suggest that the ProSeal is effective for laparoscopic cholecystectomy in non-obese patients.[49] Chatterjee et al reported the successful resuscitation of a near fatal cardiac dysrrthymia in a case of laparoscopic cholecystectomy where the PLMA was used as a sole airway device for laparoscopic cholecystectomy.[52]

Other Procedures

The PLMA has been used for antireflux surgery such as laparoscopic fundoplication, laparoscopic colectomy, laparoscopic renal cyst excision, nephrectomy and some short paediatric laparoscopic procedures at our institution (unpublished data).

DIFFICULT AIRWAY

Perhaps the greatest contribution of the LMA is its use to allow ventilation and intubation in situations where a tracheal tube cannot be placed with conventional techniques.[53] The PLMA with its bougie guided insertion technique has a role in patients who are at risk of aspiration or require controlled ventilation.[54]

The author has used it for difficult airway in both laparoscopic and non-laparoscopic surgery (abdominal hysterectomy in a patient with Cormack and Lehane grade IV). It was used successfully for a patient with ankylosing spondylitis who underwent laparoscopic cholecystectomy (unpublished data).

FAILED INTUBATION

Problems with tracheal intubation were the most frequent causes of anaesthetic deaths in the published analyses of records of the UK medical defence societies.[55,56] The laryngeal mask airway is included in the algorithm for unexpected failed intubation published and promoted by the airway societies of the US and Canada.[13, 57] The PLMA has been reported as a rescue device after failed intubation during rapid-sequence induction.[58]

COEXISTING DISEASE

The PLMA and cLMA are suitable for patients with coexisting diseases. These devices may be used in patients with bronchial asthma, chronic obstructive pulmonary disease or obesity provided high inflation airway pressures are not needed for ventilation.[59] However PLMA is superior to cLMA since the improved seal allows its use in patients with diseases that cause a reduction in pulmonary compliance and the drain tube allows its use in patients with some increased risk of regurgitation. The PLMA has been successfully used in obese patients as a temporary airway prior to tracheal intubation, for gynaecologic laparoscopy and for laparoscopic cholecystectomy. There are few studies of LMA use in obese and morbidly obese patients. The PLMA seems better suited than the cLMA for such patients. They are more likely to have reduced thoracic compliance, increased inspiratory resistance[60] and are commonly believed to be at greater risk of regurgitation. Natalini et al in a 2003 study of 60 patients

(BMI>30 kg/m²) ventilated at 7 ml/kg tidal-volume with positive end expiratory pressure of 10 cm of H_2O reported adequate ventilation in all patients.[29] Keller et al determined the efficacy of the laryngeal mask airway ProSeal™ as a temporary ventilatory device in morbidly obese patients (body mass index 35–60 kg/m²) before laryngoscope-guided tracheal intubation.[61] The laryngeal mask airway ProSeal™ is an effective temporary ventilatory device in grossly and morbidly obese patients before laryngoscope-guided tracheal intubation scheduled for elective surgery.

The release of catecholamines in plasma has been incriminated in the development of abnormal cardiovascular responses to laryngoscopy and ETT intubation. This response may be altered with the use of PLMA or LMA due to diminished catecholamine release as suggested by Lamb K et al[62] as the PLMA is relatively simple and atraumatic to insert and does not require laryngoscopy.[63,28]

The ProSeal LMA causes decreased pressor response to insertion and lesser amounts of anaesthetic agents are needed with its use and has been successfully used in high risk cases with hypertension, coronary artery disease, post renal transplant patients, cardiomyopathy and myopathy in our institution (unpublished data).

DESIRABLE MONITORING DURING LAPAROSCOPIC SURGERY WITH LMA AS AN AIRWAY

The measurement of the oropharyngeal leak pressure or the seal pressure is of vital importance since it quantifies the efficacy of the seal with the airway and is checked for the LMA and its variants.[1,59] The value of the oropharyngeal leak pressure serves as an indicator about the safety and the feasibility of positive pressure ventilation. It is lower in LMA as compared to an endotracheal tube and therefore, gastric insufflation, reflux and pulmonary aspiration cannot be ruled out with a cLMA. Therefore, in addition to the standard monitoring (pulse, NIBP, ECG, $EtCO_2$, SpO_2, IAP) for any laparoscopic surgery the following parameters need to be strictly monitored when LMA is being used for laparoscopic surgery.

1. Oropharyngeal leak pressure.
2. Neck and/or epigastric auscultation to rule out gastric insufflation.
3. Peak inspiratory pressure (PIP).
4. Fixation of device.
5. Intermittent gastric aspiration during prolonged surgery.
6. Intracuff pressure.

COMPLICATIONS

With appropriate selection of patients, proper anaesthetic technique, training, and periodic examination of equipment, problems arising from LMA use are rare. Reported problems include airway morbidity, pharyngolaryngeal discomfort and compression of the surrounding structures. The use of LMA with positive pressure ventilation may cause gastric insufflation in the event of malposition of the mask or in case the inspiratory pressure exceeds 20 cm H_2O.[64-66]

Gastric insufflation may precipitate oesophageal and pharyngeal regurgitation and pulmonary aspiration of gastric or pharyngeal contents. There may be compression of vessels, ducts and nerves in the surrounding area.

CONCLUSION

Controversy remains over the use of LMA for laparoscopic surgery. Most anaesthesiologists, including the author definitely have more experience and confidence in tracheal intubation. The PLMA is emerging as an effective alternative to tracheal intubation, its applications and safety are still being evaluated. However, it should not be taken as a substitute for a tracheal tube. It is controversial which supraglottic airway is the most appropriate for airway control for laparoscopy surgery.

We suggest that the experienced anaesthesiologists use the PLMA and correct position of the device must be ensured before embarking on the surgical procedure. There should be no hesitation in using an alternative device in case there is a problem regarding adequate ventilation or oxygenation. It has a special role in patients with difficult intubation coming for elective surgery where its use will avoid unnecessary trauma to the airway.

CLINICAL PEARLS

1. The ProSeal LMA is the best available LMA which is suitable for laparoscopic surgery. It must be perfectly positioned and have a good seal. A gastric tube should be inserted via the drain tube and left for free drainage.

2. A relaxant technique would be required to provide positive pressure ventilation during laparoscopic surgery. Patients should be paralyzed and ventilated to provide optimal surgical conditions. Use tidal-volumes of approximately 8-12 ml/kg.

3. Maintain peak inspiratory pressures within the maximum airway seal pressure, on average, 30 cm H_2O or less with the PLMA and 20 cm H_2O or less with the other LMAs™.

4. Control end-tidal CO_2 by altering respiratory rate.

5. Leaks during PPV may be attributable to light anesthesia, inadequate muscle relaxant, use of too small an LMA™ airway, a reduction in lung compliance related to the surgical or diagnostic procedure, patient factors or displacement of the LMA™ by head turning or traction.

6. During the recovery period, reverse the effects of the muscle relaxant or allow it to wear off before switching off the anaesthetic agents at the end of the procedure. With gentle, assisted ventilation, the patient should be allowed to start breathing.

REFERENCES

1. Brain AIJ. The laryngeal mask—A new concept in airway management. Br J Anaesth 1983; 55: 801–805.
2. Pelosi P, Foti G, Cereda M, Vicardi P and Gattinoni L. Effects of carbon dioxide insufflation for laparoscopic cholecystectomy on the respiratory system. Anaesthesia 1996; 51: 744-49.
3. Smith I, Benzie RJ, Gordon NLM, Kelman GR, Swapp GH. Cardiovascular effects of peritoneal insufflation of carbon dioxide for laparoscopy. BMJ 1971; 3: 410-11.
4. Puri GD, Singh H. Ventilatory effects of laparoscopy under general Anaesthesia. Br J Anaesth 1992; 68: 211-13.
5. Johannsen G, Ndersen M, Juhl B. The effect of general anaesthesia on the haemodynamic events during laparoscopy with CO_2-insufflation, Acta Anaesthesiol Scand 1989; 33: 132-36.
6. Brown DR, Fishburne JI, Roberson VO, Hulka JF. Ventilatory and blood gas changes during laparoscopy with local anesthesia. Am J Obstet Gynecol 1976; 124: 741-45.
7. Kelman GR, Swapp GH, Smith I, Benzie RJ, Gordon NLM. Cardiac output and arterial blood-gas tension during laparoscopy. Br J Anaesth 1972; 44: 1155-61.
8. Hodgson C, McClelland RMA, Newton JR. Some effects of the peritoneal insufflation of carbon dioxide at laparoscopy. Anaesthesia 1970; 25: 382-90.
9. Scott DB. Endotracheal intubation: Friend or foe (editorial). Br Med J 1986; 292: 157-58.
10. Chen P, Chiu P: Endobronchial intubation during laparoscopic cholecystectomy. Anaesth intensive care 1992; 20: 537.
11. Miller Donald M. A proposed classification and scoring system for supraglottic sealing airways: A Brief Review. Anesth Analg 2004; 99: 1553-59.

12. Brimacombe J, Brain AIJ, Berry A. The laryngeal mask airway: Review and Practical guide. London: WB Saunders, 1997.
13. Benumof J L. The laryngeal mask airway and the ASA difficult airway algorithm. Anesthesiology 1996; 84: 686-99.
14. Sood. J. Laryngeal Mask Airway and its Variants. Indian J Anaesth 2005; 49(4): 275-80.
15. Brimacombe J. The advantages of the LMA over the tracheal tube or facemask: A meta-analysis. Can J Anesth 1995; 42: 1017-23.
16. Joshi GP, Morrison SG, White PF, et al. Work of breathing in anesthetized patients: Laryngeal mask airway versus tracheal tube. J Clin Anesth 1998; 10: 268-71.
17. Faberowski, LW and Banner, MJ. Laryngeal mask airways (LMA) impose significantly less work of breathing compared to endotracheal tubes (ETT) for spontaneously breathing pediatric patients. Anesth and Analg 86, 1998; S398. (Abstract).
18. Wilkins CJ, Cramp PG, Staples J, Stevens WC. Comparison of the anesthetic requirement for tolerance of laryngeal mask airway and endotracheal tube. Anesth Analg 1992; 75: 794-97.
19. Berry A, Brimacombe J, Keller C, Verghese C. Pulmonary airway resistance with the endotracheal tube versus laryngeal mask airway in paralyzed anesthetized adult patients. Anesthesiology 1990; 90: 295-97.
20. Keller C, Brimacombe JR. Bronchial mucus transport velocity in paralyzed anesthetized patients: a comparison of the laryngeal mask airway and cuffed tracheal tube. Anesth Analg 1998; 86: 1280-82.
21. Joshi GP, Inagaki Y, White PF, et al. Use of the laryngeal mask airway as an alternative to the tracheal tube during ambulatory anesthesia. Anesth Analg 1997; 85: 573-77.
22. Brimacombe J, Berry A. The incidence of aspiration associated with the laryngeal mask airway: A meta-analysis of published literature. J Clin Anesth 1995; 7: 297-305.
23. Keller C, Brimacombe J, Raedler C, Puehringer F. Do laryngeal mask airway devices attenuate liquid flow between the esophagus and pharynx? A randomized, controller cadaver study. Anesth Analg 1999; 88: 904-7.
24. Keller C, Brimacombe J. Pharyngeal mucosal pressures, airway sealing pressures and fiberoptic position with the intubating versus the standard laryngeal mask airway. Anesthesiology 1999; 90: 1001-6.
25. Ferson DZ, Rosenblatt WH, Johansen MJ, et al: Use of the intubating LMA-Fastrach in 254 patients with difficult-to-manage airways. Anesthesiology 2001; 95:1175–81.
26. Lu PP, Brimacombe J, Yang C, Shyr M. ProSeal *versus* the classic laryngeal mask airway for positive pressure ventilation during laparoscopic cholecystectomy. Br J Anaesth 2002; 88: 824–27.
27. Maltby JR, Beriault MT, Watson NC, Liepert D, Fick GH. The LMA-ProSeal™ is an effective alternative to tracheal intubation for laparoscopic cholecystectomy. Can J Anesth 2002; 49: 857-62.
28. Sharma B, Sahai C, Bhattacharya A, Kumra V.P., Sood J. ProSeal laryngeal mask airway: A study of 100 consecutive cases of laparoscopic surgery. Indian J Anaesth 2003; 47 (6): 467-72.
29. Natalini G, Lanza G, Rosano A, Dell'Agnolo P, Bernardini A. Standard Laryngeal Mask Airway and LMA-ProSeal during laparoscopic surgery. J Clin Anesth. 2003; 15(6):428-32.
30. Garcia-Aguado R,Vivo BenllochM, Zaragoza Fernandez C, Garcia Solbes JM. Proseal Laryngeal Mask for Laproscopic Cholecystectomy. Rev Esp Anestesiol Reanim. 2003; 50 (1): 55-7.
31. Maltby JR, Beriault M,Watson NC, Liepert D, Fick GH. LMA-Classic™ and LMA-ProSeal™ are effective alternatives to endotracheal intubation for gynecological laparoscopy. Can J Anesth 2003; 50:71-7.
32. Piper SN, Triem JG, Rohm KD, Maleck WH, Schollhorn TA, Boldt J. ProSeal-laryngeal mask versus endotracheal intubation in patients undergoing gynaecologic laparoscopy. Anasthesiol Intensivmed Notfallmed Schmerzther. 2004;39 (3):132-37.
33. Roth H, Genzwuerker HV, Rothhaas A, Finteis T, Schmeck J.The ProSeal laryngeal mask airway and the laryngeal tube Suction for ventilation in gynaecological patients undergoing laparoscopic surgery. Eur J Anaesthesiol. 2005; 22(2): 117-22.
34. Brimacombe J, Keller C. The ProSeal laryngeal mask airway. A randomized, crossover study with the standard laryngeal mask airway in paralyzed, anesthetized patients. Anesthesiology 2000; 93: 104-9.
35. Keller C, Brimacombe J, Kleinsasser A, Loeckinger A. Does the ProSeal laryngeal mask airway prevent aspiration of regurgitated fluid? Anesth Analg 2000; 91: 1017-20.
36. Mitchell S, Brimacombe J, Keller C. Feasibility, accuracy and optimal location for oesophageal core temperature measurements using the ProSeal laryngeal mask airway drainage tube. Anaesth Intens Care 2003; 31: 282-85.
37. Keller C, Brimacombe J. Mucosal pressure and oropharyngeal leak pressure with the ProSeal versus the classic laryngeal mask airway. Br J Anaesth 2000; 85:262-66.
38. Brimacombe J, Vosoba Judd D, Tortely K, et al. Gastric tube-guided reinsertion of the ProSeal laryngeal mask airway. Anesth Analg 2002; 94: 1670.

39. Verghese C, Brimacombe J. Survey of laryngeal mask airway usage in 11910 patients: Safety and efficacy for conventional and nonconventional usage. Anesth Analg 1996; 82:129-33.
40. Ilzuka T, Ishii N. The efficacy of the Laryngeal mask airway during positive-pressure ventilation, 1997; 84:S240.
41. Buniatian AA, Dolbneva EL. Laryngeal mask under total myoplegia and artificial pulmonary ventilation during laparoscopic cholecystectomy. Vestn Ross Akad Med Nauk 1997; 9: 33-38.
42. Maltby JR, Beriault MT, Watson NC, Fick GH. Gastric distension and ventilation during Laparoscopic cholecystectomy: LMA-Classic vs. tracheal intubation. Can J Anesth 2000;47:622-26.
43. Tobias JD, Holcomb GW, Rasmussen GE, Lowe S, Morgan WM. General anesthesia using the laryngeal mask airway during brief, Laparoscopic inspection of the peritoneum in children. J Laparoendosc Surg. 1996;6:175-80.
44. Ilzuka T, Kinoshita K, Fukui H. Pulmonary compliance of the laryngeal mask airway during laparoscopic cholecystectomy. Anesth Analg 2000; 90: S210.
45. Haley A, Kais H, Efrati Y et al: Continuous esophageal pH monitoring during laparoscopic cholecystectomy. Surg endosc 1994; 8: 1294.
46. Lind JF, Warrian, WG, Wankling WJ. Responses of the gastro-esophageal junctional zone to increases in abdominal pressure. Can J Surg 1966; 9: 32-8.
47. Jones MJ, Mitchell RW, Hindocha N. Effect of increased intra-abdominal pressure during laparoscopy on the lower esophageal sphincter. Anesth Analg 1989; 68: 63-5.
48. Akhtar TM, Shankar RK, Street MK. Is Guedel's airway and facemask dead ? Today's Anaesthetist 1994; 9: 56-8.
49. Dingley J, Asai T. Insertion methods of the laryngeal mask airway. A survey of current practice in Wales. Anaesthesia 1996; 51: 596-99.
50. Crilly H, McLeod K. Use of the laryngeal mask airway: A survey of Australian anaesthetic practice. Anaesth Intens Care 2000; 28: 224.
51. Cunningham AJ, Brull SJ. Laparoscopic cholecystectomy. Anaesthetic implications. Anesth Analg 1993; 76: 1120-33.
52. Chatterjee R, Venugopal M, Ram K., Kapoor V. K. Successful resuscitation of a near fatal cardiac dysrrythmia in a case of laparascopic cholecystectomy: A case report. Indian J. Anaesth. 2003, 47(6): 479-80.
53. Bogetz MS. Using the laryngeal mask airway to manage the difficult airway. In: The Upper Airway and Anesthesia. Anesthesiol Clin N Am 2002; 20(4): 863-70.
54. Brimacombe J. Keller C, Vosoba Judd D. Gum elastic bougie-guided insertion of the ProSeal ™ laryngeal mask airway is superior to the digital and introducer tool techniques. Anesthesiology 2004; 100: 25-9.
55. Utting JE. Pitfalls in anaesthetic practice. Anaesthesia 1987; 59: 877-90.
56. Gannon K. Mortality associated with anaesthesia. A case review study. Anaesthesia 1991; 46: 962-66.
57. Crosby ET, Cooper RM, Douglas MJ, et al. The unanticipated difficult airway with recommendations for management. Can J Anaesth 1998; 45: 757–76.
58. Awan R, Nolan J, Cook TM. Use of the ProSeal LMA for airway maintenance during emergency Caesarean section after failed intubation. Br J Anaesth 2004; 92: 144-46.
59. Brimacombe J. Maintenance phase. Laryngeal Mask Anesthesia. Principle and Practice. London: WB Saunders, 2005.
60. Sprung J, Whalley DG, Falcone T, Warner DO, Hubmayr RD, Hammel J. The impact of morbid obesity, pneumoperitoneum, and posture on respiratory system mechanics and oxygenation during laparoscopy. Anesth Analg 2002; 94: 1345-50.
61. Keller C, Brimacombe J, Kleinsasser A, Brimacombe L. The laryngeal mask airway ProSeal™ as a temporary ventilatory device in grossly and morbidly obese patients before laryngoscopic-guided tracheal intubation. Anesth Analg 2002; 94: 737-40.
62. Lamb K, James MF, Janicki PK. Laryngeal mask airway for intraocular surgery, effects on intraocular pressure and stress responses. Br J Anaesth 1992;69:143-47.
63. Evans NR, Gardner SV, James MFM, et al. The ProSeal laryngeal mask: Results of a descriptive trial with experience of 300 cases. Br J Anaesth 2002; 88(4): 534-39.
64. Latorre F, Eberle B, Weiler N, Mienert R, Stanek A, Goedecke R, et al. Laryngeal mask airway position and the risk of gastric insufflation. Anesth Analg 1998; 86: 867-71.
65. Ho-Tai LM, Devitt JH, Noel AG, O'Donnell MP. Gas leak and gastric insufflation during controlled ventilation: face mask versus laryngeal mask airway. Can J Anaesth 1998; 45: 206-11.
66. Weiler N, Latorre F, Eberle B, Goedecke R, Heinrichs W. Respiratory mechanics, gastric insufflation pressure, and air leakage of the laryngeal mask airway. Anesth Analg 1997; 84: 1025-28.

CHAPTER 19

Anaesthesia for Laparoscopic Cholecystectomy

INTRODUCTION

Endoscopic approach to cholecystectomy was introduced in 1987, which was the beginning of explosive growth in minimally invasive surgery. Subsequently it started gaining popularity as an alternative technique to conventional cholecystectomy and is now the "gold standard" for surgical treatment of cholelithiasis.[1] Phillipe Mouret first described the technique in France in 1998 (Personal Communication). It was reported in literature later by Perissat et al[2] and was refined and popularized in US by Reddick and Oslen.[3]

The documented advantages of laparoscopic cholecystectomy over open cholecystectomy are:

1. Minimal pain associated with small, limited incision and improved cosmesis
2. Preservation of pulmonary and diaphragmatic function.
3. Reduced morbidity.
4. Early ambulation.
5. Economic benefits in context with:
   - Shorter hospital stay (mean 1-3 days) regardless of underlying medical condition.
   - Early return to work and normal activities (mean 6.5-12.8 days)

PHYSIOLOGIC CHANGES

Although they are visually "minimally invasive" to the patient (Fig. 12.1), the intraoperative requirements of laparoscopic surgery produce significant pathophysiological changes, some of which are deleterious to the patient. They are described elsewhere in the book and are due to position of patient, carboperitoneum and raised intra-abdominal pressure (IAP). Laparoscopic cholecystectomy is unique in that a change in body position from Trendelenburg when establishing carboperitoneum, to reverse Trendelenburg during dissection of gallbladder is necessary to avoid inadvertent bowel injury and to provide optimum exposure.

In brief, the pathophysiological changes produced are due to:

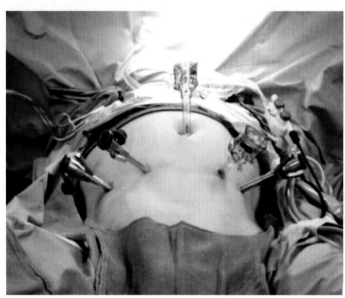

Fig. 12.1: Access for laparoscopy

POSITION OF PATIENT

Trendelenburg Position

During initial stages of laparoscopic cholecystectomy, the patient is normally placed in 10-20 degree Trendelenburg position to produce gravitational displacement of the viscera away from the blind trocar insertion. Gravity has profound physiological effects on the cardiovascular and pulmonary systems.

Cardiovascular effects: The cardiovascular changes may be influenced by the extent of the head-down tilt, patient's age, intravascular volume status, associated cardiac disease, anaesthetic drugs and ventilation techniques.[4] The head down position favours venous return, right atrial pressure, central blood volume and improves cardiac output. Pricolo et al reported a small (10%) but significant increase in cardiac index (CI) without increase in central venous pressure (CVP), pulmonary capillary wedge pressure (PCWP), heart rate (HR) or systemic vascular resistance (SVR) in normotensives in a 10-degree head down position. In contrast, CVP and PCWP increased and CI decreased significantly in normotensives with coronary artery disease (CAD) during head down positioning. The increase in venous return and myocardial oxygen demand that occurs in severe cardiovascular disease can precipitate acute heart failure.[5]

Respiratory effects: Pulmonary function changes associated with head down position will depend upon patient's age, weight, preoperative lung function, degree of head down tilt, the anaesthetic agents used and intraoperative ventilatory techniques. Vital capacity (VC) and functional residual capacity (FRC) decrease because of increased weight of abdominal viscera on the diaphragm – exaggerated in obese, elderly or debilitated patients. Decreased compliance, increased ventilation – perfusion abnormalities and cephalad displacement of mediastinum commonly occur. [6]

A reduction in functional residual capacity (FRC) relative to closing volume may be associated with development of intraoperative atelectasis and intrapulmonary shunting. These changes may occur during general anaesthesia because of a variety of factors i.e.

i. Cephalad shift of diaphragm associated with supine position.[7]
ii. Loss of inspiratory muscle tone.
iii. Appearance of end-expiratory muscle tone in the abdominal expiratory muscles.
iv. Changes in intrathoracic blood volume associated with induction of anaesthesia.
v. Influence of muscle relaxants on diaphragmatic excursion.[8]

This reduction in FRC associated with GA may be compounded by carboperitoneum during laparoscopic cholecystectomy. A reduced cardiac output (CO) secondary to reduction in venous return or drug induced myocardial depression may reduce mixed-venous oxygen tension.

Frazee et al claimed that there occurs 20-25 per cent less reduction in FEV_1, FVC and forced expiratory flow (FEF) of preoperative baseline values in patients undergoing laparoscopic cholecystectomy in comparison to open cholecystectomy due to minimal abdominal wall disruption as it requires only four small skin incisions for insertion of trocars leading to less postoperative pain. This difference in pulmonary functions were present despite longer anaesthetic and operative time in the laparoscopic group.[9]

Wittgen et al compared the ventilatory effects of laparoscopic cholecystectomy in 20 patients with normal cardiopulmonary status (ASA I) to 10 patients with documented cardiac and pulmonary disease (ASA II, III). ASA I patients had increased end-tidal CO_2 and $PaCO_2$ and decreased arterial pH after CO_2 insufflation but no significant change in minute volume and peak inspiratory pressure. In contrast, significant decrease in arterial pH and increase in arterial carbon dioxide, minute volume and peak inspiratory pressure was observed in patients with cardiovascular disease after CO_2 insufflation.[10]

Reverse Trendelenburg Position

This is accompanied by respiratory advantages and cardiovascular disadvantages. It improves diaphragmatic function and respiratory status but results in decrease in venous return (VR), right atrial pressure (RAP) and pulmonary capillary wedge pressure (PCWP) resulting in a fall in mean arterial pressure (MAP) and cardiac output (CO), reflected by changes in left ventricular end diastolic area. These cardiovascular changes get exacerbated by compression of inferior venacava during carboperitoneum. The cardiac output changes in this position are insignificant in healthy patients, but may not be so benign in patients with pre-existing cardiorespiratory disease.[11] Adequate hydration to replace expected preoperative fluid deficit prior to changes in position prevents hypotension from these causes.

A steep head up position causes venous stasis in the legs predisposing these patients to deep vein thrombosis (DVT) particularly in obese patients and in procedures of long duration.[12]

CREATION OF CARBOPERITONEUM (FIG. 12.2)

Creation of carboperitoneum has generalized systemic effects. CO_2 has remained the insufflation gas of choice because of its ready availability, low cost, and properties (odourless, relatively inert, non-combustible) and high Ostwald's blood-gas partition co-efficient (0.48). Due to its high solubility, the incidence of fatal gas embolism is rare (0.001-0.0017%). The extent of cardiovascular changes associated with the creation of carboperitoneum depend on IAP, volume of carbon dioxide absorbed, intravascular volume, ventilatory strategy, surgical conditions and anaesthetic agents.[13]

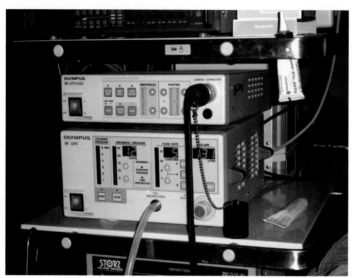

Fig. 12.2: Insufflator

INTRA-ABDOMINAL PRESSURE (IAP)

Increased IAP has two opposite effects on the cardiovascular system : it forces blood out of the abdominal organs and inferior vena-cava into the central venous reservoir, while at the same time it increases peripheral blood pooling in the lower extremities and thus tends to decrease the central blood volume.[14]

An increased cardiac output at lower IAP may result from increased cardiac filling pressures due partly to mechanical factors and partly to sympathetically mediated constriction of capacitance vessels and CO_2 induced effects on cardiac efferent sympathetic activity.[15]

An inadvertent right main stem bronchial intubation and hypoxaemia may occur as the endotracheal tube, firmly secured at its proximal end, does not always move along with the trachea as the diaphragm displaces the lung and carina cephalad.[16]

PRE-ANAESTHETIC ASSESSMENT

Conversion to laparotomy is always a possibility and must be considered during the pre-anaesthetic assessment. The cardiac and pulmonary status of all patients should be carefully assessed on priority and optimised preoperatively.

Some patients may present with deranged liver function which requires consideration in investigation and choice of the pharmacological agent. As haemorrhage is more difficult to control laparoscopically, the patient should have a coagulopathy corrected prior to laparoscopy.

Basic tests should include complete blood count (CBC), urine analysis, base-line electrolytes, renal function tests, clotting functions and electrocardiogram. Baseline chest films are necessary not only to rule out active disease, but also for postoperative comparison of acute changes such as subcutaneous or mediastinal emphysema, pneumothorax, interstitial or pulmonary oedema.

Recent case reports and studies documenting profound intraoperative hypoxaemia and respiratory acidosis in patients with pre-existing chronic obstructive and restrictive lung disease suggest that pre-operative arterial blood gas analysis and pulmonary function tests are appropriate in patients with cardiopulmonary disease for laparoscopic cholecystectomy.[17]

PREMEDICATION

A short acting anxiolytic allays anxiety and ensures a rapid recovery. An antiemetic and a gastroprokinetic reduces incidence of postoperative nausea and vomiting as well as incidence of pulmonary aspiration. A H_2-receptor antagonist decreases the volume and modifies the pH of gastric secretions. Pre-emptive analgesia may be achieved with non-steroidal anti-inflammatory drugs (NSAIDs). Deep vein thrombosis (DVT) prophylaxis is recommended for patients prone to DVT.[12]

MONITORING (FIG. 12.3)

Mandatory monitoring includes heart rate, pulse oximetry, NIBP, $EtCO_2$, ECG and IAP, while the desirable ones are indicators of inspired O_2 fraction, minute volume, peak airway pressure and precordial stethoscope. $EtCO_2$ monitors ventilation, helps in diagnosis of CO_2 embolism and cautions against risk of arrhythmias in the setting of hypercapnia. $EtCO_2$ is most commonly used as a non-invasive substitute for $PaCO_2$ in evaluating the adequacy of ventilation during laparoscopic cholecystectomy. However, $EtCO_2$ may differ considerably from $PaCO_2$ because of ventilation – perfusion (V/Q) mismatching and increased alveolar arterial CO_2 gradient. Therefore, arterial blood gas analysis should be considered in patients with preoperative severe cardiorespiratory disease and in situations where intraoperative hypoxaemia, high airway pressure or elevated $EtCO_2$ are encountered.[10]

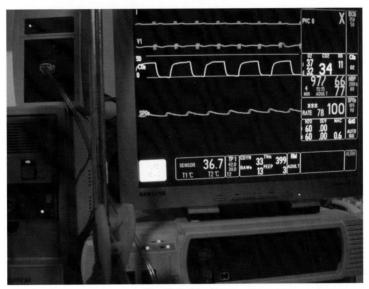

Fig.12.3: Monitor

ANAESTHETIC TECHNIQUE

The anaesthetic considerations for laparoscopic cholecystectomy are similar to those for other laparoscopic procedures. It depends upon the preoperative condition of the patient and anaesthesiologist's evaluation. The basic aim of anaesthesia is respiratory and haemodynamic stability of the patient, so the choice of anaesthetic technique should enable satisfactory analgesia, amnesia, muscular relaxation, faster recovery and shorter hospital stay.[18]

GENERAL ANAESTHESIA (FIG. 12.4)

The recommended anaesthesia technique for laparoscopic cholecystectomy is general anaesthesia with a cuffed tracheal tube and controlled ventilation. This enables adequate muscle relaxation, good surgical conditions, protection against aspiration of gastric contents and analgesia. Adequate carboperitoneum is achieved at lower IAP with adequate muscle relaxation. Muscle relaxation and paralysis are necessary because the increase in IAP and splinting of diaphragm makes spontaneous breathing difficult. It also provides a quieter surgical field, better surgical exposure and controlled ventilation can compensate for hypercarbia and respiratory acidosis that results from absorption of CO_2.[18]

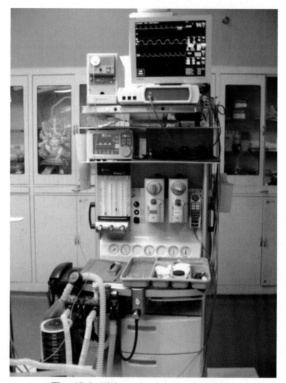

Fig. 12.4: High end anaesthesia set up

A vagolytic drug such as atropine may be required because vagal stimulation due to stretching of peritoneum during insufflation may cause reflex bradycardia.[19] Preloading with 5-10 ml/kg of crystalloid solution is recommended to prevent the haemodynamic changes during carboperitoneum, however, moderation is required in high risk cardiac cases.[19] Thiopentone sodium is the standard induction agent, however, propofol is gaining popularity for its quick, clear-headed recovery and central anti-emetic properties, especially in case of out patient laparoscopy.[20] A considerable choice of non-depolarising muscle relaxants is available.

In laparoscopic cholecystectomy total intravenous anaesthesia (TIVA) with short acting anaesthetics like propofol and remifentanil is characterized by stability of haemodynamic and gas exchange parameters at all stages of the operation and a better recovery profile.[21] Therefore, it has become increasingly popular, as it is advantageous also from a cost minimization standpoint.[22]

Single breath vital capacity rapid inhalational induction technique with sevoflurane (5%) and N_2O 65 per cent in oxygen and maintenance with sevoflurane 1-1.5 per cent and N_2O 65 per cent in oxygen can cause prolongation of QT interval and dysrhythmia in comparison with induction and maintenance with propofol in laparoscopic cholecystectomy.[23] Ventilatory response to CO_2 does not occur under inhalational anaesthesia. Halothane is to be avoided for its negative inotropic and chronotropic action and it may also produce arrhythmia in the presence of hypercarbia. Sevoflurane or isoflurane (Fig. 12.5) is preferred because of its direct vasodilating action by decreasing systemic vascular resistance, rapid recovery with minimal PONV and its least sensitivity to arrhythmia in presence of increased catecholamines due to hypercarbia.[24]

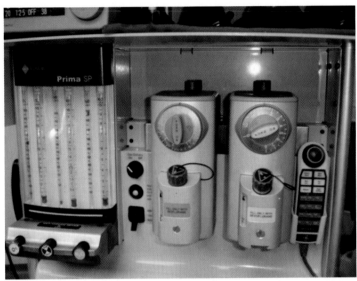

Fig.12.5: Voporizers

N_2O is a commonly used adjuvant because of its physical properties for rapid uptake and elimination with advantages of additional analgesia and less risk of awareness. The use of N_2O during laparoscopic cholecystectomy produces no clinically significant effect on surgical conditions owing to bowel distention nor an increase in the incidence of postoperative emesis.[25] However, if large volumes of air is present in the bowel because of air swallowing or mask assisted ventilation or significantly longer surgical procedures (70-75 mins), N_2O might impair operating conditions during laparoscopic cholecystectomy.[26]

Intraoperative gastric decompression by naso/orogastric tube reduces risk of visceral puncture at the time of trocar insertion, improves laparoscopic visualization and facilitates retraction of the right quadrant structures. Urinary bladder catheterization after induction of anaesthesia avoids bladder injury.

The problems of pulmonary atelectasis, decrease FRC and high peak airway pressure associated with carboperitoneum can be ameliorated by careful adjustment of ventilatory patterns to maintain $EtCO_2$ at approximately 35 mmHg, which requires a 15-25 per cent increase of minute volume. Increase of respiratory rate rather than tidal volume is preferable because of reduced lung compliance and especially in patients with COPD or history of pneumothorax or bullous emphysema to avoid increased alveolar inflation and to reduce risk of pneumothorax. IAP should be monitored and kept as low as possible to reduce haemodynamic and respiratory changes. Threshold pressure that has minimal effects on haemodynamic is ≤ 10-12 mmHg.[27] Pressure points should be padded with great care to prevent nerve injuries.

The use of PLMA (laryngeal mask airway with ProSeal) and LMA show similar air-tight efficiency during laparoscopy. The frequency of sore throat (early, in recovery room and late, after 1 week) does not show any difference in both groups.[28] However, LMA has its limitations, since it does not protect against aspiration of gastric contents at airway pressure >20 cm of H_2O.[29,30]

Perioperative Narcotics

Narcotics as premedication or intraoperatively cause spasm of sphincter of Oddi – which may create cholangiographic findings indistinguishable from those produced by an impacted CBD stone, causing unnecessary exploration of CBD. However, this narcotic induced spasm of sphincter of Oddi may be antagonized by naloxone, glucagon and nalbuphine.

Fentanyl, a potent narcotic analgesic with rapid onset of action, relative cardiovascular stability and negligible histamine release, is used widely in balanced anaesthesia technique. In a human study comparing equianalgesic doses of intravenous fentanyl, morphine, meperidine and pentazocine on CBD pressures, Radney et al demonstrated an intrabiliary pressure increase of 99.5 per cent, 52.7 per cent, 61.3 per cent and 15.1 per cent respectively. So the advent of parenteral perioperative NSAIDs, like diclofenac/ketorolac and the tendency for less postoperative pain with laparoscopic approach may obviate the need for perioperative narcotics.[31]

REGIONAL ANAESTHESIA (FIG. 12.6)

General anaesthesia as the only suitable technique for laparoscopic cholecystectomy is a concept of the past. A problem with modern general anaesthesia is that even though patients can be oriented and awake shortly after cessation of anaesthetic, these agents do not facilitate postoperative analgesia or an emesis-free recovery, two most important problems associated with laparoscopy.[32] There is a growing body of evidence that epidural anaesthesia has an important role to play in the care of patients undergoing laparoscopic cholecystectomy and its scope depends upon the creativeness of the surgeons, anesthesiologists and patient acceptance. A low level of IAP with less degree of patient tilt is recommended for such procedures.

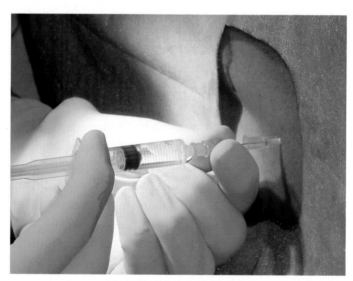

Fig. 12.6: Regional anaesthesia

Laparoscopic cholecystectomy has been performed safely and successfully under epidural anaesthesia in patients in their third trimester of pregnancy, COPD patients and patients with cystic fibrosis who are deemed high risk for general anaesthesia.[33] The goal of anaesthesia management in a COPD patient includes avoidance of anaesthetic that depresses mucociliary transport, provision of postoperative pain relief adequate to prevent deterioration of respiratory mechanics and ambulation as early as possible. Epidural anaesthesia fulfills all of the above criteria and provides excellent operative conditions with a quick and uneventful postoperative recovery.

Preloading with 15 ml/kg of normal saline over 20 minutes prevents hypotension during the procedure. Throughout surgery patient oxygenation is maintained by 100 per cent oxygen by mask at a rate of 2 L /min. Hypotension is corrected by decreasing the IAP, increasing crystalloid infusion or using vasopressor drugs. Intraoperative sedation is provided with titrated doses of midazolam/propofol infusion/fentanyl or alfentanil. Epidural block is achieved via an epidural catheter, 3 cm cephalad inserted at T_9–T_{10} or T_{10}–T_{11} intervertebral space. Drugs used are an initial bolus of 8 ml of 0.5 per cent bupivacaine with incremental doses of 2 ml of 0.5 per cent of bupivacaine to achieve a block up to T_4-T_5.[34]

To avoid vagal stimulation, slow CO_2 insufflation at 2 L /min to an IAP of less than 10 mmHg is preferred. Mild to moderate brachioscapular pain, possibly due to irritation of subdiaphragmatic peritoneum or traction of the mesentery, may occur during surgery. Intraoperative shoulder tip or abdominal pain does not seem to be a major deterrent and can be effectively controlled with small doses of opioids. Under regional anaesthesia, since the patient is awake, there is an early detection of complications. The excellent postoperative analgesia and lower incidence of PONV accelerate the discharge process, and so is cost effective.

However, there are several disadvantages of the regional technique. Sympathetic denervation of high regional block may exaggerate vagal reflexes leading to bradycardia, hypotension and decreased cardiac output. There has been no record of laparoscopic cholecystectomy done under subarachnoid block because of the haemodynamic effects of high level of block required in the reverse Trendelenburg position.

LOCAL ANAESTHESIA

Local anaesthesia seems unsuitable for laparoscopic cholecystectomy because of requirement of multiple puncture sites, considerable organ manipulation, steep tilt and voluminous carboperitoneum making spontaneous breathing difficult. CO_2 causes direct peritoneal irritation and pain under local anaesthesia because it forms carbonic acid in contact with moist peritoneum.

POSTOPERATIVE MORBIDITY

The vitals should be monitored in recovery room since haemodynamic changes induced by carboperitoneum outlast the release of carboperitoneum. All patients should be administered oxygen postoperatively since slow release of CO_2 from the tissues may result in hypoxia.

Although laparoscopic cholecystectomy is associated with minimal morbidity, postoperative pain, nausea and vomiting are common problems.

POSTOPERATIVE PAIN

Laparoscopic surgery, although less painful than open surgery, is far from pain-free. Various causes of pain implicated are an acidic milieu due to formation of carbonic acid, and referred shoulder pain due to phrenic nerve stimulation. Persistent abdominal or shoulder-tip pain is one of the reasons for failure to achieve same day discharge. Pre-emptive and multimodal analgesia and careful evacuation of residual CO_2 after desufflation can minimize postoperative pain.[35]

Pre-emptive low dose ketamine (0.7 mg/kg) is able to produce an adequate postoperative analgesia at awakening despite short duration (approximately 1 hour) and increases the analgesic effects of tramadol.[36]

Furthermore, the adverse effects of ketamine (hallucinations, nystagmus, photophobia, psychomotor excitation and psychotic symptoms) can be reduced by intra-operative administration of benzodiazepines, anti-emetic drugs or by the association of ketamine and a peripheral analgesic (keterolac).[36]

Applying local anaesthetic (0.5% bupivacaine) to skin, subcutis, fascia and parietal peritoneum through trocar sites reduces the pain intensity and postoperative analgesic requirement. This approach is more effective when applied at the end of surgery than at the start.[37] Right sided subdiaphragmatic instillation with local anaesthetic reduces shoulder-tip pain.[38] Short-acting opioids may be used for rescue analgesia.

POSTOPERATIVE NAUSEA AND VOMITING (PONV)

The incidence of PONV after laparoscopy has been reported to be as high as 42 per cent by Stanton et al.[39] Patients undergoing general anaesthesia for laparoscopic cholecystectomy are at higher risk for postoperative emetic symptoms (nausea, vomiting and retching) which is unpleasant and the most important factor in causing an overnight admission after ambulatory surgery. Some of the causal factors leading to activation of neurogenic pathways such as peritoneal gas insufflation, CO_2 peritoneal irritation and bowel manipulation are essentially unavoidable, so propofol based anaesthesia and a variety of anti-emetic medications like antihistaminics (hydroxyzine, promethazine), butyrophenones (droperidol), dopamine receptor antagonists, gastrokinetics (metoclopramide) and selective serotonin receptor antagonists (SSRAs) have been investigated for the prevention and treatment of emetic symptoms.[40] However, these drugs are associated with undesirable adverse effects such as excessive sedation, hypotension, dry mouth, dysphoria, hallucinations and extra-pyramidal signs.

Prophylactic dixyrazine (10 mg), an alternate neuroleptic drug to droperidol, is an effective, safe and cheap anti-emetic drug for laparoscopic cholecystectomy without any significant adverse effects.[41] The combination of metoclopromide (10 mg) and droperidol (1.25 mg) decreases incidence of PONV significantly whereas metoclopramide alone proved inefficient. Droperidol should be given early in the procedure because it potentiates sedation, is long-acting, and as an α–blocker, it counteracts the hypertensive effect of systemic CO_2.

Ondansetron (5 HT_3-antagonist) has a sustained and more effective anti-emetic effect in the postoperative period if administered at the end of surgery than as a single dose before induction or as a split dose at induction and end of surgery because of its relatively short elimination half life of 2.8 $\pm$ 0.6 hours.[42] Granisetron hydrochloride, a newer SSRA in a dose of 20 mcg/kg is effective for the treatment of established postoperative emetic symptoms.[43] Dexamethasone (10 mg IV) reduces PONV in first 24 hours without having any adverse effects from this single dose of steroid.[44]

COMPLICATIONS OF LAPAROSCOPIC CHOLECYSTECTOMY

Although surgical complications can occur any time, they are also related to patient position, carboperitoneum and increased IAP.

TROCAR INSERTION

Traumatic injuries sustained during blind trocar insertion include bleeding from abdominal wall vessels and major vessels, gastrointestinal tract perforations, hepatic and splenic tears, avulsion of adhesions, omental disruption and herniation at the trocar insertion site.

CARBOPERITONEUM AND INCREASED IAP

The most frequent complications include pneumothorax, pneumomentum, subcutaneous or mediastinal emphysema, cardiac dysrhythmias and CO_2 embolism. Tension pneumothorax has been reported during laparoscopic cholecystectomy following trocar insertion and intraperitoneal CO_2 insufflation. A congenital defect of the diaphragm (patent pleuroperitoneal canal) through which the insufflated gas passes into the thoracic cavity has been suggested as the underlying mechanism for pneumothorax and pneumomediastinum.[45]

EXOGENOUS CO$_2$

Hypercarbia causes sympathetic nervous system stimulation as demonstrated by two to three fold increase in plasma catecholamine concentration. The systemic effects of CO_2 may manifest as hypertension, tachycardia, cerebral vasodilation, increased cardiac output, hypercarbia and respiratory acidosis. Mild hypercarbia causes sympathetic stimulation while severe hypercarbia exerts a negative inotropic effect on the heart and reduces left ventricular function.

The differential diagnosis for intraoperative hypoxemia during laparoscopic cholecystectomy includes:
1. Pre-existing conditions - cardiopulmonary disease, morbid obesity.
2. Hypoventilation—patient position, carboperitoneum, endotracheal tube obstruction and inadequate ventilation – spontaneous /controlled
3. Intrapulmonary shunting—Reduced FRC (carboperitoneum induced), endobronchial intubation, pneumothorax, emphysema (mediastinum /subcutaneous), bowel distension (N_2O induced) and pulmonary aspiration of gastric contents.
4. Reduced cardiac output—haemorrhage; trocar injury, inferior vena cava compression, dysrrthymias-hypercarbia/ volatile anaesthetic agents, myocardial depression- drug induced / acidosis, CO_2 venous embolism
5. Technical/Equipment failure—circuit disconnection, delivery of hypoxic mixture.

VENOUS CO$_2$ EMBOLISM

It can occur when carbon dioxide enters a vessel during attempts of creation of carboperitoneum and may present as profound hypotension, cyanosis, momentary rise in endtidal CO_2 followed by fall in endtidal CO_2 and asystole.[46] It may also occur in the immediate post-operative period and must be considered in the differential diagnosis of cardiovascular collapse.[47] Management is with immediate cessation of insufflation, release of carboperitoneum, administration of 100 per cent oxygen, intravenous atropine, Durant's position (head low 20°-30°, left lateral) and inotropic support. [46]

CONCLUSIONS
CLINICAL PEARLS

1. Laparoscopic cholecystectomy is a 'gold standard' for all laparoscopic procedures.
2. It is often being performed as a day care procedures due to the advantages of laparoscopy and newer anaesthestic agents.
3. Vigilant monitoring essential.

REFERENCES

1. Way LW. Changing therapy for gall stone disease. N Engl J Med 1990; 323:1273-4.

2. Perissat J, Collet DR, Belliard R. Gall stones: Laparoscopic treatment, intracorporeal lithotripsy followed by cholecystostomy or cholecystectomy – a personal technique. Endoscopy 1989; 21: 373-4.

3. Reddick EJ, Olsen DO. Laparoscopic laser cholecystectomy. A comparison with mini-lap cholecystectomy. Surg Endosc 1989; 3: 131-3.

4. Cunningham AJ, Brull SJ. Laparoscopic cholecystectomy: Anaesthetic implications. Anaesth Analg 1993; 76: 1120-33.

5. Pricolo VE, Burchard KW, Singh AK, et al. Trendelenburg versus PASU application: haemodynamic response in man. J Trauma 1986; 26: 718-26.

6. Case EH, Stiles JA. The effect of various surgical positions on vital capacity. Anaesthesiology 1946; 7: 29-31.

7. Craig DB. Postoperative recovery of pulmonary function. Anaesth Analg 1981; 60: 46-52.

8. Froese AB, Bryan AC. Effects of anaesthesia and paralysis on diaphragmatic mechanics in man. Anaesthesiology 1974; 41: 242-55.

9. Frazee RC, Roberts JW, Okeson GC, et al. Open versus laparoscopic cholecystectomy: a comparison of postoperative pulmonary function. Ann Surg 1991; 213: 651-3.

10. Wittgen CM, Andrus CH, Fitzgerald SD, et al. Analysis of the haemodynamic and ventilatory effects of laparoscopic cholecystectomy. Arch Surg 1991; 126: 997-1001

11. Cunningham AJ et al. TEE assessment of haemodynamic function during laparoscopic cholecystectomy. Br J Anaesth 1993; 70: 621.

12. Beebe DS et al. Evidence of venous stasis after abdominal insufflation for laparoscopic cholecystectomy. Anaesthesiology 1992; 77 suppl 3A, A 148.

13. Liu SY, Leighton T, Davis I, et al. Prospective analysis of cardiopulmonary responses to laparoscopic cholecystectomy. J. Laparoendosc Surg 1991; 1: 241-6.

14. Kelman GR, et al. Cardiac output and arterial blood gas tension during laparoscopy. Br J Anaesth 1972; 44: 1155-62.

15. Rasmussen JP, Dauchot PJ, Depalma RG, et al. Cardiac function and hypercarbia. Arch Surg 1978; 113: 1196-200.

16. Heinonen J, Takki S, Tammisto T. Effect of the Trendelenburg tilt and other procedures on the position of endotracheal tubes. Lancet 1969; 1: 850-3.

17. Jones DB, Soper NJ, Brunt LM, et al. Effect of age and ASA status on outcome of laparoscopic cholecystectomy. Surg Endosc 1996; 10: 238.

18. Andrus C. H. & Wittgen C.M. Anaesthetic considerations. Operative Laparoscopy and Thoracoscopy edited by MacFadyen B.V. Lippincott publishers. Chap 2 page 18.

19. Brichant J.F. Anaesthesia for minimally invasive abdominal surgery. Recent advances in Anaesthesia and Analgesia Vol 19. pg 33-49.

20. Borgeat A et al. Subhypnotic doses of propofol possess direct antiemetic properties. Anaesth Analg 1992; 74 : 339-41.

21. Vincenzo F, Caterina P, Marco T, et al. Comparative cost-analysis of a propofol – cisatracurium- based anaesthesia with Remifentanil or Fentanyl for laparoscopic surgery. Surg Laparosc Endosc Percutan Tech 2005; 15(3): 147-52.

22. Smith, Ian. Total intravenous anaesthesia: Is it worth the cost? CNS Drugs, 2003; 17(9): 609-19.

23. Sen S, Ozmort G, Booan N, et al. Comparison of single breath vital capacity rapid inhalation with sevoflurane 5% and propofol induction on QT interval and haemodynamics for lap surgery. Eur J Anaesth 2004; 21(7): 543-6.

24. Kenefick JP, Leader A, Malthy Jr, et al. Laparoscopy: Blood gas values and minor sequelae associated with 3 tech based on isoflurane. Br J Anaesth 1987; 59: 189-94.

25. Ellis Taylor et al. Anaesthesia for laparoscopic cholecystectomy. Is nitrous oxide contraindicated? Anaesthesiology 1992; 76: 541-43.

26. Eger EI II, Saidman LJ. Hazards of nitrous oxide anaesthesia in bowel obstruction and pneumothorax. Anaesthesiology 1965; 26: 61-6.

27. Ishizaki Y, et al. Changes in splanchnic blood flow and cardio-vascular effects following peritoneal insufflation of carbon dioxide. Surg Endosc 1993; 7: 420-3.

28. Natalini, Lanze, Roscino, et al. Standard LMA & LMA-proSeal during laparoscopic surgery. J Clin Anaesth 2003; 15(6): 428-32.

29. Brimacombe JR., Berry AM. The Laryngeal Mask Airway. In: The Difficult Airway I. Anesthesiol Clin N Am 1995; 13(2): 411-37.

30. Rosenblatt WH. Airway Management. In: Barash PG, Cullen BF, Stoelting RK.(eds) Clinical Anesthesia (4th Edn) 2001; 23: 599-605.

31. Radney PA, Brodman E, Mankikar D, et al. The effect of equi-analgesic doses of fentanyl, morphine, meperidine and pentazocine on common bile duct pressure. Anaesthesiology 1980; 29: 26-9.

32. Ian Smith anaesthesia for laproscopy with emphasis on outpatient laproscopy. Anaesthesiology clinics of North America. 2001;19(1): 21-41.

33. Gramatica L et al. Laparoscopic cholecystectomy performed under regional anaesthesia in patients with chronic obstructive pulmonary disease. Surg Endosc 2002; 16: 472-5.

34. Pursnani KG, Bazza Y, Calleja M, et al. Laparoscopic cholecystectomy under epidural anaesthesia in patients with chronic respiratory disease. Surg Endosc 1998; 12: 1082-4.

35. Alexander JI. Pain after laparoscopy. Br J Anaesth 1997; 79: 369-78.

36. Launo C et al. Pre-emptive ketamine during general anaesthesia for postoperative analgesia in patients undergoing laparoscopic cholecystectomy. Minerva Anesthesiol 2004; 70(10): 727-34, 734-8.

37. Inan A, Sen M, Dener C. Local anaesthesia use for laparoscopic cholecystectomy. World J Surg 2004; 28(8): 741-4. E pub 2004, Aug '03.

38. Narchi P, et al. Intraperitoneal local anaesthetic for shoulder pain after day care laparoscopy. Lancet 1991; 338: 1569.

39. Stanton JM. Anesthesia for laparoscopic cholecystectomy. Anaesthesia 1991; 46: 317.

40. Scott DM. Some effects of peritoneal insufflation of carbon dioxide at laparoscopy. Anaesthesia 1970; 25: 590-3.

41. Glaser C et al. Dixyrazine for prevention of PONV after laparoscopic cholecystectomy. Acta Anaesthesiol Scand 2004 Nov; 48(10): 1287-91.

42. Tang J, Wang B, White PF, et al. The effect of timing of ondansetron administration on its efficacy, cost-effectiveness and cost-benefit as a prophylactic anti-emetic in the ambulatory setting. Anaesth Analg 1998; 86: 274.

43. Fujii Y, Tanaka H, Kawasaki T. Effects of granisetron in the treatment of nausea and vomiting after laparoscopic cholecystectomy: a dose-ranging study. Clin Therapeutics 2004; 26(7): 1055-60.

44. Wang JJ, Ho ST, Liu HS, et al. Prophylactic antiemetic effect of dexamethasone in women undergoing ambulatory laparoscopic surgery. Br J Anaesth 2000; 84: 459.

45. Calverley RK, Jenkins LC. The anaesthetic management of pelvic laparoscopy. Can Anaesth Soc J 1973; 20: 679-86.

46. Clarke CC, Weeks DB, Gusdon JP. Venous carbon dioxide embolism during laparoscopy. Anaesth Analg 1977; 56: 650-2.

47. Root B, Levy MN, Pollack S, et al. Gas embolism death after laparoscopy delayed by "trapping" in the portal circulation. Anaesth Analg 1978; 57: 232-7.

Laparoscopic Repair of Abdominal Hernias: Anaesthetic Considerations

CHAPTER 13

INTRODUCTION

Repair of inguinal hernia is one of the most common operations performed today.[1] The conventional surgical approach to groin hernias has been to ligate or reduce the herniac sac and perform suture reconstruction of the inguinal floor through an open incision. As the experience with laparoscopic cholecystectomy increased, it provided an impetus to use the laparoscope to perform other laparoscopic procedures. Initial enthusiasm for laparoscopic herniorrhaphy was driven by dissatisfaction with pain, disability and recurrence following traditional hernia repair. Laparoscopic herniorrhaphy allows identification of contralateral hernias while offering a safer repair of recurrent hernia by avoiding cord structures and regional nerves in the previous operative site.

The first approach to the problem of groin hernia is credited to Ger who intra-abdominally stapled the neck of hernial sac.[2] The different approaches in use today are:

1. Laparoscopic Intraperitoneal Onlay Mesh (IPOM)- Placement of onlay mesh over peritoneal defects in the lower abdominal wall.
2. Transabdominal Preperitoneal Mesh (TAPP)- The preperitoneal space is opened transabdominally and the target posterior inguinal wall is covered with a prosthetic mesh.
3. Total Extraperitoneal Mesh (TEP) - A total extraperitoneal technique for placement of mesh into the preperitoneal space (Table 13.1).

Table 13.1: Indications for repair techniques[3] (TAPP, TEP, OPEN)

	Unilateral, Bilateral, Recurrent	Large scrotal, Incarcerated, diagnostic laparoscopy, Previous Pelvic incision-transverse	H/O Suprapubic prostatectomy, H/O pelvic radiation, H/O severe pelvic infection, Cardiopulmonary insufficiency, Previous Pelvic Incision-midline
TEP	⊕		
TAPP		⊕	
OPEN (Fig. 13.1) (Tension free)	⊕		⊕

⊕ Indicates preferred approach

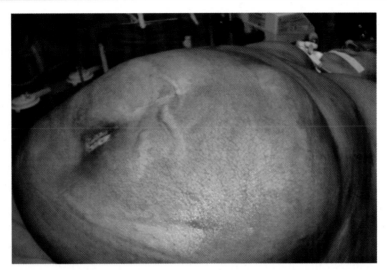

Fig.13.1: Incisional hernia with morbid obesity (for open surgery)

From Table 13.1 we see that the TEP technique may be preferred if the patient has a simple unilateral, bilateral or recurrent hernia. TAPP approach can help the surgeon approach large scrotal incarcerated and complex recurrent hernias with a higher margin of safety and ease. TAPP approach allows a concomitant diagnostic laparoscopy.

An open repair may be prudent in a patient with a history of pelvic radiation or severe pelvic infection with adhesions. Laparoscopic herniorrhaphy is an excellent technique but it is not minimally invasive. It may be too stressful an operation for the young patient with a unilateral hernia or an older patient who is better served with a less invasive operation performed under local anaesthesia.

Laparoscopic hernia repair requires a general anaesthetic with its associated risks, for a procedure that can be done conventionally under local anaesthesia. There is a small, but finite risk of serious injury to abdominal organs that is not associated with traditional inguinal herniorrhaphy. Also, costs may be higher because of the need for expensive equipment and other supplies related to laparoscopic instrumentation. Unlike those for laparoscopic cholecystectomy these increased costs are not offset by decreased hospital charges, since hernia operations are routinely outpatient procedures regardless of method of repair. A comparison of conventional with laparoscopic herniorrhaphy indicated an average increase in cost of 135 per cent with the laparoscopic approach. Whether these direct costs may be partially offset by an earlier return to employment is not known.[4]

THE LEARNING CURVE

Several studies have shown that the complication rate after laparoscopic hernioplasty is reduced by experience.[3] An experienced laparoscopic surgeon late in the learning curve can safely handle complex, recurrent, incarcerated hernias laparoscopically whereas a surgeon early in the learning curve could begin with simple, unilateral or bilateral, recurrent laparoscopic hernioplasties and use the open approach for difficult hernias.

PATHOPHYSIOLOGICAL CHANGES DURING ENDOSCOPIC HERNIA REPAIR

During laparoscopic procedures the normal homeostasis is disturbed due to patient positioning, introduction of several litres of gas (CO_2) into the abdominal cavity to produce carboperitoneum and raised intra-abdominal pressure that ensues from it. All these produce several pathophysiological changes some of which are unique to laparoscopy.

POSITION OF THE PATIENT

The patient is positioned with arms tucked at the side for TAPP/TEP repair of hernias and with arms extended for ventral hernia. Extending the arms on arm boards may not allow enough room for the surgeon to comfortably operate. The patient is placed in the Trendelenburg position (15-20°) for initial introduction of the Veress needle to produce carboperitoneum for, both, transabdominal preperitoneal (TAPP) repair of inguinal hernia and intraperitoneal onlay mesh (IPOM) repair of umbilical hernia. This position may be retained for a longer period in total extraperitoneal repair (TEP) of inguinal hernia. While doing a TAPP/TEP repair the surgeon stands on the opposite side of the table from the hernia. A Foley catheter is placed for continuous decompression of the bladder, unless the patient voids immediately preoperatively. The videomonitor is placed at the foot end of the operating table (Fig. 13.2). The height of the monitor is adjusted for comfortable viewing by, both, surgeon and the assistants. For most midline hernias the surgeon stands on either the patient's left or right side so that the surgeon's view on the screen is parallel and in line with the laparoscopic repair of the hernia within the abdomen. The assistant stands opposite the surgeon and a second monitor is placed in a suitable position.

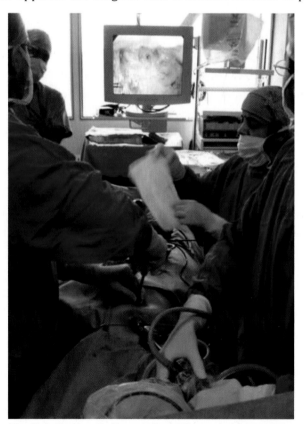

Fig. 13.2: Position of video monitor at foot end of the operating
table for TAPP-TEP repair of hernia

Patient tilt should be reduced as much as possible and should not exceed 15 to 20 degrees. Tilting must be slow and progressive to avoid sudden haemodynamic and respiratory changes. The position of the endotracheal tube must be checked after any change in patient position. Induction and release of pneumoperitoneum must be slow and progressive. Mask ventilation before intubation can inflate the stomach with gas, which must be aspirated before trocar placement to avoid gastric perforation particularly for supramesocolic laparoscopy.

In the Trendelenburg position there is an increase in the venous return (VR), right atrial pressure (RAP), central blood volume and cardiac output. However the vital capacity (VC), functional residual capacity (FRC) and lung compliance are reduced. [5,6,7] These changes are more marked in obese, elderly or debilitated patients. Central blood volume and pressure changes are greater in patients with coronary artery disease, particularly with poor ventricular function leading to a potentially deleterious increase in myocardial oxygen demand.[20]

The reverse Trendelenburg position (20-30°), which may be adopted for IPOM procedures, improves diaphragmatic function and is considered more favourable for respiration. However, it reduces the central blood volume and cardiac output.[8] This decrease in cardiac output compounds the haemodynamic changes produced by pneumoperitoneum. The steeper the tilt, the greater the fall in cardiac output. Venous stasis in the legs occurs during the head up position and since pneumoperitoneum further increases blood pooling in the legs, any additional factor contributing to circulatory dysfunction should be avoided.

INSUFFLATION OF EXOGENOUS GAS

Carbon dioxide is the insufflation gas of choice as it is readily available. It is relatively inert and non-combustible and has a high Ostwald blood/gas partition coefficient (0.48).[9]

Absorption of CO_2 from the peritoneal cavity is the mechanism for hypercarbia and a rise in end-tidal CO_2 ($EtCO_2$).[10] Absorption of CO_2 following extraperitoneal insufflation is more than that in intraperitoneal insufflation (Fig. 13.3).[11] This is probably because the resorptive surface is much larger when gas is insufflated directly into the extraperitoneal tissue.[12] The absorption of CO_2 steadily increases in TEP repair, while it tends to reach a plateau in TAPP (Fig. 13.4)[13]

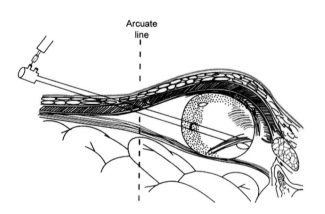

Fig.13.3: Extraperitoneal insufflation of gas for TEP repair

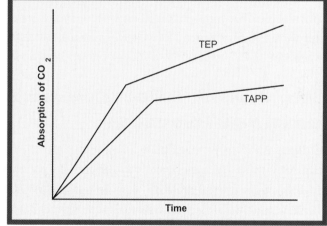

Fig. 13.4: Comparison of absorption of CO_2 in TEP and TAPP

Another mechanism suggested by Glascock et al. is the direct intravascular absorption of CO_2 which may be facilitated by the disruption of microvascular and lymphatic channels during the development of the TEP working space.[14] The resorptive surface can increase with time as subcutaneous emphysema develops and spreads, which would explain why one observes a steady increase in CO_2 absorption during insufflation period in the TEP procedures.

In an animal model, absorption from peritoneum decreases after insufflation pressure increases above a certain level. It is less at the commonly used pressure of 14-18 mmHg (TAPP, IPOM repair) than at 12-15 mmHg (TEP repair) probably due to a reduction in the capillary blood flow.[15] The resulting acidosis lowers the threshold for arrhythmias. However, haemodynamic alteration occurs only when partial pressure of CO_2 ($PaCO_2$) is increased by 30 per cent above the normal limit.[10]

In patients undergoing TAPP hernioplasty the total CO_2 elimination increased during the first 20 minutes after beginning of insufflation by a mean of 46 per cent more than baseline and then remained constant. VE had to be increased by an average of 35 per cent to maintain normocapnia.[13]

Endtidal CO_2 often underestimates arterial CO_2 during laparoscopic surgery and the inaccuracy increases with the duration of insufflation.[16,17]

The data of Sumpf et al show that CO_2 absorption can vary widely both intra and inter individually in patients undergoing TEP hernioplasty.[13] They recorded two instances when it was so rapid, that it was not possible to maintain normocapnia without incurring risk of barotrauma. In these patients airway pressures reached 50 mmHg at VE of 30L/min at which point they did not increase ventilation any further but accepted hypercapnia instead. In patients with restrictive or obstructive lung disease such an upper limit could be reached even earlier. During the period from the end of insufflation to tracheal extubation there is a rapid decrease in CO_2 elimination. The apparent CO_2 absorption was only 30 ml/min 30-50 minutes after terminating insufflation even in patients with extensive subcutaneous emphysema. The rapid reduction of CO_2 elimination to such low levels was probably not caused solely by decrease in absorption or terminal elimination of residual CO_2 and it probably underestimates the true amount of CO_2 absorption. CO_2 retention was observed with an increase in arterial pCO_2 because of residual sufentanil effect. The increase was not however sufficient to pose a clinical risk.

CARBOPERITONEUM AND INCREASED INTRA-ABDOMINAL PRESSURE

An increase in the intra-abdominal pressure is the most important factor contributing to circulatory instability during laparoscopy.[18] Since TEP is performed without establishing carboperitoneum, the adverse effects of a raised IAP are not seen; unlike in TAPP and IPOM, which necessitate the establishment of carboperitoneum.[19]

REPERCUSSIONS OF PNEUMOPERITONEUM IN SPECIAL PATIENT GROUPS

PATIENT WITH CARDIAC DISEASE (TABLE 13.2)

The demonstration of significant haemodynamic changes during pneumoperitoneum raises the question of tolerance of these changes by cardiac patients. In patients with mild to severe cardiac disease the pattern of the change in mean arterial pressure, cardiac output and systemic vascular resistance is qualitatively similar to that in healthy patients.[20-26] Quantitatively, these changes appear to be more marked. In a study including ASA III-IV patients, SvO_2 decreased in 50 per cent of patients despite perioperative haemodynamic optimisation using a pulmonary artery catheter.[23] Patients who experienced the most severe haemodynamic changes with inadequate oxygen delivery were patients with low preoperative cardiac output and central venous pressure and high mean

Table 13.2: Anaesthetic considerations in patients with cardiac disease

1.	Haemodynamic consequences of ↑ IAP seen in TAPP, IPOM; not seen in TEP
2.	Change in mean arterial pressure, cardiac output and systemic vascular resistance more marked in patients with cardiac disease.
3.	Right atrial pressure and pulmonary artery occlusion pressures are not reliable indices of cardiac filling pressures during pneumoperitoneum.
4.	Congestive heart failure can develop in early postoperative period.
5.	Low intra-abdominal pressure and low insufflation rates cause minimal haemodynamic changes.

arterial pressure and systemic vascular resistance (a profile suggesting depleted intravascular volume). The author suggests preoperative preload augmentation to offset the haemodynamic effects of pneumoperitoneum. Intravenous nitroglycerin and nicardipine have been used to manage the haemodynamic changes induced by increased IAP in selected patients with heart disease.[22,25,27] Nitroglycerin was chosen to correct reduction in cardiac output associated with increased pulmonary capillary occlusion pressures and systemic vascular resistance. The administration of nicardipine may be more appropriate than that of nitroglycerin. Right atrial and pulmonary capillary occlusion pressures are not reliable indices of cardiac filling pressures during pneumoperitoneum. Increased afterload is a major contributor to the altered haemodynamics seen during pneumoperitoneum in cardiac patients. Nicardipine acts selectively on arterial resistance vessels and does not compromise venous return.[28] Finally this drug is beneficial in case of congestive heart failure.[29,30] Since normalisation of haemodynamic variables does not occur for at least 1 hour postoperatively in certain patients, congestive heart failure can develop in the early postoperative period,[21,26] Dhoste et al did not observe impaired haemodynamics in elderly ASAIII patients but used low intraperitoneal pressures (10 mmHg) and low insufflation rates (1L/min).[31]

PULMONARY DISEASE (TABLE 13.3)

Many adult patients requiring hernia repair have either chronic obstructive or restrictive lung disease, which can impair increase in alveolar ventilation required to eliminate additional CO_2.[4] Upper abdominal surgery results in postoperative changes in pulmonary function. Greater reductions in volumes and slower recovery of pulmonary function after laparoscopy are reported in older, obese patients, smokers and patients with COPD than in healthy patients.[32] Postoperative pulmonary function of these patients however is improved after laparoscopy as compared with laparotomy.[34-40]

Table 13.3: Anaesthetic considerations in patients with pulmonary disease

1. Postoperative pulmonary dysfunction is more significant in patients with COPD, smokers, obese, elderly
2. Postoperative pulmonary dysfunction less after laparoscopy as compared with open surgery.
3. TEP can be performed under regional anaesthesia.
4. Patients with pulmonary disease at risk of significant hypercapnia acidosis and barotrauma.
5. CO_2 absorption less with TAPP approach but greater reduction in pulmonary compliance

The TEP approach to inguinal hernias offers the advantages that the peritoneum is not opened and the procedure is often faster and can be performed under regional anaesthesia. The data of Sumpf at al shows that CO_2 absorption is much higher with this approach and that patients with pulmonary pathology can be at a risk of significant hypercapnia. The increase in VË to prevent hypercapnia particularly in the presence of subcutaneous emphysema, might be impossible to sustain or achieve even with mechanical ventilation especially in patients with preoperative pulmonary dysfunction. In case, regional anaesthesia is given then the increase in VË to prevent hypercapnia would be unpleasant for the spontaneously breathing patient. If opioids are used for sedation then the VE may not match the hypercapnia due to the reduced sensitivity of the respiratory centre to CO_2 (opioid effect). CO_2 absorption is consistently lower in the TAPP approach. However, the technique has the disadvantage that it is an intra-abdominal operation requiring general anaesthesia and that the reduction in the pulmonary compliance is greater than in the TEP technique.

PAEDIATRIC PATIENTS

Endohernia repair has been performed in paediatric patients especially in recurrent inguinal hernia and for evaluation of contralateral hernia. The various anaesthetics concerns are discussed in detail in the chapter on laparoscopy in paediatric patients

CHOICE OF ANAESTHETIC TECHNIQUE

Endohernia repair has been performed under general, regional (spinal, epidural, combined spinal epidural) and local anaesthesia. All the standards for inpatient anaesthesia should be followed.

A thorough pre-anaesthetic assessment with optimisation of the cardiac and pulmonary status is essential. The aim of the anaesthesiologist is to provide excellent intraoperative condition, ensure patient safety, decrease the incidence of adverse effects and to ensure rapid recovery and early return to daily activities.

PREMEDICATION

A short acting anxiolytic allays anxiety and speeds recovery. The medications the patient is receiving for co-existing diseases are continued till the morning of the surgery. An antiemetic and H_2 receptor antagonist reduce post-operative nausea and vomiting (PONV) [41], as well as the volume and pH of gastric secretions. Pre-emptive analgesia may be achieved with non-steroidal anti-inflammatory drugs (NSAIDs), as opioids are associated with PONV.

MONITORING (TABLE 13.4)

Meticulous monitoring is essential for safe conduct of laparoscopic procedures. With the growing trend towards minimally invasive procedures and their potential benefits in the postoperative period (less pain and early return to normal activity) more and more of ASA III-IV patients are presenting for laparoscopic procedures. Mandatory monitoring is done of the following: - pulse oximetry, noninvasive blood pressure, electrocardiogram, $EtCO_2$, insufflation pressure and airway pressure. In patients with chronic obstructive pulmonary disease and asthma estimation of arterial blood gas may be required.[42] A sizeable $PaCO_2$-$PetCO_2$ does not obviate the value of $PetCO_2$ for physiologic monitoring. A rise in $PetCo_2$ still indicates a rise in $PaCO_2$, but one cannot equate the numerical value of $PetCO_2$ with $PaCO_2.$ If one or two comparisons are available between $PetCO_2$ and $PaCO_2,$ the difference between the two values can be established and provided the patient remains clinically stable, the $PetCO_2$ reflects the $PaCO_2$.

Table 13.4: Monitoring for laparoscopic repair of hernias

Mandatory	Desirable	Optional
Pulse oximetry (SpO_2),Non-invasive blood pressure (NIBP), Electrocardiogram Capnography ($EtCO_2$), Insufflation pressure and airway pressure	ABG (COPD, long procedures) Urine output] Long procedures Temperature Side-stream spirometry with breath by breath analysis of dynamic compliance BIS (Bispectral Index) Esophageal stethoscope	Pulmonary capillary wedge pressure (PCWP).

Side stream spirometry when available is most useful in detecting complications during laparoscopy. It illustrates breath-by-breath changes of dynamic compliance as a transformation of a graphic loop. It is very useful in detection of pneumothorax.

Finally one cannot underscore the importance of clinical monitoring of reduced an entry, hyper-resonance, swelling or crepitus to diagnose tube migration, pneumothorax or emphysema.

GENERAL ANAESTHESIA

As for all laparoscopic procedures general anaesthesia with endotracheal intubation and controlled ventilation remains the preferred technique for endoscopic hernia repair. The technique provides good muscle relaxation, ability to control hypercarbia, protection from aspiration of gastric contents and optimal surgical conditions.[43] Atropine is administered at induction to prevent bradycardia, which may occur due to peritoneal stretching at insufflation (during TAPP, IPOM repair).

Propofol is a popular induction agent since it is associated with rapid, clear headed recovery and reduced incidence of PONV. The muscle relaxants are chosen from the intermediate or short acting group depending upon the patients coexisting problems. Intra-operative analgesia may be provided with short acting opioids; however NSAIDs are suitable alternatives.

Recovery from anaesthesia should be rapid with minimal residual effects. Sevoflurane or isoflurane ensure rapid recovery with minimal PONV. They show the least tendency to produce arrhythmias in the presence of increased catecholamines due to hypercapnia. Intraoperative administration of intravenous metoclopramide, droperidol or ondansetron before completion of surgery prevents PONV.[45] All patients should be administered O_2 postoperatively since slow release of CO_2 from tissues may result in hypoxia.[46]

In cases a difficult airway is encountered, the proseal LMA offers an alternative to endotracheal intubation. Due to an additional channel for drainage of the stomach it provides better protection from aspiration than the classical LMA.[47]

REGIONAL ANAESTHESIA

Although general anaesthesia is the preferred technique for endoscopic procedures they may also be conducted under regional anaesthesia.[48,49] Creation of carboperitoneum in patients breathing spontaneously under epidural anaesthesia results in an increase in minute ventilation with an unchanged $EtCO_2$.[50] Epidural anaesthesia provides excellent postoperative analgesia, lower incidence of PONV and no sequelae of general anaesthesia such as sore throat, muscle pain and airway trauma. Therefore, it may be the anaesthesia of choice for patients in whom general anaesthesia is contraindicated.

However, laparoscopic procedures under regional anaesthesia may cause problems. Sympathetic block may enhance the development of vagal reflexes. Anaesthesia is required upto T_8 dermatomal level and referred shoulder tip pain is often present, adequate intraoperative sedation is essential, which may be achieved with midazolam, fentanyl or propofol infusion (4-6 ml/kg/hr) titrated as per the patients response. Sedation given in conjunction with regional block, decreases the sensitivity of the respiratory centre to hypercarbia. The combined effect of carboperitoneum and sedation can lead to respiratory acidosis and finally to disorientation and hypoxia.[51]

Nitrous oxide (N_2O) is better as an insufflation gas when the procedure is to be conducted under regional anaesthesia, since it produces minimal irritation of the peritoneal cavity.[52] Helium insufflation is a reasonable alternative in patients at risk for CO_2 retention.[53]

Since TEP is an entirely extraperitoneal procedure with infraumbilical ports, it can be successfully accomplished under regional anaesthesia (Fig. 13.5).

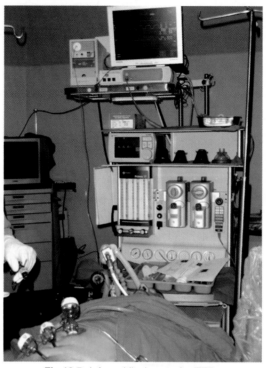

Fig.13.5: Infraumblical ports for TEP

Spinal, epidural or combined spinal-epidural anaesthesia may be given as per patient's condition and duration of the procedure.

SPINAL ANAESTHESIA

It is quick in onset and provides excellent analgesia. However, urinary retention or delay in the return of normal lower urinary sensations may delay discharge from the hospital. Spinal anaesthesia with a low dose of lignocaine or bupivacaine along with a small dose of fentanyl citrate provides adequate analgesia with minimal motor blockade.

EPIDURAL ANAESTHESIA

It is slow in onset. Since the epidural local anaesthetic is given in titrated doses and a segmental block can be achieved, the magnitude of sympathetic blockade is less as compared to spinal anaesthesia. The ability to extend the duration of the block with epidural supplementation is an advantage.

COMBINED SPINAL AND EPIDURAL ANAESTHESIA

Offers advantages of both, the spinal and the epidural injection.

LOCAL ANAESTHESIA

Ilioinguinal and iliohypogastric block can be used for inguinal herniorrhaphy. Supplementation with a genitofemoral nerve block may be necessary (Fig. 13.6).

Repair of small direct inguinal hernia (TEP) can be performed under local block. Since the patient may experience discomfort during manipulation of the contents of the hernial sac, a very gentle surgical technique is essential.[54] A relaxed cooperative patient is essential for the procedure to be conducted under local anaesthesia.[55]

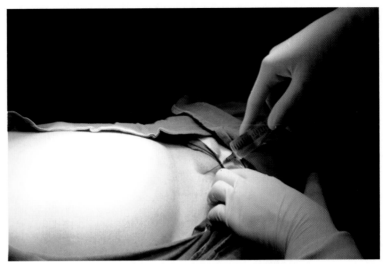

Fig. 13.6: Bilateral Inguinal block for TEP repair

COMPLICATIONS

Some complications that commonly occur during endoscopic repair of hernia are described below.

SUBCUTANEOUS EMPHYSEMA

Subcutaneous emphysema can develop as a complication of accidental extraperitoneal insufflation but can also be considered as an effect of certain laparoscopic surgical procedures that require intentional extraperitoneal insufflation such as inguinal hernia repair and pelvic lymphadenectomy. In these circumstances $\dot{V}CO_2$ and consequently $PaCO_2$ and $PetCO_2$ increase. Therefore, any increase in $PetCO_2$ occuring after $PetCO_2$ has plateaued should suggest this complication.[56] The increase in VCO_2 may be such that prevention of hypercapnia by adjustment of ventilation becomes almost impossible. In this case laparoscopy must be temporarily interrupted to allow CO_2 elimination and can be resumed after correction of hypercapnia using a lower insufflation pressure. CO_2 pressure determines the extent of the emphysema and the magnitude of CO_2 absorption. CO_2 emphysema will readily resolve once insufflation has ceased. CO_2 subcutaneous emphysema, even cervical, does not contraindicate tracheal extubation at the end of surgery. It is recommended to keep the patient under controlled mechanical ventilation until hypercapnia is corrected, particularly in COPD patients to avoid an excessive increases in work of breathing.

Mediastinal cervical, subcutaneous and pharyngeal emphysema may result if CO_2 tracks along inguinal blood vessels, through the retroperitoneum, into the mediastinum and is then decompressed into the soft tissues of the neck.

PNEUMOTHORAX

Pneumothorax is a rare complication of laparoscopic herniorrhaphy.[57,58] It may be related to high insufflation pressure and duration of the procedure. However it has also been reported after 35 minutes of surgery when the insufflation pressure was kept at 12 mm of Hg.[59]

When pneumothorax is caused by a highly diffusible gas such as N_2O or CO_2 without associated pulmonary trauma, spontaneous resolution occurs within 30 to 60 minutes after exsufflation. The following guidelines are provided when pneumothorax develops during laparoscopy:

1. Stop N$_2$O administration
2. Adjust ventilator settings to correct hypoxaemia
3. Apply positive end expiratory pressure
4. Reduce IAP as much as possible
5. Maintain close communication with the surgeon
6. Avoid thoracocentesis unless necessary, as pneumothorax will spontaneously resolve after exsufflation

In case of pneumothorax secondary to rupture of pre-existing bullae, PEEP must not be applied and thoracocentesis is mandatory. [20]

Complications that may occur after any general laparoscopic procedure may also be seen during endohernia repair. Vascular injuries particularly to large vessels (aorta, inferior vena cava and iliac vessels) and gastrointestinal organs may occur during Veress needle insertion or trocar placement. Unrecognised gastrointestinal injuries can lead to potentially lethal septic complications. Other complications include gas embolism, arrhythmias, aspiration, endobronchial intubation, etc.

CONCLUSIONS

CLINICAL PEARLS

1. Extraperitoneal absorption more than intraperitoneal
2. Recommended anaesthesia technique is GA with controlled ventilation
3. TEP may be conducted under regional anaesthesia

REFERENCES

1. Nathaniel J. Soper, L Michael Brunt, Kurt Kerbl. Laparoscopic General surgery. The New England Journal of Medicine. 1994 Volume 330: 409-419.
2. Ger R. The management of certain abdominal herniae by intra-abdominal closure of the neck of the sac. Ann R Coll Surg Eng 1982; 64:342-44.
3. David L. Crawford and Edward H. Phillips. Laparoscopic hernia repair-Indications and Contraindications In: Bruce V. Macfadyen Jr ed. Laparoscopic surgery of the abdomen. Springer 273-9.
4. Gill BD, Traverso LW, Continuous quality inventory; open versus laparoscopic groin hernia repair. Surg Endosc 1993; 7:116-116. (Abstract)
5. Cunningham AJ, Brull SJ. Laparoscopic cholecystectomy. Anaesthetic implications. Anesth Analg 1993; 76:1120-33.
6. Safran DB, Orlando R. Physiological effects of pneumoperitoneum. Am J Surg 1994; 167:281.
7. Makinen MT, Yli-Hankala A. Respiratory compliance during laparoscopic hiatal and inguinal hernia repair. Can J Anaesth 1998; 45:865.
8. Joris JL, Noirot DP, Legrand MJ, Jacquet NJ, Lamy ML. Haemodynamic changes during laparoscopic cholecystectomy. Anesth Analg 1993; 76:1067-71.
9. Uhlich GA. Laparoscopy. The question of the proper gas. Gastrointest Endosc 1982; 28: 212-13.
10. Magno R, Medegard A, Bengtsson R, Tronstad SE. Acid-base balance during laparoscopy. Acta Obstet Gynecol Scand 1979; 58:81.
11. Mullet CE, Viale JP, Sagnard PE, Miallet CC, Ruynat LG, Counioux HC. Pulmonary CO$_2$ elimination during surgical procedures using intra- or extraperitoneal CO$_2$ insufflation. Anesth Analg 1993; 76:622-6.
12. Wolf JS Jr, Monk TG, McDougall EM, McClennan BL, Clayman RV. The extraperitoneal approach and subcutaneous emphysema are associated with greater absorption of carbon dioxide during laparoscopic renal surgery. J Urol 1995; 154:959-63.
13. Sumpf E, Crozier TA, Ahrens D, Brauer A, Neufang T, Braun U. Carbon dioxide absorption during extra peritoneal and transperitoneal endoscopic hernioplasty. Anesth Analg 2000; 91:589-95.

14. Glascock JM, Winfield HN, Lund GO, Donovan JF, Ping ST, Griffiths DL. Carbon dioxide homeostasis during transperitoneal or extraperitoneal laparoscopic pelvic lymphadenectomy. Endourology 1996; 10: 319-23.

15. Blobner M, Bogdanski R, Jelen Esselborn S. Visceral absorption of intra-abdominal insufflated carbon dioxide in swine. Anaesthesiol Intensivmed Notfallmed Schmerzther 1999; 34:94-9.

16. Wahba RW, Mamazza J. Ventilatory requirements during laparoscopic cholecystectomy. Can J anaesth 1993; 40(3): 206-10.

17. Reid CW, Martineare RJ, Miller DR et al. A comparison of transcutaneous, end-tidal and arterial measurements of carbon dioxide during general anaesthesia. Can J Anaesth 1992; 39:31-6.

18. Ishizaki Y, Bandai Y, Shimomura K, Abe H, Ohtomo Y, Idezuki Y. Changes in splanchnic blood flow and cardiovascular effects following peritoneal insufflation of carbon dioxide. Surg; Endosc 1993; 7:420-3.

19. Andrus CR, Naunheim KS, Wittgen CM. Anaesthetic considerations. In: MacFadyen BV Jr (ed). Operative laparoscopy and thoracoscopy. Philadelphia: Lippincott-Raven and Ponsky JL Publishers; 1996; 18-20.

20. Jean L, Joris. Anesthesia for laparoscopic surgery In: Ronald D. Miller ed. Anesthesia. Philadelphia. Churchill Livingstone. 2000; 2003-23.

21. Harris SN, Ballantyne GH, Luther MA et al. Alterations of cardiovascular performance during laparoscopic colectomy: A combined haemodynamic and electrographic analysis Anesth Analg 1996; 83: 482.

22. Feig BNW, Berger DH, Dougherty TB et al. Pharmacologic intervention can establish baseline haemodynamic parameters during laparoscopy Surgery 1994; 116: 733.

23. Safran D, Sgambati S, Orlando R. Laparoscopy in high risk cardiac patients. Surg Gynecol Obstet 1993; 176; 548.

24. Iwase K, Takenaka H, Yagura A et al. Haemodynamic changes during laparoscopic cholecystectomy in patients with heart disease. Endoscopy 1992; 24:771.

25. Hein HA, Joshi GP, Ramsay MA et al. Haemodynamic changes during laparoscopic cholecystectomy in patients with severe cardiac disease. J Clin Anesth 1997; 9: 261.

26. Portera CA, Compton RP, Walters DN et al. Benefits of pulmonary artery catheter and transesophageal echo cardiographic montorines in laparoscopic cholecystectomy patients with cardiac disease. Am J Surg 1995; 169: 202.

27. Duale C, Bazin JE, Ferrier C et al. Haemodynamic effects of laparoscopic cholecystectomy in patients with coronary disease. Br J Anaesth 1994; 72 (Suppl 51): A31.

28. Pepine CL, Lambert CR. Cardiovascular effects of nicardipine Angiology 1990; 41: 978.

29. Aroney CN, Semigran MJ, Dec GW et al. Inotropic effect of nicardipine in patients with heart failure. Assessment by left ventricular end-systolic pressure volume analysis. J Am Coll Cardiol 1989; 14: 1331.

30. Burlew BS, Gheorghiade M, Jafri SN et al. Acute and chronic hemodynamic effects of nicardipine hydrochloride in patients with heart failure Am Heart J. 1987; 114: 793.

31. Dhoste K, Lacoste L, Karayah J et al. Haemodynamic and ventilatory changes during laparoscopic cholecystectomy in elderly ASA III patients. Can J Anaesth 1996; 43: 783.

32. Wilcox S, Vandam LD. Poor Trendelenberg and his position. Anaesth Analg 1988; 67:574.

33. Lumb AB, Nunn JF. Respiratory function and ribcage contribution to ventilation in body position commonly used during anesthesia. Anesth Analg 1991; 73:422.

34. Joris J, Cigarini I, Legrand Met al. Metabolic and respiratory changes after cholecystectomy performed via laparotomy or laparoscopy. Br J Anaesth 1992; 69:341.

35. Wahba RWM, Beique F, Kleiman SJ. Cardiopulmonary function and laparoscopic cholecystectomy. Can J Anesth 1995; 42:51.

36. Mealy K, Gallagher H, Barry M et al. Physiological and metabolic responses to open and laparoscopic cholecystectomy. Br J Surg 1992; 79:1061.

37. Putensen-Himmer G, Putensen C, Lammer H et al. Comparison of postoperative respiratory function after laparoscopy or open laparotomy for cholecystectomy. Anesthesiology 1992; 77: 675.

38. McMohon AJ, Russell IT, Ramsay G et al. Laparoscopic and minilapartomy cholecystectomy. A randomized trial comparing postoperative pain and pulmonary function. Surgery 1994; 115:533.

39. Frazee R, Roberts J, Okeson G. Open versus laparoscopic cholecystectomy. A comparison of postoperative pulmonary function. Ann Surg 1991; 213:651.

40. Freeman J, Armstrong I. Pulmonary function tests before and after laparoscopic cholecystectomy. Anaesthesia 1994; 49: 579.

41. Chui PT, Oh TE. Anaesthesia for laparoscopic general surgery. Anaesth Intensive Care 1993; 21:163.

42. Wittgen CM, Andrus CH, Fitzgerald SD. Analysis of the haemodynamic and ventilatory effects of laparoscopic cholecystectomy. Arch Surg 1991; 126:997.

43. Brichant JF. Anaesthesia for minimally invasive abdominal surgery. In: Adams AP, Cashman IN (eds). Recent advances in anaesthesia and analgesia, Vol. 19. London: Churchill Livingstone; 1995: 33-49.

44. Harris MNE, Plantevin OM, Crowther A. Cardiac arrhythmias during anaesthesia for laparoscopy. Br J Anaesth 1984; 56: 1213-17.

45. Raphael JH, Norton AC. Antiemetic efficacy of prophylactic ondansetron in laparoscopic surgery: Randomized double-blind comparison with metoclopramide. Br J Anaesth 1993; 71:845.

46. Vegfors M, Cederholm I, Lenmarken C, Lofstrom JB. Should oxygen be administered after laparoscopy in healthy patients? Acta Anaesthesiol Scand 1988; 32:350-2.

47. Maltby JR, Beriault MT, Watson NC, Leipert DJ, Fick GH. LMA-Classic and LM-ProSeal are effective alternatives to endotracheal intubation for gynaecological laparoscopy. Can J Anaesth 2003; 50:71-7.

48. Pursnani KG. Laparoscopic cholecystectomy under epidural anaesthesia in patients with chronic respiratory disease. Surg Endosc 1998; 12:1082-4.

49. Chowbey PK, Sood J, Vashistha A, Sharma A, Khullar R, Soni V, et al. Extraperitoneal endoscopic groin hernia repair under epidural anaesthesia. Surg Laparosc Endosc Percutan Tech 2003; 13: 185-90.

50. Ciofolo MJ, Clergue F, Seebacher J, Lefebvre G, Viars P. Ventilatory effects of laparoscopy under epidural anaesthesia. Anesth Analg. 1990; 70:357-61.

51. Brady CE, Harkleroad LE, Pierson WP. Alteration in oxygen saturation and ventilation after IV sedation for peritoneoscopy. Arch Intern Med 1989; 149:1029.

52. Ferzli GS, Dysarz FA. Extraperitoneal endoscopic inguinal herniorrhaphy performed without carbon dioxide insufflation. J Lap Surg 1994; 4:301-4.

53. Fitzgerald SD, Andrus CH, Baudendistal LJ, Dahms TE, Kaminski DL. Hypercarbia during carbon dioxide pneumoperitoneum. Am J Surg 1992; 163:186-9.

54. Ferzli GS, Massad A, Albert P. Extraperitoneal endoscopic inguinal hernia repair. J Laparoendosc Surg 1992; 2:281-6.

55. Collins LM, Vaghadia H. Regional anaesthesia for laparoscopy Anesthesiology Clinics of North America. Number I, Vol. 19. WB Saunders Company; 2001:44-7.

56. Klopfenstein CE, Mamie C, Forster A. Laparoscopic extraperitoneal inguinal hernia complicated by subcutaneous emphysema. Can J Anaesth 1995; 42:523-5.

57. Chien GL, Soifer BE. Pharyngeal emphysema with airway obstruction as a consequence of laparoscopic inguinal herniorrhaphy. Anesth Analg 1995; 80:201-3.

58. Ferzli GS, Kiel T, Hurwitz JB, Davidson P, Piperno B, Fiorillo MA, et al. Pneumothorax as a complication of laparoscopic inguinal hernia repair. Surg Endosc 1997; 11: 152-3.

59. Toyoshima Y, Tsuchida H, Namiki A. Pneumothoran during extrapentoneal heniorrhaphy. Anaesthesiology 1998; 89:4.

Anaesthesia for Ambulatory Laparoscopic Surgery

INTRODUCTION

Laparoscopy has now become a common surgical procedure to be carried out on a day care basis. Inspection of the abdominal cavity through an endoscope was initially started by the gynecologists but greater application of laparoscopy has taken place since general surgeons adopted this procedure for diagnostic and therapeutic purposes. To this was later added the facility of using video camera which enabled the use of instruments with both hands while an assistant controlled the camera. The use of more efficient lighting techniques is helping to reduce surgical trauma /discomfort thereby widening the scope of laparoscopy. The potential of laparoscopic surgery has expanded exponentially with the development of specialized instruments and greater acceptability of laparoscopic procedures and has even led to the development of the speciality called "Minimal Invasive Surgery" or more preferably "Minimal Access Surgery."

Laparoscopic surgery performed on a day care basis presents several challenges for the anaesthesiologist. There are the usual problems of preoperative evaluation, rapid recovery, early ambulation, postoperative pain relief, and control of adverse side effects that are associated with any outpatient procedure. Postoperative nausea and vomiting (PONV) can be especially problematic after laparoscopic surgery, after rapid ambulation.

Laparoscopic procedures require the establishment of a pneumoperitoneum to assist trocar insertion and provide an adequate view. This can compromise cardiovascular and respiratory function and contribute to postoperative pain. Most laparoscopic procedures also require that the patient be tilted either head down (for pelvic procedures) or head up (for upper abdominal surgery). These patient positions can further compromise cardiac and respiratory function, increase the risk of regurgitation, and even result in nerve injuries.[1] These complications occur mostly with the prolonged duration of surgery and are relatively rare when laparoscopy is mainly confined to brief gynaecologic procedures in healthy patients. The complications are more likely with longer and more complex surgery performed in older and less fit patients.

PREOPERATIVE EVALUATION

The preoperative evaluation of the patient for laparoscopy should encompass the same elements as for an open procedure (Fig. 14.1).

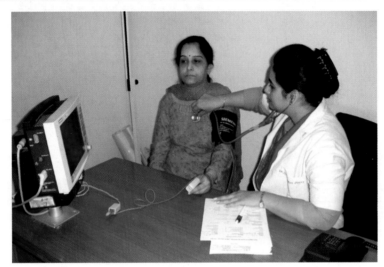

Fig. 14.1: Preoperative assessment clinic

Many patients scheduled for laparoscopic surgery will be admitted a few hours before the scheduled time for surgery. Some of these patients may have been assessed earlier, while others are seen for the first time by the attending anaesthesiologist.

As laparoscopy has moved from the young, healthy patient to a more diverse population, the presence of chronic medical conditions has increased. For certain groups of patients, like those with increased intracranial pressure, ventricular or peritoneal shunts, pneumoperitoneum and laparoscopy are contraindicated on ambulatory basis. Again, patients with congestive heart failure may not be good candidates for day care laparoscopy.

Patients with cardiac disease need to be assessed about the capacity to withstand the haemodynamic changes seen with pneumoperitoneum and this must be weighed against the possibility of a more benign postoperative course offered by a laparoscopic procedure in comparison to an open procedure. Cardiac consultation, as well as echocardiography should be done where appropriate. In patients with reduced left ventricular ejection fraction, the option of invasive monitoring should be considered. Such patients will require continued monitoring postoperatively and probably not be candidates for same day discharge.

Laparoscopy is occasionally indicated for pregnant patients. The likelihood of first trimester miscarriage increases with surgery. The incidence of premature delivery also increases with surgery in late pregnancy. These risks should be fully explained to the patients and recorded.

HIGH-RISK GROUP FOR DAY CARE LAPAROSCOPY

Patients who are marginal candidates or high risk for open laparotomy are now being offered laparoscopic surgery. These are clinical conditions, which pose greater risk for laparoscopic surgery, therefore should be assessed preoperatively for suitability for day care surgery. Chest diseases and ischaemic heart disease need a special mention here.

Respiratory Diseases

In chronic obstructive disease $EtCO_2$ and $PaCO_2$ do not correlate. The changes in $PaCO_2$ are much larger than the changes $EtCO_2$, due to increasing V/Q mismatch. There is increased shunt as well as physiological dead space with pneumoperitoneum.[2,3] Increase in dead space also occurs when airway pressure becomes high in the presence of *severe chest disease* or when cardiac output is reduced.[4] Such patients may be good candidates for laparoscopy but may not be suitable as day care patients as they require continued monitoring in the post operative period.

Ischaemic Heart Disease

Coronary artery disease is associated with higher morbidity.[5,6] Preoperative evaluation is of paramount importance to identify major risk factors. Only patients with stable coronary disease should be considered for day care laparoscopy. Those who have undergone coronary revascularization with absence of symptoms are usually considered suitable. They have a much lower complication rate compared with their matched counterparts.[7,8] The management of ischaemic heart disease patients rests on prevention of myocardial ischaemia and cardiac dysfunction. Oxygen desaturation and hypotension are detrimental to myocardial O_2 supply and should be avoided.

Pneumoperitoneum reduces venous return and cardiac output, which is further aggravated by reverse Trendelenburg position. Patients with limited cardiac reserve may not be able to compensate for these maneuvers.[9]

High intraabdominal pressure during pneumoperitoneum has adverse haemodynamic effects in patients with coronary artery disease. This can be circumvented to an extent by using low pressure during pneumoperitoneum, not exceeding 10 cms H_2O, or by using laparo lift whereby the anterior abdominal wall is lifted up by specially designed retractors without the use of pneumoperitoneum. The major drawback of this gasless method of laparoscopy is diminished visibility, which could prolong surgical time. But this does have beneficial post operative respiratory and haemodynamic effects.[10,11]

Obesity

Laparoscopy may offer the surgeon a better view in obese patients compared with that obtained during laparotomy. The other advantage of laparoscopy is rapid recovery and quick return of respiratory functions to preoperative levels. However, intraoperative problems are possible due to reduced cardiac and respiratory reserve which these patients possess.[12] The intra-abdominal pressures required to raise the abdominal wall of a morbidly obese patient is significantly higher, which may result in gross reduction in cardiac output besides reduction in functional residual capacity and elevation in dead space. Intraoperatively these patients may require intensive monitoring of respiratory and haemodynamic functions which should be continuous and invasive.

Pregnancy once thought to be a contraindication for laparoscopic surgery may actually be better because of the improved view of structures with laparoscopic approach. Uteroplacental blood flow may be compromised due to reduction in venous return related to raised intra-abdominal pressure and reverse Trendelenburg position. Continuous maternal and fetal monitoring is mandatory during laparoscopic procedures. Major surgery in presence of pregnancy is contraindicated as a day care procedure, as there is need to monitor fetus postoperatively for a variable period.

PREMEDICATION

As a rule, sedative premedication is avoided except in the very young and in apprehensive patients. Agent to be used is selected with rapid emergence and early discharge in mind. Of the benzodiazepines, midazolam is a better choice because of the short elimination half-life (Table 14.1).

Table 14.1: Benzodiazepines for anxiolysis

Drug	Half life (hours)
Alprazolam	12-15
Diazepam	48
Lorazepam	10-22
Midazolam	1.7-2.6
Temazepam	10-21

Narcotics are used in painful conditions only, and that too in smaller dosages thereby reducing the incidence of nausea and prolonged emergence. An antisialagogue is often helpful, if not contraindicated. Atropine and scopolamine cross the blood-brain barrier and can cause postoperative delirium. Glycopyrrolate is preferred as it does not cross the blood brain barrier, but atropine remains the drug of choice for the treatment of severe bradycardia.

In patients with an increased risk of regurgitation, consider the preoperative administration of antacids, H_2 receptor antagonists such as ranitidine and gastroprokinetic agents like metoclopramide. Prophylactic use of medications for decreasing the risk of aspiration in all patients is controversial. This does entail cost as well as possibility of side effects of the drugs themselves. Inspite of this, most anaesthesiologists still use medications for aspiration prophylaxis to avoid possibility of legal action in the event of adverse outcome. In high risk group of patients like hiatus hernia, obesity, pregnancy, these medications must be used. Most antihypertensive drugs are taken preoperatively with sips of water on the morning of surgery.

PNEUMOPERITONEUM

The creation of a pneumoperitoneum gives rise to several considerations unique to laparoscopic surgery. The abdominal cavity is insufflated with carbon dioxide (CO_2) and the patient is in a Trendelenburg position, both of which create respiratory and haemodynamic changes. In other surgical procedures like cholecystectomy, reverse Trendelenburg position is used, which can cause pooling of blood and thereby lowering cardiac output.

Misplacement of the *Veress* needle or trocar can produce acute hemorrhage, perforation of bowel or bladder, pneumothorax, pneumopericardium or gas embolism.[13,14] Prompt detection is obviously important but can be hindered by the significant physiologic changes that normally accompany laparoscopy. Understanding these changes helps in distinguishing normal from abnormal responses.

To achieve a pneumoperitoneum, CO_2 is insufflated at abdominal pressures of 10 to 15 mmHg. The increased intra-abdominal pressure leads to a decrease in total lung compliance and functional residual capacity (FRC), resulting in basal atelectasis and increased airway pressure. The *result is mismatch in ventilation/perfusion* (V/Q) in many lung units. In addition, insufflation of CO_2 also increases CO_2 absorption.[15] In a study of the ventilatory effects of laparoscopic surgery on patients under general anaesthesia,[16] it was found that there was an increase in CO_2 elimination after insufflation that continued until 10 minutes postdeflation of the abdomen. There was a corresponding rise in arterial CO_2 (PaCO$_2$) concentration. The PaCO$_2$ declined in the recovery period, which was consistent with a decrease in CO_2 production and an increase in the ability of a spontaneously breathing patient to eliminate CO_2. A mean difference between arterial and end-tidal CO_2 (EtCO$_2$) tension of 0.44 kPa has been reported with general and epidural anaesthesia.[17] The respiratory changes are less evident when laparoscopy is performed with the patients under regional anaesthesia. An increase in CO_2 concentration was not observed during laparoscopy in patients breathing spontaneously during epidural anaesthesia.[18] The creation of the pneumoperitoneum resulted in an increase in minute ventilation with an unchanged EtCO$_2$.[18] In contrast to general anaesthesia, the Trendelenburg position during epidural anesthesia did not lead to significant changes in ventilatory parameters. Despite the increase in respiratory work and V/Q mismatch, alveolar ventilation was not compromised, because the increase in minute ventilation reduced the respiratory effects of laparoscopy. Multiple studies have confirmed that arterial blood gases during laparoscopy under regional anaesthesia are maintained within normal limits.

Haemodynamic changes during laparoscopy have been studied mainly after induction of general anaesthesia and following CO_2 insufflation.[19] Increase in systemic vascular resistance and mean arterial pressure, and a decrease in cardiac index with minimal changes in heart rate is seen with pneumoperitoneum with CO_2. No change in mean arterial pressure or heart rate during Trendelenburg positioning or insufflation is found in patients undergoing epidural anaesthesia.

Haemodynamic effects of pneumoperitoneum are exaggerated if it is performed in Trendelenburg or reverse Trendelenburg position.[20] The patient's positioning should therefore be done after establishing pneumoperitoneum.

PATIENT POSITIONING

Great care should be taken in positioning patients in order to prevent nerve injuries. Adequate padding, especially of arms tucked at the patient's side, is needed to prevent ulnar nerve injury, and care must be taken in raising the foot of the operating room table at the conclusion of surgery to avoid entrapment of the fingers. If shoulder braces are used, they should be placed facing the coracoid process. Patients placed in the lithotomy position should not have their legs placed in exaggerated attitudes. The peroneal nerve must be adequately padded to protect from compression injury.

ANAESTHETIC TECHNIQUE

A variety of anaesthetic drugs are available for use in laparoscopic procedures, each offering various advantages. For procedures conducted on an outpatient basis, the choice of maintenance agent is likely to be reduced to shorter-acting drugs such as sevoflurane, desflurane, and infusions of propofol, fentanyl, remifentanil, sufentanil, etc.

The advantage with propofol is that it produces less postoperative nausea and vomiting (PONV) compared with inhalation anaesthetics. The PONV can interfere with fast –track recovery, although sevoflurane and desflurane were found to be superior to propofol, even when PONV was considered.[21] On the other hand, propofol has been used to treat PONV in intractable nausea and vomiting.

Intravenous anaesthetics though accepted to be the preferred route for induction of anaesthesia, can be more difficult to titrate compared with inhalation anaesthetics for maintenance of anaesthesia. Use of bispectral index (BIS), a possible monitor of depth of hypnosis, can help to reduce occurrence of awareness and titrate the depth of anaesthesia. This monitor has been used to titrate intravenous and inhaled anaesthetic drugs. Similarly BIS has been used to reduce the consumption of inhalational agents and facilitate early postoperative recovery.

Analgesia is an integral part of the general anesthetic technique and opioids are the most potent analgesics in use. Opioids are associated with significant PONV and are likely to result in perioperative awareness if the technique is predominantly opioids based.[22] Hence, supplementation of intravenous or inhalation-based anaesthesia with opioids is more appropriate. Morphine, though time tested has a prolonged duration of action and therefore is not ideal for short procedures. Remifentanil has the advantage that doses sufficient to produce analgesia and to modify cardiovascular responses to anaesthesia and surgery can be used without affecting the recovery. The risk of postoperative depression is minimal but it does not provide postoperative analgesia.

Table 14.2: Pharmacokinetic profile of common intravenous anaesthetic agents

	Propofol	Thiopentone	Methohexitone
VDss	2.09 L/kg	2.5 L/kg	2.2 L/kg
Cl (e)	28.3 ml/kg/min	3.4 ml/kg/min	7.0 ml/kg/min
α ½ **life**	1.81 min	2.4 min	2.2 min
β ½ **life**	24.2 min	11.6 hr	3.9 hr

INTRAVENOUS TECHNIQUES IN AMBULATORY ANAESTHESIA

In contrast to in- patients, day care patients are expected to return to the pre-operative state soon after surgery and every effort is made to make this period, from the end of surgery to getting back to the pre-operative state, as short as possible. Anaesthetic techniques should aim to provide patient comfort, reduce recovery time and length of stay. Intravenous agents can be used for induction and maintenance of anaesthesia as well.

Total intravenous anaesthesia (TIVA) involves induction and maintenance of anaesthesia with intravenous drugs alone. In TIVA, hypnosis can theoretically be achieved with many agents (barbiturates, benzodiazepines, etomidate, ketamine or propofol). Because of its superior pharmacokinetic and pharmacodynamic properties, propofol has gained increased popularity for TIVA in ambulatory surgery (Table 14.2). Propofol TIVA provides the ability to enhance patient satisfaction when compared with inhalational techniques, and results in a clinically relevant reduction in PONV when compared with isoflurane/nitrous oxide anaesthesia.[23] Intravenous anaesthesia is often associated with the administration of nitrous oxide; which does not delay recovery and may be used to decrease the requirement for the more expensive intravenous drugs. Nitrous oxide has been accused of increasing the incidence of PONV, but this assertion has been challenged.[24] Because nitrous oxide inhibits the NMDA receptor, it might reduce tolerance and hyperalgesia caused by opioid administration and thus improve postoperative pain control.[25]

TARGET-CONTROLLED INFUSION (TCI)

Computerized infusion systems are designed to achieve and to maintain any desired target blood concentration of drug appropriate for an individual patient and the level of surgical stimulation.[26] It takes into consideration the pharmacokinetic data of distribution and elimination of the intravenous agents. The agents commonly used for TCI are propofol and remifentanil. TCI rapidly achieves and maintains a predefined plasma or effect site concentration of the anesthetic drug. Appropriate target concentrations change with inter individual pharmacodynamic variability and the nature of the surgery. When an appropriate target concentration for achieving the desired clinical endpoint is chosen, TCI delivery systems perform better than manual systems.[27] For propofol, target concentration of 6 mcg/ml is required to prevent movement in response to surgical incision in 50 per cent of individuals when patient is breathing oxygen which is reduced to 4.5 mcg/ml when 67 per cent N_2O is used instead.

LIMITS OF INTRAVENOUS TECHNIQUES IN AMBULATORY PATIENTS

Intravenous techniques in ambulatory anaesthesia have limitations that need to be clearly understood to prevent their consequences.

The use of specific equipment, such as pumps able to deliver very low and very high infusion rates, is mandatory to ensure a proper titration of anaesthesia. Dead space between the stopcock and the indwelling catheter should be as small as possible, and a one-way valve will best avoid a backflow of the anaesthetic agent in the main infusion line. It is not possible with intravenous agents to keep the same syringe for successive patients and therefore wastage of drugs will frequently occur.

Other limitations are mainly the result of pharmacokinetic properties of the agents and to the fact that direct drug concentration measurements are not available. The relationships between infusion rates and adequate effect-site concentrations are not readily available and, even in the presence of predicted concentrations, a good understanding of the pharmacokinetic model implemented in the device is necessary to adapt the dosage to the individual patient. A good example is the elderly patient, in whom initial distribution of drugs is impaired, leading to concentrations higher than expected, and therefore to an increased incidence of overdosage at induction of anesthesia. This overdosage may increase the incidence of haemodynamic unwanted side effects.[28] Therefore, propofol induction doses should be reduced in elderly patients by approximately 40 per cent, even for achieving conscious sedation.[29] When using TCI, if age is not a covariate incorporated in the model used, the initial predicted concentrations will be grossly underestimated in elderly patient. One way to overcome this problem is to monitor spontaneous or evoked EEG parameters like Bispectral Index monitoring when titrating intravenous hypnotics.

In obese patients, changes in volume of distribution and redistribution of drugs after prolonged continuous infusions may lead to a significant accumulation. This may result in delay in awakening after prolonged surgery and therefore, continuous infusion of propofol may not be the optimal anaesthesia regimen for this group of patients.[30]

Table 14.3: Inhalational agents: Partition Coefficients of Inhalational agents at 37°C

	Blood / Gas	Brain / Blood	Fat / Blood
Nitrous oxide	0.47	1.1	23
Halothane	2.5	1.9	51
Isoflurane	1.49	1.6	45
Sevoflurane	0.69	1.7	48
Desflurane	0.42	1.3	27

Volatile anaesthetics are convenient in short day care procedures when compared to intravenous agents. The depth of anaesthesia can be varied rapidly and rapid elimination of the vapour provides faster recovery. Comparing blood gas (B/G) solubility of various agents, desflurane with B/G solubility of 0.42 has faster onset and recovery from its effect on discontinuation[31] (Table 14.3). With fat/blood solubility also much lower than other inhalational agents, there is less likelihood of accumulation of this vapour in fatty tissue on longer exposure. Intermediate recovery after desflurane is comparable with propofol based anaesthesia.[32] There is a greater incidence of headache after inhalational agents in laparoscopy patients when compared with narcotic and nitrous oxide based anaesthesia.[21] Postoperative nausea and vomiting is definitely more after inhalational agents compared with propofol based anaesthesia. It is mandatory therefore, that all patients undergoing laparoscopy using inhalational agents, have antiemetics given prophylactically irrespective of the duration of surgery.

AIRWAY CONTROL FOR LAPAROSCOPY IN DAYCARE

Most laparoscopy procedures are performed using controlled ventilation because pneumoperitoneum elevates the diaphragm compromising its movement. The effect is further aggravated if head down tilt and lithotomy position is used, as in pelvic surgery.

LARYNGEAL MASK AIRWAY (LMA) FOR LAPAROSCOPY

Compared with the tracheal tube, the LMA is easy to place, does not require muscle relaxation and laryngoscopy, and may prevent complications associated with tracheal intubation.[33] The LMA is tolerated at lower anaesthetic concentrations than the tracheal tube and therefore, allows titration of anaesthetic concentrations to the surgical stimulus rather than for airway tolerance. With the patient breathing spontaneously, opioid requirements can be based on the respiratory rate. Dosing requirements of hypnotic anaesthetics (IV or the inhaled) can be based on BIS values or recommended end-tidal concentrations of inhaled anaesthetics known to prevent awareness. This allows earlier emergence from anaesthesia and improved perioperative efficiency.

It has become very widely used for outpatient surgical procedures, it provides a superior airway compared to a facemask and is less traumatic compared with a tracheal tube. The safety of LMA has been established in a large series reported by Verghese C et al.[34] The use of the LMA during gynecologic laparoscopy still is considered by some to be controversial. The major concern with the LMA is the possible risk of aspiration of regurgitated gastric contents. The LMA does not offer any protection to the trachea from aspiration of regurgitated material.

A new variety of laryngeal mask, The ProSeal LMA, overcomes the disadvantage of potential risk of regurgitation by providing a tube for drainage of gastric contents.

Laparoscopy is thought to increase the risk of regurgitation by means of an increase in intra-abdominal pressure (during pneumoperitoneum) and by head-down tilt. Pneumoperitoneum certainly increases intra-abdominal pressure, and this is transmitted as raised intragastric pressure.[35] However, the lower oesophageal pressures increases to a greater degree than does the rise in intragastric pressure thereby increasing the barrier pressure.[35] Head-down tilt to 15° has no measurable effect on either intragastric or lower oesophageal pressure[36] and so should not alter the risk of regurgitation. Increasing the tilt to 30° does raise the intragastric pressure, but again, lower esophageal pressure increases to a greater degree, strengthening the barrier pressure.[36] So none of these maneuvers increases the possibility of regurgitation.

This physiologic evidence is strengthened by an old series of approximately 5000 patients having gynecologic laparoscopies managed by a facemask, none of who aspirated.[36] More recently, a small randomized comparison of LMA with tracheal intubation during pelvic laparoscopy showed similar perioperative conditions in both groups (despite the avoidance of neuromuscular block in the LMA group) and no cases of aspiration. Another small study showed no cases of aspiration using the LMA with spontaneous ventilation in association with either inhalation or intravenous anaesthesia.[37] Continuous esophageal pH monitoring failed to detect gastro-esophageal reflux in a series of 30 women undergoing pelvic laparoscopy with the LMA[38], while the same technique revealed no regurgitation in 100 female patients.[39] Clinically significant aspiration was not detected in two large series of 1469 and 3000 gynecologic laparoscopies performed with the LMA.[34,40]

This combined evidence suggests that the incidence of aspiration is low when the LMA is used for pelvic laparoscopy. Aspiration can still occur before tracheal intubation or after extubation, and the incidence of this is probably similar to that of aspiration during LMA usage.[40] Tracheal intubation (ideally combined with cricoid pressure and other measures to prevent aspiration) is advisable for individuals at especially high risk, such as obese patients and those with significant symptomatic reflux. Tracheal intubation is also advisable when steep head-down tilt is required, and for prolonged procedures.

MUSCLE RELAXANTS

Endotracheal intubation is still preferred by many for securing the airway and preventing aspiration in laparoscopy. Muscle relaxants are required to facilitate this and to provide good operating conditions. Muscle relaxants can still be used if the laryngeal mask is used to secure control of the airway. For diagnostic laparoscopies and short procedures like tubal ligation, muscle relaxation can be accomplished with suxamethonium. The disadvantage with suxamethonium is postoperative muscle pains, which is more apparent in ambulatory patients. Muscle pains lasting upto 4 days have been reported.[41,42]

The use of muscle relaxants may be required in outpatient anaesthesia to facilitate endotracheal intubation and to optimise the surgical conditions. In addition, their use can decrease the anaesthetic requirement and recovery time.[43]

With shorter-acting nondepolarising muscle relaxants- atracurium and vecuronium, prompt reversal of neuromuscular blockade can be achieved even after brief surgical procedures.[44] With mivacurium, the rate of spontaneous recovery appears to be even more rapid than with atracurium and vecuronium. For reversal of neuromuscular block, edrophonium (0.5 mg/kg) may offer an advantage in the outpatient setting because of its quicker onset of action than neostigmine.[45] There is a relationship between postoperative emetic symptoms and the antagonism of neuromuscular blockade by neostigmine and atropine.[46]

REGIONAL ANAESTHESIA FOR LAPAROSCOPY

Regional anaesthesia has been used successfully in laparoscopy for minor procedures and for cholecystectomy. Still, it has not gained popularity when compared to general anaesthesia techniques. The potential advantages of regional anaesthesia include - quicker recovery, decreased PONV, less postoperative pain, shorter postoperative stay, cost effectiveness, improved patient's satisfaction, overall safety, early diagnosis of complications, and fewer haemodynamic changes[47,48] Sequelae of general anaesthesia such as sore throat, muscle pain, and airway trauma can be avoided. Regional anaesthesia, however requires a willing operator and a relaxed and co-operative patient. Besides, there is need to have reduced tilt, low intra-abdominal pressure (IAP), gentle surgical technique to reduce pain and ventilatory disturbances. A block from T_4 to L_5 is necessary for surgical laparoscopy and the local anaesthetic dose needs to be adjusted accordingly. Any compromise may result in increased patient anxiety, pain, and discomfort, necessitating supplementation with intravenous sedation. This combined effect of pneumoperitoneum and sedation can lead to hypoventilation and arterial oxygen desaturation, offsetting the advantages offered by regional technique. Regional anaesthesia can also be used as a supplement to general anaesthesia.

In a report by Ciofolo et al respiratory changes were less evident when laparoscopy was performed in awake patients under regional anaesthesia, and arterial blood gases were maintained within normal limits.[49]

SPINAL ANAESTHESIA

Spinal anesthesia is reliable among the regional anaesthesia techniques and can be used for many outpatient procedures, including laparoscopy.[50] The introduction of fine gauge spinal needles has popularised the use of spinal anaesthetic for short duration outpatient laparoscopy. The important issues with spinal anesthesia are risk of postdural puncture headache (PDPH) and backache.

Spinal anaesthesia, as the primary technique for laparoscopy, offers many benefits over general anaesthesia; however, conventional dose hyperbaric drugs used in spinal anaesthesia might not be ideal for laparoscopy. In fact, the Trendelenburg position predisposes administration of reduced doses of the local anaesthetics or hypobaric solutions to minimise side effects.[51,52] In ambulatory gynecologic laparoscopy, small-dose spinal anaesthesia is an effective alternative to a desflurane general anaesthetic. It results in less postoperative pain, cost, and faster recovery.[53]

The risk of PDPH has been reduced to fewer than 2 per cent with the advent of fine gauge (25-G-27-G) noncutting (or pencil-point) spinal needles. Back pain does not seem to be associated with needle size or type.

The transient radicular irritation (TRI) varies with the local anaesthetic used and the criteria used for diagnosis. It was seen more often with 5 per cent lignocaine with dextrose.

With hyperbaric spinal anaesthesia, there is a tendency for the level of block to migrate in the cephalad direction during the Trendelenburg position, thus increasing the magnitude of sympathectomy and predisposing to the development of hypotension and bradycardia. Conversely, low-dose hypobaric solutions do not migrate cephalad in the Trendelenburg position, and the risk of hypotension is reduced.

The optimal dose of fentanyl for use with low-dose hypobaric lidocaine-fentanyl spinal anaesthesia was found to be 25 mcg.[54] Substitution of fentanyl with sufentanil 10 mcg facilitates reduction of the lignocaine dose from 25 mg to 10 mg without compromising surgical conditions.[55]

Surgical procedures, such as laparoscopic inguinal hernia repair with extra peritoneal gas insufflation, have also been accomplished safely and comfortably with spinal anaesthesia.[56]

EPIDURAL ANAESTHESIA

Epidural anaesthesia is another option to general anaesthesia for daycare laparoscopy as it retains the ability to keep the respiratory control mechanism intact. This allows the patient to adjust the minute ventilation and therefore maintain near normal $EtCO_2$.[49]

Oxygenation during the period of pneumoperitoneum is adequate, and results in a shortened recovery period and fewer postoperative complications. In addition, surgeon, anesthesiologist and patient acceptance were excellent.[57]

There is increase in respiratory work but alveolar ventilation is not compromised even in the Trendelenburg position, and the time to discharge is significantly reduced using epidural compared with general anaesthesia. Shoulder pain, secondary to diaphragmatic irritation that results from abdominal distension, is incompletely alleviated using epidural anesthesia alone. The epidural administration of opiates and/or clonidine might help to provide adequate analgesia.[58] In case of gasless laparoscopy for gynecologic surgery, epidural anaesthesia can provide comfort and more adequate pain relief, while avoiding most of the side effects of carbon dioxide pneumoperitoneum. Furthermore, no significant difference in cardiorespiratory function is present in gasless gynecologic laparoscopy whenever general or epidural anaesthesia is performed.[59] Chronic obstructive pulmonary disease (COPD) is a high-risk group to be taken up on a day care basis. In patients with COPD, epidural anaesthesia has been used for laparoscopic cholecystectomy, therefore, avoiding general anesthesia in such patients.[60,61]

Laparoscopic extraperitoneal herniorrhaphy can be performed effectively under epidural anaesthesia, obviating the need for general anaesthesia.[62]

COMBINED SPINAL-EPIDURAL ANAESTHESIA (CSEA)

The disadvantage of epidural anaesthesia is the relatively slow onset of anaesthesia.

Potential advantages of CSEA include rapid onset of anaesthesia and the ability to administer minimally effective doses of intrathecal agents initially with a resultant decrease in recovery time. The technique involves location of the epidural space with an epidural needle followed by insertion of a spinal needle though the epidural needle.

An epidural catheter is left in place for extending the duration and height of the block if required. This catheter can be utilised for the postoperative pain relief as well.

LOCAL ANAESTHETIC INFILTRATION

Local anesthesia could be used as a reliable and affordable alternative to general anaesthesia. It is safe, effective, less costly and has been primarily used for patients with infertility, chronic pelvic pain and tubal ligation[63,64] The advances in optical fiber technology have now produced laparoscopes with external diameters of as little as 1.2 to 2.2 mm. These instruments allow "microlaparoscopy" to be performed with local anesthesia alone or supplemented by sedation. Therefore, office microlaparoscopy for female sterilisation under local anaesthesia is cost-effective and safe[65] with less postoperative analgesic requirement as compared with conventional laparoscopic sterilisation.[66] In the therapy for polycystic ovarian syndrome, ovarian drilling in minilaparoscopy under local anaesthesia has similar therapeutic results to those achieved by traditional laparoscopy. It offers a less-invasive technique with an early hospital discharge that can be carried out in an outpatient service without the need for general anesthesia and postoperative additional analgesia.[67] Microlaparoscopy is not suitable for obese for technical reasons. The short instruments are likely to end up in the extraperitoneal space, and the low insufflation pressure is insufficient to lift the weight of the abdomen and provide a good view. Patients with multiple adhesions from previous surgery are also less suitable. Further developments in optics and small instruments could increase the indications for microlaparoscopy.

Almeida et al[68] assessed the safety of diagnostic and surgical microlaparoscopy performed in the office setting in patients presenting with chronic pelvic pain.

The use of laparoscopy with local anaesthesia has been reported for the diagnosis of suspected appendicitis and been found beneficial in avoiding unnecessary laparotomy in over 70 per cent of the cases.[69] In trauma patients, laparoscopy with local anaesthesia was found to be useful in improving the management of stab wounds and blunt injuries. In selected patients, in conjunction with diagnostic peritoneal lavage, it allows further diagnosis and potentially the treatment of injuries without laparotomy.[70]

Laparoscopic zygote intrafallopian transfer (ZIFT) procedure also can be performed with patient under local anaesthesia, augmented with intravenous anaesthesia. Significant discomfort can be minimised by transferring zygotes to one tube only.[71]

In a randomized study, Peterson et al[72] compared laparoscopic tubal sterilisation performed with the patient under either general or local anaesthesia. Haemodynamic stability was greater in the local anesthetic group. Satisfaction was equal among patients in each group (80%).

Local anaesthesia also has an important role in reducing morbidity in patients under general anaesthesia. Haldane et al[73] found that a pouch-of-Douglas block was an effective method of postoperative pain relief in patients undergoing laparoscopic sterilisation.

The pharmacokinetics and pharmacodynamics of lignocaine and bupivacaine were investigated by Spielman et al[74] when used for laparoscopic sterilisation under local anaesthesia. Either 240 mg of lignocaine or 100 mg of bupivacaine were sprayed onto the fallopian tubes. Venous blood samples were assayed, the peak concentrations of each agent were well below the convulsive level.

Patient Safety and Satisfaction

In a study of 1200 laparoscopic sterilisations on patients under local anaesthesia, Penfield et al[75] reported no complications. In 8509 laparoscopic sterilisations on patients under local anaesthesia, Pattinson et al[76] reported major complications (anaphylactic shock after local anaesthetic injection) in 1 per cent and a technical failure rate of 1.15 per cent. Poindexter et al[77] reported on 3000 outpatient laparoscopic sterilizations under local anaesthesia and found no major complications, a technical failure rate of 0.14 per cent, and reduction in hospital costs by 68 to 85 per cent.

With the increasing emphasis on office-based laparoscopic sterilisation using local anaesthesia with sedation, Miller et al[78] retrospectively studied the safety of performing this procedure in that environment and proposed that there was no evidence of increased risk of life-threatening complications.

MONITORING

The other area of major change has come with improved noninvasive monitoring of cardiovascular status. This enables sicker patients with more complex medical conditions to be safely cared for in an ambulatory setting. Biosensor development will eliminate the need for arterial catheters, central lines, and pulmonary artery catheters. It will probably become possible to measure blood flow to end organ systems to be able to protect the patient from injury during anaesthesia.[79] Eventually, closed-loop systems will deliver anaesthetic agents by pumps or vaporizers controlled by intelligent systems that measure and predict a patient's response to anaesthesia.[80] Similarly monitoring of the ventilatory functions is desirable for patients undergoing laparoscopy. Capnography helps to detect air embolism early before haemodynamic instability appears. Capnography is also useful in detecting endotracheal tube migration to the bronchus which may result from pneumoperitoncum (Fig. 14.2).

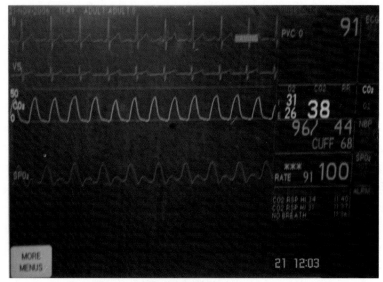

Fig. 14.2: Monitor

RECOVERY AFTER LAPAROSCOPY

The driving force behind the increased number of patients in day care surgery is the earlier return to pre-surgery status with little physical disability and earlier return to normal activities. Recovery from the anaesthesia is a continuous process and the first phase commences with discontinuation of the anaesthetic agent. Aldrete score or its modifications[81] are used to monitor the recovery in this stage. A score of 9 ensures safe discharge of the patient to step down recovery. Phase II recovery is till the patient achieves discharge criteria, whereas Phase III extends from discharge upto the resumption of normal activities (Fig. 14.3).

Fast tracking from theatre to phase II recovery is possible in shorter laparoscopic procedures. In a study by Song et al[21], desflurane anaesthesia for maintenance was accompanied by a higher percentage of patients eligible for fast tracking.

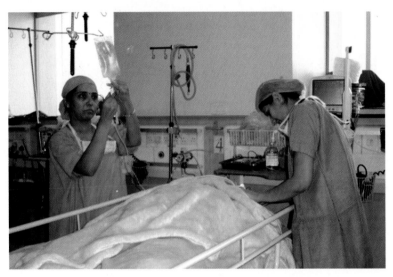

Fig.14.3: Post anaesthesia care unit (PACU)

During the early postoperative period, respiratory rate and $EtCO_2$ of patients breathing spontaneously are higher after laparoscopy as compared with open surgery. The additional carbon dioxide load can lead to hypercapnia even in the postoperative period. This causes an increased ventilatory requirement, when the ability to increase ventilation is impaired by residual anaesthetic drugs and diaphragmatic dysfunction. Patients with respiratory disease can have problems excreting an excessive carbon dioxide load, which results in increasing hypercapnia and eventually respiratory failure. Patients with cardiac disease are more prone to haemodynamic changes and instability caused by the hyperdynamic state developing after laparoscopy.

As compared with other outpatient procedures, laparoscopic surgery still produces substantial morbidity.

Telephone follow-up revealed incisional pain in about 50 per cent of laparoscopic patients, double the overall incidence of pain in outpatients. Drowsiness (36%) and dizziness (24%) were also more common after laparoscopic surgery than after any other ambulatory procedure.[82] A high incidence of minor morbidities is noticed: abdominal pain (71%), shoulder pain (75%), sore throat (26%), headache (12%) and nausea (3%), and only 8 per cent of the patients would have preferred an overnight stay.[83] Although morbidity is considerable, most symptoms resolve within a week.[84] The anesthesiologist must deal with these postoperative problems and address them adequately.

The return of CO_2 levels to pre-induction levels can take upto 45 minutes after deflation of the abdomen.[85] The diaphragmatic activity may take upto 24 hours to return to normal (Fig. 14.4).[86]

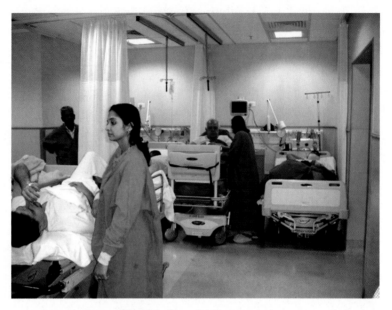

Fig.14.4: Step down recovery

POSTOPERATIVE NAUSEA AND VOMITING

PONV is extremely common after laparoscopic surgery; the symptoms are unpleasant and can delay discharge after outpatient surgery.[87] Some of the causal factors, such as peritoneal gas insufflation, bowel manipulation, and pelvic surgery are essentially unavoidable. Some aspects of the anaesthetic technique could influence the incidence of PONV, however, and a low-risk technique obviously should be used whenever possible. In addition, a variety of antiemetic medications can be used to prevent or treat PONV.

Propofol is associated with the lowest incidence of PONV. Maintenance of anaesthesia for laparoscopic surgery with propofol resulted in a lower incidence of PONV compared with enflurane,[88] desflurane alone,[90] or desflurane with ondansetron.[90] Although propofol anaesthesia appears to reduce PONV associated with isoflurane-N_2O anaesthesia,[91] nevertheless, omission of N_2O failed to reduce the occurrence of PONV after laparoscopic cholecystectomy or pelvic laparoscopic surgery[91,92] In addition, omission of N_2O is not without hazard and resulted in at least one case of perioperative awareness.[93] Opioids are potent causes of PONV, and substituting ketorolac for fentanyl reduced the number of patients requiring antiemetic treatment after gynecologic laparoscopy, while also providing superior pain relief.[94] The routine use of neostigmine to reverse residual neuromuscular block has been reported to increase the incidence of PONV compared with spontaneous recovery from mivacurium[95], however, others have failed to confirm an adverse effect of neostigmine in a similar study.[96]

A wide range of antiemetic medications is available, including droperidol, metoclopramide, and a variety of 5-HT$_3$ receptor antagonists. Some of the older antiemetics can be associated with significant side effects. Droperidol in particular can produce adverse effects, although it is suggested that these are avoided by lowering the dose. Following outpatient laparoscopy, the incidence of restlessness was close to 30 per cent with either 10 or 20 mcg/kg of droperidol.[97] The lower doses also failed to reduce the incidence of anxiety or dysphoria; it was equally effective as an antiemetic, but was associated with more severe pain in the early postoperative period. The authors concluded that there was no advantage in reducing the dose of droperidol below 20 mcg/kg.[97] Antagonists of the 5 HT$_3$ receptor, such as ondansetron, avoid most of the side effects associated with traditional antiemetics. These drugs were initially thought to be more effective than older antiemetics, although ondansetron is apparently no more successful in preventing PONV than either droperidol[98] or cyclizine.[99] The timing of ondansetron is important, however, with administration at the end of surgery producing a significantly greater antiemetic effect compared to preinduction dosing.[100] Various other 5-HT3 antagonists, such as dolasetron and granisetron, are also available. These have mostly been evaluated against placebo,[101] but indirect comparisons show that they are no better than ondansetron.

Other novel forms of antiemetic therapy have also been evaluated. Dexamethasone, 10 mg IV, reduced PONV in the first 24 hours following laparoscopic sterilisation from 73 to 34 per cent, compared with a control group.[102] PONV in the first 4 hours was reduced from 63 to 27 per cent and the requirement for rescue antiemetics, from 28 to 7 per cent. No adverse effects were apparent from this single dose of steroid.[102] Following gynaecologic laparoscopy, acupuncture at the PC6 point reduced the incidence of PONV in hospital from 65 to 35 per cent and at home from 69 to 31 per cent compared with placebo.[103] Ginger powder (2 gm) failed to prevent PONV following laparoscopy.[104]

Although less intense and less prolonged compared with open procedures, these symptoms can be quite severe relative to other outpatient procedures, particularly in the early postoperative period.

POSTOPERATIVE PAIN

Postoperative pain is a significant factor in the PACU, 35 to 40 per cent of patients report moderate to severe pain at home in the first 24 hours after hospital discharge.[105,106] Many patients reported pain significant enough to interfere with daily activities.[107] The most significant predictor of severe pain during this period of recovery was insufficient pain control during the first several hours after surgery.[106] With this in mind, investigators have attempted to improve on intraoperative and postoperative pain control and minimize the side effects that typically lead to delayed discharge from the PACU. Opioids have been the most widely used drugs for pain control, and many studies have been done comparing shorter-acting to longer-acting agents. When equianalgesic amounts of morphine or fentanyl were given, patients who received fentanyl (a short-acting agent when compared with morphine) had higher pain scores in the PACU and required more oral analgesics. The patients given morphine had better pain control but a greater incidence of PONV, most of which occurred after discharge. There was no significant difference in the duration of PACU stay or time to home readiness between the two groups.[108]

Nonsteroidal anti-inflammatory agents (NSAIDs) such as ketorolac and the newer COX-2 inhibitors have also become important adjuncts in ambulatory anaesthesia. Their use has resulted in a decreased use of opioids (and thus opioid-related side effects), longer duration of analgesia, and lower postoperative pain scores.[109-111] Studies have consistently shown a shorter time to home readiness and an improved recovery profile, with little to no PONV in patients given these agents.[112,113]

In laparoscopic cholecystectomy under general anaesthesia, injection of local anaesthetic before trocar insertion, significantly reduces postoperative pain and decreases medication usage costs.[114] Moreover, intraperitoneal spray of local anaesthetic significantly decreases postoperative pain.[115] The extraperitoneal laparoscopic repair of inguinal hernia is feasible under local anaesthesia in the population where general anesthesia is contraindicated.[116]

Although the discomfort following laparoscopic surgery is less severe compared with the corresponding open procedure; postoperative pain still can be considerable. Prevention and treatment of pain relies on local anesthesia, nonsteroidal anti-inflammatory drugs, and opioid analgesics, often used in combination.

Because nonsteroidal anti-inflammatory drugs (NSAIDs) have analgesic properties comparable with opioid compounds without opioid-related side effects, these drugs are often administered as adjuvants during and after surgery. There is no significant difference between the various NSAIDs in their efficacy, provided that an adequate dose is used and sufficient time is allowed for the onset of effect. There could be minor differences between drugs in the pattern of side effects, but most patients tolerate short-term administration of NSAIDs remarkably well.[117] Opioid analgesics are obviously effective in treating pain after laparoscopic procedures; however, these drugs are associated with numerous side effects, including nausea, respiratory depression, and sedation, which are especially undesirable in outpatients.

The most effective pain relief can be obtained by combining opioids, local anesthetics, and NSAIDs into balanced analgesia. This approach at least allows the opioid dose to be reduced by the use of other modalities, thereby limiting side effects, reducing postoperative pain and analgesic requirements, and facilitating an earlier return to normal activities.[112,118]

CONCLUSIONS

Because expertise and equipment have improved, laparoscopy has become one of the most common surgical procedures performed on an outpatient basis. Now sicker patients are being offered day care services and rendering anaesthesia for laparoscopy is becoming technically difficult and more challenging.

Laparoscopy was introduced as a safe and simple procedure that could be performed on an outpatient basis. It does compromise the cardiovascular and respiratory function and extreme caution regarding the anaesthetic technique is required in the present expanding scope of laparoscopic surgery.

CLINICAL PEARLS

1. Role of daycare laparoscopy has increased
2. Laparoscopic approach is associated with early recovery
3. Use of multimodal strategies to prevent postoperative pain and PONV allow early emergence

REFERENCES

1. Romanowski L, Reich H McGlynn F et al: Brachial plexus neuropathic after advanced laparoscopic surgery. Fertil Sterile 1993; 60: 729.
2. Witten CM, Andrus CH, Fitzgerald SD, et al. Analysis of the haemodynamic and ventilatory effects of laparoscopic cholecystectomy. Arch Surg 1991; 126: 997-1001.
3. Fitzgerald SD, Andrus CH, Baudendistel LJ. Hypercarbia during carbon dioxide pneumoperitoneum. Am J Surg 1992; 163: 186-90.
4. Brompton WJ, Watsor RJ. Arterial to end tidal carbon dioxide tension difference during laparoscopy. Anaesthesia 1990; 45: 210-4.
5. Detsky A, Abrams H, McLaughlin J, et al. Predicting cardiac complications inpatients under-going non-cardiac surgery. J Gen Intern Med 1986; 1: 211-90.
6. Mangano DT. Perioperative cardiac morbidity. Anesthesiology 1990; 72:153-84.

7. Eagle KA, Rihal CS, Mickel MC, et al. Cardiac risk of noncardiac surgery: influence of coronary disease and type of surgery in 3368 operations. CASS investigations and University of Michigan Heart care program. Coronary artery surgery study. Circulation 1997; 96:1882-7.

8. Posner KL, Van Norman GA, Chan V. Adverse cardiac outcomes after noncardiac surgery in patients with prior percutaneous transluminal coronary angioplasty. Anesth Analg 1999; 89: 553-60.

9. Reid CW, Martineu RJ, Hull KA, Miller DR. Haemodynamic consequences of abdominal insufflation with CO_2 during laparoscopic cholecystectomy. Can J Anaesth 1992; 39: A132.

10. Lindgren L, Koivusalo AM, Kellkumpu I. Conventional pneumoperitoneum compared with abdominal wall lift for laparoscopic, cholecystectomy. Br J Anesthesia 1995; 75: 567.

11. Ninoyima K, Kitano S, Yoshida T, et al. Comparison of pneumoperitoneum and abdominal wall lifting as to hemodynamic and surgical stress response during laparoscopic cholecystectomy. Surg Endosc 1998; 12:124.

12. Shankman Z, Shir Y, Brodsky JB. Perioperative management of obese patient. Br J Anaesth 1993; 70: 349-59.

13. Lew JKL, Gin T, Oh TE: Anaesthetic problems during laparoscopic cholecystectomy. Anaesth Intens Care 1992; 20: 91.

14. Skelly AM, Whitwam JG. Laparoscopy and its complications. In Whitwam JG (ed): Day-case Anaesthesia and sedation. London Blackwell Scientific, 1994; 202.

15. Brown DR, Fishburne JI, Robertson VO, et al. Ventilatory and blood gas changes during laparoscopy with intraperitoneal carcinomatosis using a new optical catheter. Gynecol Oncol 1992; 47: 337.

16. Puri GD, Singh H. Ventilatory effects of laparoscopy under general anesthesia. Br J Anesth 1992; 68: 211.

17. Brampton WJ, Watson RJ. Arterial to end-tidal carbon dioxide tension difference during laparoscopy: Magnitude and effect of anaesthetic technique. Anaesthesia 1990; 45:210.

18. Ciotolo MJ, Clergue F, Seebacher J. Ventilatory effects of laparoscopy under epidural anaesthesia. Anaesth Analg 1990; 70: 357.

19. Johannes G, Andersen M, Juhl B. The of general anaesthesia on the hemodynamic events during laparoscopy with CO_2 insufflation. Acts Anesthesiol Scand 1989; 33: 132.

20. William MD, Murr PC. Laparoscopic insufflation increase the abdomen depresses cardiopulmonary function. Surg Endosc 1993; 7: 12.

21. Song D, Joshi GP White PF. Fast-track eligibility after ambulatory anesthesia: A comparison of desflurane, and propofol. Anesth Anal 1998; 86: 267.

22. Rising S, Dodgson Ms Steen PA. Isoflurane v fentanyl for out patient laparoscopy. Acta Anaesthesiol Scand 1985; 29: 251.

23. Apfel CC, Kranke P, Katz MH, et al. Volatile anaesthetic may be the main cause of early but not delayed postoperative vomiting: randomized controlled trial of factorial design. Br J Anaesth 2002; 88:659-68.

24. Arellano RJ, Pole Ml, Rafuse SE, et al. omission of nitrous oxide from a propofol-based J Anesthetic does not affect the recovery of women undergoing outpatient gynecologic surgery. Anesthesiology 2000; 93: 332-9.

25. Jevtovic-Todorovic V, Todorovic SM, Mennerick S, et al. nitrous oxide is an NMDA antagonist, neuroprotectant and neurotoxin. Nat Med 1998; 4:460-3.

26. Van den Nieuwenhuyzen MC, Engbers FH, Vuyk J, Burm AG. Target-controlled infusion systems: role in anaesthesia and analgesia. Clin Pharmacokinet 2000; 38: 181-90.

27. Passot S, Servin F, Allary R, et al. target-controlled versus manually- controlled infusion of propofol for direct laryngoscopy and postoperative recovery after desflurane, propofol, or isoflurane anaesthesia among morbidly obese patients: a prospective, randomized study. Anesth Analg 2000; 91: 714-9.

28. Kazama T, Takeuchi K, Morita K, et al. comparison of the effect-site of propofol for blood pressure and bispectral index in elderly and younger patient. Anesthesiology 1999; 90:1517-27.

29. Kazama T, Ikeda K, et al. Optimal propofol plasma concentration during upper gastrointestinal endoscopey in young, middle-aged, and elderly patients. Anesthesiology 2000; 93: 662-9.

30. Juvin P, Vadam C, Malek L, et al. postoperative recovery after desflurane, propofol, or isoflurane anaesthesia among morbidly obese patients: a prospective, randomized study. Anesth Analg 2000; 91: 714-9.

31. Rapp SE, Conahan TJ, Paulin DJ, et al. Comparison of desflurane with propofol in outpatients undergoing peripheral orthopaedic surgery. Anesth Analg 1992; 75: 572.

32. Van Hemecrick J, Smith I, White PF. Use of desflurane for outpatient anaesthesia – comparison with propofol and nitrous oxide. Anesthesiology 1991; 75: 197.

33. Joshi GP. The use of laryngeal mask airway devices in ambulatory anesthesia. Seminars in Anesthesia, Perioperative Medicine and Pain 2001; 20: 257-63.

34. Verghese C, Brimacombe JR. Survey of laryngeal mask airway usage in 11910 patients: Safety and efficacy for conventional and nonconventional usage. Anesth Analg 1996; 82: 129.

35. Jones MJ, Mitchell RW, Hindocha N: Effect of increased intra-abdominal pressure during laparoscopy on the lower esophageal sphincter. Anesth Analg 1989; 68: 63.

36. Heijke SAM, Smith G, Key A. The effect of the Trendelenburg position on lower esophageal sphincter tone. Anaesthesia 1991; 46:185.

37. Goodwin APL, Rowe WL, Ogg TW. Day-case laparoscopy; A comparison of two anaesthetic techniques using the laryngeal mask during spontaneous breathing anaesthesia 1992; 47: 892.

38. Ho BYM, Skinner HJ, Mahajan RP. Gastro-esophageal reflux during day-case gynaecological laparoscopy under positive pressure ventilation: Laryngeal mask vs tracheal intubation. Anaesthesia 1998; 53: 921.

39. Bapat PP, VergheseC. Laryngeal mask airway and the incidence of regurgitation during gynaecological laparoscopies. Anesth Analg 1997; 85: 139.

40. Malins AF, Cooper GM. Laparoscopy and the laryngeal mask airway {letter}. Br J Anesth 1994; 73: 121.

41. Brindle GF, Soliman MG. Anaesthetic complications in surgical outpatients. Can Anaesth Soc J 1975; 22: 613.

42. Urbach GM, Edelist G. An evaluation of the anaesthesia techniques used in an outpatient unit. Can Anaesth Soc J 1977; 24: 401.

43. Herbert M, Healy TEJ, Bourke JB, et al. Profile of recovery after general anaesthesia. Br Med J 1983; 286: 1539.

44. Fragen RJ, Shanks CA. Neuromuscular recovery after laparoscopy. Anaesth Analg 1984; 63: 51.

45. Cronnelly R, Morris RB. Antagonism of neuromuscular blockade. Br J Anaesth 1982; 54: 183.

46. King MJ, Milazkiewicz R, Carli F, Deacock AR. Influence of neostigmine on postoperative vomiting. Br J Anaesth 1988; 62:403.

47. Mazdisnian F, Palmieri A, Hakakha B, Hakakha M, Cambridge C, Lauria BJ. Office microlaparoscopy for female sterilization under local anesthesia. A cost and clinical analysis. Reprod Med 2002; 47: 97-100.

48. Collins LM, Vaghadia H. Regional anesthesia for laparoscopy. Anesthesiol Clin North America 2001; 19:43-55.

49. Ciofolo ML, Clergue F, Seebacher J, Lefebvre G, Viars P. Ventilatory effects of laparoscopy under epidural. Anaesthesiol 2004; 21: 489-95.

50. Vaghadia H. Spinal anaesthesia for out patients: controversies and new techniques. Can J Anesth 1998; 45: 64.

51. Vaghadia H, McLeod DH, Mitchell GW, Merrick PM, Chilvers CR. Small-dose hypobaric lidocaine-fentanyl spinal anesthesia solution of 10 mg lidocaine with 10 mg of sufentanil provides adequate analgesia.

52. Vaghadia H, Viskri D, Mitchell GW, Berrill A, Selective spinal anesthesia for outpatient laparoscopy. Characteristics of three hypobaric solutions. Can J Anaesth 2001; 48: 256-60.

53. Lennox PH, Vaghadia H, Henderson C, Martin L, Mitchell GW. Small-dose selective spinal anesthesia for short-duration outpatient.

54. Chilvers CR, Vaghadia H, Mitchell GW, et al: Small-does hypobaric lidocaine- fentanyl spinal anesthesia for short duration outpatient laparoscopy. Optimal fentanyl dose. Anesth Analg 1997; 84:65.

55. Viskri D, Berrill A, Waghadia H: Walk-in/walk out spinal Anesthesia for out laparoscopy: Evaluation of three hypobaric solutions. Can J Anaesth 1997; 44 A26-B.

56. Spivak H Nudelman I, Fuco V, et al. Laparoscopic extraperitoneal inguinal hernia repair with spinal anesthesia and nitrous oxide insufflation. Surg Endosc 1999; 10:1026.

57. Bridenbaugh LD, Soderstrom RM. Lumbar epidural block anesthesia for out patient laparoscopy. J Record Med 1979; 23: 85.

58. Collins LM, Vaghadia H. Regional anesthesia for laparoscopy. Anesthesiol Clin North America 2001; 19: 43-55.

59. Vofsi O, Barak M, Moscovici R, Bustan M, Katz Y. Cardio respiratory parameters during conventional or gasless gynecological laparoscopy under general or regional anesthesia. Med Sci Monit 2004; 10: CR152-CR155.

60. Gramatica L, Jr, Brasesco OE, Mercado Luna A. Laparoscopic cholecystectomy performed under regional anesthesia in patients with chronic obstructive pulmonary disease. Surg Endosc 2002; 16:472-5.

61. Pursnani KG, Bazza Y, Calleja M, Mughal MM. Laparoscopic cholecystectomy under epidural anesthesia in patients with chronic respiratory disease. Surg Endosc 1998; 12:1082-4.

62. Azurin DJ, Go LS, Cwik JC, Schuricht AL. The efficacy of epidural anesthesia for endoscopic preperitoneal herniorrhaphy: a prospective study. J Laparoendosc A Surg 1996; 6:369-73.

63. Zupi E, Marconi D, Sbracia M, et al. Is local anesthesia an affordable alternative to general anesthesia for minilaparoscopy? J Am Assoc Gynecol Laparosc 2000; 7:111-4.

64. Palter S.F. Office microlaparoscopy under local anesthesia. Obstet Gynecol Clin North Am 2002; 26: 109-20.

65. Mazdisnian F, Palmieri A, Hakakha B, Hakakha M, Cambridge C, Lauria B. Office microlaparoscopy for female sterilization under local anesthesia. A cost and clinical analysis. J Reprod Med 2002; 47: 97-100.

66. Tiras MB, Gokce O, Noyan V, et al. Comparison of microlaparoscopy and conventional laparoscopy for tubal sterilization under local anesthesia with mild sedation. J Am Assoc Gynecol Laparsc 2001; 8:385-8.

67. Zullo F, Pellicano M, Zupi E, Guida M, Mastrantonio P, Nappi C. Minilaparoscopic ovarian drilling under local anesthesia in patients with polycystic ovary syndrome. Fertile Steril 2000; 74: 376-9.

68. Almeida OD Jr, Val-Gallas JM. Office microlaparoscopy under local anesthesia in the diagnosis and treatment of chronic pelvic pain. J Am Assoc Gynecol Laparoscopic 1998; 5: 407.

69. Kuster GG, Gilroy SB. The role of laparoscopy in the diagnosis of acute appendicitis. Am Surg 1992; 58: 627.

70. Salvino CK, Esposito TJ, Marshal WJ, et al. The role of diagnostic laparoscopy in the management of trauma patients: A preliminary assessment's. Trauma 1993; 34: 513.

71. Waterstone JJ, Bolton VN, Wren M. Laparoscopic zygote intrafallopian transfer using augmented local anesthesia. Fertil Steril 1992; 57:442.

72. Peterson HB, Hulka JF, Spielman FJ. Local versus general anesthesia for laparoscopic sterilization: A randomized study. Obstet Gynecol 1987; 70:903.

73. Haldane G, Stott S, Mc Menemin I. Pouch of Douglas block for laparoscopic sterilization. Anesthesia 1998; 53: 589.

74. Spielman FJ, Hulka JF, Ostheimer GW. Pharmacokinetics and pharmacodynamics of local analgesia for laparoscopic tubal ligation. Am J Obstet Gynecol 1983; 146: 821.

75. Penfield AJ. Laparoscopic sterilization under local anesthesia: 1200 cases. Obstet Gynecol 1977; 49: 725.

76. Pattinson RC, Louw NS, Engelbrecht B, et al. Complications in 8509 laparoscopic Falope ring sterilizations performed under local anesthesia. S Afr Med J 1983; 64: 975.

77. Poindexter AN, Abdul Malak M, Fast JE. Laparoscopic tubal sterilization under local anesthesia. Obstet Gynecol 1990; 75: 5.

78. Miller GH. Office single puncture laparoscopy sterilization with local anesthesia. J soc Laparoendosc Surg 1997; 1:55.

79. Lindahi SG. Future anesthesiologists will be as much outside as inside operating theaters. Acta Anesthesiol Scand 2000; 44: 906-9.

80. Reader JC. Anesthesiology into the new millennium. Acta Anesthesiol Scand 2000; 44:3-8.

81. Aldrete JA. The post anaesthesia score revisited (letter) J Clin Anesth 1995; 7:89-91.

82. Chung F, Un V, Su J. Postoperative symptoms 24 hours after ambulatory anaesthesia. Can J Anaesth 1996; 43:1121-7.

83. Ratcliffe F, Lawson R, Millar J. Day-case laparoscopy revisited: have postoperative morbidity and patient acceptance improved? Health Trends 1994; 26: 47-9.

84. Swan BA, Maislin G, Traber KB. Symptom distress and functional status changes during the first seven days after ambulatory surgery. Anesth Analg 1998; 86:739-45.

85. Girardis M, Broi UD, Antonutto G, et al. The effect of laparoscopic cholecystectomy on cardiovascular function and pulmonary gas exchange. Anesth Analg 1996; 83: 134.

86. Ericef, Fox GS, Salib YM, et al. Diaphragmatic function before and after laparoscopic cholecystectomy. Anaesthesiology 1994; 79: 966.

87. Kapur PA. The big "little" problem. Anesht Analg 1991; 73: 243.

88. Ding Y, White PF: Recovery following outpatient anesthesia: Use of enflurane versus propofol. J Clin Anesth 1993; 5: 447.

89. Green G Jonsson L. Nausea: The most important factor determining length of stay after ambulatory anesthesia: A comparative study of isoflurane and propofol techniques. Acta Anesthesiol Scand 1993; 37: 742.

90. Eriksson H, Korttila K. Recovery profile after desflurane without ondansetron compared with propofol in patients undergoing outpatient gynecological laparoscopy. Anesht Analg 1996; 82: 533.

91. Scuderi PE, D Angelo R, Haris L, et al. Small-does propofol by continues infusion does not prevent postoperative vomiting in female under going out patient laparoscopy. Anesth Analg 1997; 84: 71.

92. Sukhani R, Vasquez J, Pappas AL, et al. Recovery after propofol with and without intraoperative fentanyl in patients undergoing ambulatory gynecologic laparoscopy. Anaesth Analg 1996; 83: 975.

93. Segupta P, Planetevin OM. Nitrous Oxide and day-case laparoscopy: Effects on nausea, vomiting and return too normal activity. Br J Anaesth 1988; 60:750.

94. Chassard D, Berrada K, Tournade J-P, et al. The effect of neuromuscular block on peak airway pressure and abdominal elastance during pneumoperitoneum. Anaesth Analg 1996; 82:525.

95. Ding Y, White PF. Comparative effects of ketorolac dezocine, and fentanyl as adjuvant during outpatient anaesthesia. Anaesth Analg 1992; 75:566.

96. Nelskyla K, Yli-Hankala A , Soikkeli A, et al. Neostigmine with glycopyrrolate does not increase the incidence or severity of postoperative nausea and vomiting in out patients undergoing gynaecological laparoscopy. Br J Anaesth 1998; 81: 757.

97. Lim BSL, Pavy TJG, Lumsden G. The antiemetic and dysphoric effects of deroperidol in the day surgery patient. Anaesth Intens Care 1999; 27: 371.

98. Fortney JT, Gan TJ, Graczyk S, et al. A comparison of the efficacy, safety, and patient satisfaction of ordansetron versus droperidol as antiemetics for elective outpatient surgical procedures. Anaesth Analg 1998; 86: 731.

99. Cholwill JM, Wright W, Hobbs GJ, et al. Comparison of ondansetron and cyclizine for prevention of nausea and vomiting after day-case gynaecological laparoscopy. Br J Anaesth 1999; 83: 611.

100. Tang J, Wang B, White PF, et al. The effect of timing of ondansetron administration on its efficacy, cost-effectiveness, and cost-benefit as a prophylactic in the ambulatory setting. Anaesth Analg 1998; 86: 274.

101. Ding Y, White PF. Recovery following outpatient anesthesia: Use of enflurane versus propofol. J Clin Anesth 1993; 5:447.

102. Wang JJ, Ho ST, Liu HS, et al. Prophylactic antiemetic effect of Dexamethasone in women undergoing ambulatory laparoscopic surgery. Br J Anaesth 2000; 84: 459.

103. Al-Sadi M, Newman B, Julious SA. Acupuncture in the prevention of postoperative nausea and vomiting. Anaesthesia 1997; 52: 658.

104. Visalyaputra S, Petchpaisit N, Somcharoen K, et al. The efficacy of ginger root in the prevention of postoperative nausea and vomiting after outpatient gynaecological laparoscopy. Anaesthesia 1998; 53: 506.

105. Rawal N, Hylander J, Nydahl PA, et al. Survey of postoperative analgesia following ambulatory surgery. Acta Anaesthesiol Scand 1997; 41(8): 1017-22.

106. Beauregard L, Pomp A, Choiniere M. Severity and impact of pain after day-surgery. Can J Anaesth 1998; 45(4): 304-11.

107. Chung F, Mezei G. Adverse outcomes in ambulatory anesthesia. Can J Anaesth 1999; 46(5 Pt 2): R18-34.

108. Carroll NV, Miederhoff PA, Cox FM, et al. Costs incurred by outpatient surgical center in managing postoperative nausea and vomiting. J Clin Anesth 1994; 6(5): 364-9.

109. Watcha MF, Smith I. Cost-effectiveness analysis of antiemetic therapy for ambulatory surgery. J Clin, Anesth 1994; 6(5): 370-7.

110. Ben-David B, Baune-Goldstein U, Goldik Z,et al. Is preparative ketorolac a useful adjunct to regional anesthesia for inguinal herniorrhaphy? Acta Anaesthesiol Scand 1996; 40(3): 358-63.

111. Gimbel JS, Brugger A, Zhao W, et al. Efficacy and tolerability of celecoxib versus hydrocodone/acetaminophen in the treatment of pain after ambulatory orthopedic surgery in adults. Clin Ther 2001; 23(2): 228-41.

112. Eriksson H, Tenhunen A, Korttila K. Balanced analgesia improves recovery and outcome after outpatient tubal ligation. Acta Anaesthesiol Scand 1996; 40(2): 151-5.

113. Ramirez-Ruiz M, Smith I, White PF. Use of analgesics during propofol sedation: a comparison of ketorolac, dezocine, and fentanyl. J Clin Anesth 1995; 7(6): 481-5.

114. Hasaniya NW, Zayed FF, Faiz H, Severino R. Preinsertion local anesthesia at the trocar site improves perioperative pain and decreases costs of laparoscopic cholecystectomy. Surg Endosc 2001; 15:962-4.

115. Labaille T, Mazoit JX, Paqueron X, Franco D, Benhamou D. The clinical efficacy and pharmacokinetics of intraperitoneal ropivacaine for laparoscopic cholecystectomy. Anesth Analg 2002; 94:100-5.

116. Frezza E.E, Ferzli G. Local and general anesthesia in the laparoscopic preperitoneal hernia repair. JSLS 2000; 4:221-4.

117. Gotzche PC. Extracts from "clinical evidence." Non-steroidal anti-inflammatory drugs. BMJ 2000; 320:1058-61.

118. Michaloliakou C, Chung F, Sharma S. Preoperative multimodal analgesia facilitates recovery after ambulatory laparoscopic cholecystectomy. Anesth Analg 1996; 82: 44-51.

CHAPTER 15

Anaesthesia for Gynaecologic Laparoscopy

INTRODUCTION

Gynaecologists continue to perform laparoscopic procedures in greater volume than their peer surgeons. Interestingly, continual recent improvements in anaesthetic techniques, laparoscopy instruments and training methodology have resulted in greater patient acceptance for various laparoscopic surgical interventions.

Although these procedures are 'minimally invasive' to patients and the surgeons, significant physiologic perturbations may occur during the perioperative period. Minimally invasive surgery warrants focussed observation and possible modifications in the anaesthetic technique to ensure safety with minimal complications and rapid recovery.

HISTORY[1]

The twentieth century formed the 'age of laparoscopy'. Inspite of the lukewarm response of the prevailing medical fraternity during the early half of century, laparoscopic surgery evolved unprecedentally over the period, especially, in the last decade. It has got tremendous impact on the medical care and has wide-ranged legal, social and economic ramifications. Dimitri Ott, (Russian gynaecologist) has been credited for first laparoscopy in 1901 when he inspected the abdominal cavity with a speculum and a head lamp which he termed 'ventroscopy'. George Kelling (German surgeon) is touted by many as the originator of laparoscopy owing to the procedural similarity to the present day laparoscopy. This was followed by first publication on laparoscopy in 1910 by Hans Christian Jacobaeus.

Later, Orndoff (first to divise pointed trocar), Rocavilla (light source from outside abdomen), H. Kalk (1927; system of lenses; dual trocar technique), Ianos Veress (1938; spring loaded needle) and Hasson (1971; first reported the laparoscopic canula and technique to introduce it in 'an' abdomen) added to development of laparoscopy over the period of time.

PROCEDURES

The range of gynaecologic surgery that can be undertaken by laparoscopy is varied (Table 15.1) and is expected to encompass more procedures in time to come.

Table 15.1: Gynaecologic laparoscopic procedures

Non-operative Laparoscopy	Operative Laparoscopy
Diagnostic laparoscopy	Total laparoscopic hysterectomy
Endometriosis	Laparoscopy assisted vaginal hysterectomy
Ovarian cyst aspiration	Tubal re-canalisation
Fibroid uterus confirmation	Laparoscopic fibro-myomectomy
Fallopian tube patency	Ectopic pregnancy
Metastasis localisation & biopsy	Oopherectomy
Hematoma aspiration	Wertheim's procedure
Mini-lap tubal ligation	Adhesionolysis

MANAGEMENT OF ANAESTHESIA

Most of the laparoscopic procedures are performed under standard general anaesthesia (GA) including controlled ventilation with a secured upper airway.

PATIENT PREPARATION

Routine explanation of the procedure, a written informed consent from the patient and reassurance are carried out. Co-morbities [hypertension, diabetes, thyroid disease, anaemia, elderly, obesity, chronic obstructive pulmonary disease (COPD), bronchial asthma, seizures, etc.] are adequately addressed and optimised prior to the procedure. Premedication include aspiration prophylaxis (P.O. ranitidine and metoclopramide), anxiolysis (alprazolam / diazepam) and other medications (for associated medical illnesses).

MONITORING

Alongwith the routine monitoring (SpO$_2$, NIBP, EKG, temperature and precordial / esophageal stethoscope)[2] certain augmented monitoring aides are desirable. Exhaled end-tidal carbon dioxide (EtCO$_2$) is essential for all patients especially if CO$_2$ is employed as insufflating gas, serial arterial blood gas (ABG)[3] monitoring is desirable in patients having COPD (because EtCO$_2$ may underestimate serum CO$_2$ levels) to enhance accurate CO$_2$-estimation.[4] Half hourly urine output monitoring via transurethral drainage catheters are recommended to ascertain hydration status of the patient as well as to exclude any inadvertent iatrogenic bladder injury (during trocar placement, intraoperative handling). Bispectral index (BIS) monitoring is useful if total intravenous anaesthesia (TIVA) technique is utilized. Neuromuscular monitoring remains optional as in any other surgery.

ANAESTHESIA TECHNIQUE

General anaesthesia with inhalational (isoflurane, halothane, sevoflurane), or intravenous (thiopentone, propofol, etomidate, midazolam, ketamine) drugs with a secured airway is the preferred technique for gynaecologic laparoscopy. Various modifications, such as, TIVA with propofol and inhalation agents without nitrous oxide (N$_2$O) are being increasingly used and investigated further. While the former results in more rapid and clear recovery from anaesthesia with less incidence of postoperative nausea and vomiting (PONV); the latter technique avoids potential N$_2$O induced effects of intestinal motility, distension and postoperative emesis in this subset of patients. Furthermore, in outpatients a balanced anaesthesia technique (N$_2$O : O$_2$: inhalational agent; fentanyl) has failed to demonstrate any advantage offered by propofol-TIVA method.[5]

Neuromuscular blockade with an optimal anaesthetic depth is required for laparoscopic procedures[6] as inadequate muscle relaxation may resist abdominal distension and visualization and uncontrolled diaphragmatic movement may preclude finer manoeuvers during laparoscopy. The effect of a variety of non-deplolarising blocking drugs (pancuronium, vecuronium, atracurium) towards providing an appropriate field for surgery have been equivocal. Currently, a propofol based TIVA – atracurium relaxation technique seems to suffice for gynaecologic laparoscopy.

Since many short gynaecologic laparoscopy procedures are undertaken in a day care setting, an appropriately balanced anaesthesia technique is desirable. This promotes adverse effects free recovery and an awake, agile patient fit to get discharged thereby negating any potential for re-admission. A TIVA technique (etomidate, ketamine, midazolam, propofol) is considered most suitable, especially when propofol is employed.[7] A propofol based TIVA ensures rapid recovery from anaesthesia along with diminished nausea and vomiting.

Anaesthetic Induction

It is preferably carried out by utilizing propofol because of its favourable recovery characteristics along with its antiemetic effects. Made available commercially in 1986, propofol or 2,6-di-isopropylphenol is lipid soluble but almost insoluble in water. Anaesthetic induction (dose 2-2.5 mg-kg^{-1}) is rapid (within 20-40 sec) upon IV administration marked by loss of verbal contact. It can also be used to maintain state of anaesthesia by means of IV anaesthesia (IVA) alongwith oxygen-nitrous oxide mixture or TIVA. Relevant doses for IVA/TIVA are as given under:

i. Manual infusion: bolus – 1mg kg^{-1} $\rightarrow$ 10 mg kg^{-1}hr^{-1} $\times$ 10 min $\rightarrow$ 8 mg kg^{-1}hr^{-1} $\times$ 10 min $\rightarrow$ 6 mg kg^{-1}hr^{-1} thereafter
ii. Computer driven infusion technique
iii. Closed loop system

by programming the computer with appropriate pharmacokinetic data and equations to ensure a target – controlled infusion that closely titrates anaesthetic depth.

Muscle Relaxation

Although procedures are of short duration, yet adequate abdominal and diaphragmatic relaxation is mandatory during most laparoscopies to avoid problems of inadequate abdominal distention and uncontrolled diaphragmatic movements, which may hinder delicate laparoscopic manoeuvers. Short acting nondepolarizers (atracurium, vecuronium) are useful and can be readily reversed. These neuromuscular blockers have shown to be applicable to laparoscopies conducted under same day laparoscopy setting.[8]

Gynaecologic laparoscopy, particularly involving day-case patients is provided by short acting muscle relaxants including vecuronium (95% twich depression in 180 sec) and atracurium (95% twitch depression in 110 sec). Atracurium is more often resorted to for having more rapid onset after initial bolus (0.5 mg kg^{-1} IV) and can easily be reversed (after 25-40 min) by an anticholinesterase drug. Its unique metabolism in body, i.e., "Hoffman degradation" (dependant upon temperature and body pH) is an useful safety margin for patients with hepatic or renal comorbidity. The prime metabolite, laudanosine, has epileptogenic activity although it is never reported in humans. An adequate sized vein should be used to avoid flare and wheal reaction and fall in blood pressure secondary to histamine release upon atracurium administration.

Inhalational Agents

Sevoflurane, a newer inhalational agent, is a methyl-propyl ether available for some time now. It is non-flammable, has a pleasant odour with a MAC value ~ 2% [blood-gas coeff. 0.6 / oil-partition coeff. 55) and is stored in amber coloured bottles. Because of its favourable odour and non-irritant property, the rate of induction is much faster than other readily available agents (halothane, isoflurane) as is the recovery indices (exception being desflurane). It has a mean peak fluoride ion concentration higher than equivalent amount of isoflurane and hence should be used with caution in patients having compromised renal function.

Alternative Airway

Use of laryngeal mask airway (LMA) and ProSeal-LMA (PLMA) as a dedicated airway during GA has increased over the period of time.[9] It is very useful in day care setting owing to its unique advantages; easy to use, no pharyngolaryngeal morbidity (secondary to direct laryngoscopy and intubation), suited to different ventilatory methods (spontaneous, assist, positive pressure) and safer in patients with a difficult airway. Specially designed LMAs,[10] such as PLMA [institution of positive pressure ventilation (PPV)], intubating fasttrach-LMA (easy to insert, conversion to ETT possible, usefulness in difficult airway situations), and soft-seal disposable-LMA (no pharyngeal irritation) have largely taken over as dedicated airway gadgets in outpatients replacing conventional tracheal intubation methodology.[11,12] The author recommends this device for use in outpatients undergoing gynaecologic laparoscopy.

Since the first reported use of LMA for gynaecologic laparoscopy (Brain, 1983)[13] various studies have reported successful use of LMA for these procedures. LMA has been considered a safe and effective airway device for gynaecologic laparoscopy owing to short operating time, improved experience of anaesthesiologist with the use of this device and availability of close intraoperative monitoring backup.[14,15] However, if possible, a PLMA should be preferred. The classic-LMA (c-LMA) is suitable for shorter duration procedure involving IAP of upto 15 cmH$_2$O and less than 15° of head down Trendenlenberg tilt. Currently, over one-fifth of the anaesthesiologists utilize LMA device for gynecologic laparoscopy.

Gynaecologic laparoscopic surgery generally requires the patient to be placed in lithotomy, Trendelenberg and reverse-Trendenlenberg position. Sometimes a combination of above stated positions is required. Despite reports of reflux and aspiration,[16,17] LMA as a sole airway is increasingly being used.[18] One need to address potential problems[19,20] of these patient positions[21] [lithotomy (increased IAP, displacement), Trendelenberg (increase in IAP)] before using LMA. Currently, c-LMA (fasting patients) and PLMA (for head down tilt >15°) are considered safe and effective for use in gynaecologic laparoscopy.

Analgesia

Fentanyl, a synthetic opioid with analgesic potency 100 times that of morphine, is a lipid soluble drug which reaches opioid receptors rapidly (onset of action 1-2 min). After a single IV dose of 2-4 µg kg^{-1}, the duration of action may be 20-30 minutes. Prolonged effect may be seen after high dose or infusion. Early and late respiratory depression is likely, particularly when used in higher dose range. Sedation is poor but incidence of nausea and vomiting may be at par with morphine. A rare complication, chest wall rigidity, may occur following high doses. Transdermal/ intravenous fentanyl may also be utilized for postoperative analgesia.

Special Situations

Mini-laparoscopic tubal ligation (Fig. 15.1), a common procedure that is usually performed in a day-case scenario needs special mention. Procedural events such as fallopian tube handling and clamping with a falope ring can give rise to unbearable PONV and pain in the perioperative period. Adequate intraoperative analgesia (with fentanyl, sufentanil) and anti-emetic (ondansetron, dixamethon, metoclopramide) curtails morbidity in the immediate postoperative period, which consequently leads to uneventful and early hospital discharge.

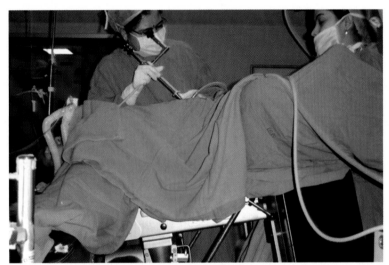

Fig. 15.1: Typical minilaparoscopic tubal ligation

A unique situation springs up during outpatient gynaecologic laparoscopy, that is, the combination of diagnostic /minor laparoscopy procedure with hysteroscopy and /or dye instillation. During hysteroscopy fluid administration must be judicious to avoid overloading. Dye instillation may lead to allergic phenomena and the anaesthetist should be aware and prepared for the event in anticipation. Importantly, a balanced analgesic regimen and deeper plane of anaesthesia is required for situations wherein cervical dilatation and uterine distension (vagal hypertonia, hypotension, patient awareness) is contemplated.

POSTOPERATIVE RECOVERY AND ANALGESIA

Diminished postoperative pain, patient discomfort, shorter length of hospital stay and early return to routine activities have made laparoscopic surgery more popular and preferred technique. Although postanaesthetic morbidity is significantly less as compared to open laparotomy, incisional and shoulder tip pain, PONV, constipation and urinary retention still exist and add to overall morbidity.

If required, short-acting opioid (fentanyl, tramodol) and non-opioids (NSAIDs; diclofenac, ketorolac, ketoprofen; COX-2 inhibitors–roficoxib) generally suffice. For PONV, 5HT-3 antagonists (ondansetron, granisetron) and dexamethasone have shown promising results. Rectus sheath block (with 0.25% bupivacaine) at termination of laparoscopy have shown to decrease postoperative analgesia requirements.[22] At the same time the concept of pre-emptive analgesia to decrease postoperative pain has been largely unsuccessful. In addition, local infiltration (with 0.25% plain bupivacaine) of the larger ports (>5mm) helps in relieving pain that occurs secondary to increase in intraabdominal pressure (coughing, belching, turning position, sneezing) in the postoperative period.

The choice of drugs to treat commonly encountered side effects in the post-laparoscopic intervention period remains attending anaesthesiologist's prerogative, but judicious selection is desirable in order to avoid problems inherent to them.

CRITICAL ISSUES

PROCEDURE RELATED

Use of Nitrous Oxide

In elective, prolonged (>90 min) laparoscopic surgery, the use of nitrous oxide has been debated owing to its effect on haemodynamics, surgical reasons (gut oedema) and postoperative effects (diffusion hypoxia).

Nitrous oxide-induced bowel distension during laparoscopy is unpredictable and many surgeons request routine avoidance of this agent.[23,24] Its effect on intestinal motility and distension seems to correlate well to the increased incidence of emesis after laparoscopic surgery.[25]

Alternatively, compressed air in oxygen is utilized to avoid nitrous oxide related ill effects. However, the use of compressed air needs to be coupled with use of inhalational agent or TIVA, probably under cover of BIS monitoring and adequate opioid analgesia.

Position

Women placed in a Trendenlenberg position have a shift of great vessels antero-superiorly, which makes them more vulnerable to air entry; therefore, the insufflating needle and trocar should always be inserted in accordance with patient's body type and orientation of their body position to horizontal.

Prolonged Gynaecologic laparoscopic surgery brings about complex patient positioning (Fig. 15.2) in tandem with concurrent stage of surgery. On a particular occasion patient can be placed in steep Trendenlenberg position while on the other, a reverse-Trendenlenberg position may be needed to focus upon surgery involving pelvic part. Notwithstanding, lithotomy position that remains consistently coupled with above-stated patient positions adds to complexities.

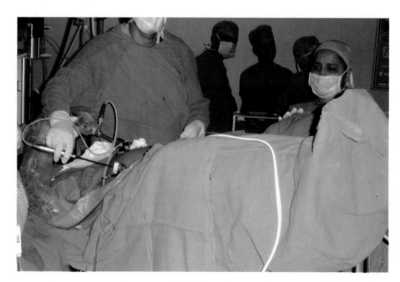

Fig. 15.2: Complex patient position

To offset any negative effect arising out of complex positioning changes intraoperatively, one must apply basic preventive measures including fluid balance (avoid haemodynamic perturbations), padding of bony points (prevent nerve injury), a secured airway, ventilatory adjustment (changing diaphragmatic positions) and maintaining a clear communication with the surgeon.

Gastric Tube Insertion

It is not very uncommon that some gases enter stomach during airway management. Generally, gastric tube insertion is warranted to evacuate the stomach of residual fluid or gases that is present initially or gets accumulated over the course of procedure.[26,27] Gastric tube insertion is deemed mandatory before institution of carboperitoneum and trocar insertion to avoid inadvertent trauma to the stomach. Ideally, a gastric tube of size greater than 16 Fr (lesser size ineffective in suctioning out residue) is inserted orally after intubation. It may be removed once the procedure is over (prior to tracheal extubation).

Urine Output Monitoring

Urine output monitoring is mandatory for lengthy gynaecologic laparoscopies that involve complicated surgical manipulations. It signifies the status of fluid balance as an indicator of tissue trauma (reflected by change in urine colour) perioperatively. However, in absence of any contraindication the catheter should be removed the morning after the surgery.

ANAESTHESIA RELATED

The management of anaesthesia during gynaecologic laparoscopy is similar to that for other laparoscopic procedures apart from few noted exceptions.

Regional and Local Anaesthesia for Laparoscopy

Peritoneal irritation secondary to CO_2-insufflation to create carboperitoneum, risk of visceral and tissue injury owing to patient movement, potential for hypercapnia and hypoxia and related cardiovascular perturbations, and emesis with subsequent aspiration potential negates the use of laparoscopy in conscious, unintubated patients.[28] Therefore, laparoscopic procedures are seldom undertaken with any LA or regional anaesthetic techniques.[29]

General anaesthesia scores over regional / LA method for laparoscopic gynaecologic surgery. Use of epidural anaesthesia (pelvic laparoscopy procedures) and local anaesthesia (abdominal diagnostic procedures) have not shown any definitive physiologic advantage over standardized GA. These techniques may however become important if a genetic problem, patient refusal, debilitated condition or previous adversity (failed difficult airway, prolonged recovery from anaesthesia) preclude a general anaesthetic.

If the laparoscopic procedure is needed to be carried out under an LA due to above-stated reasons; adequate conscious sedation and N_2O (diminished systemic absorption, minimal local irritation) as insufflating gas should be utilized. However, use of N_2O as insufflating gas precludes the use of thermal or laser cautery because it supports oxidation while being non-inflammable.

Advantages and disadvantages of different anaesthetic techniques are summarised in Table 15.2.

Table 15. 2: Anaesthesia techniques

Anaesthetic Technique	Advantage(s)	Disadvantage(s)
Local Anaesthesia[30,31]	Rapid recovery Can be combined with sedation Cost effective	Awake patient Carboperitoneum related problems Breathing difficulty Shoulder tip pain Poor muscle relaxation Risk of visceral injury (patient movement)
Regional Anaesthesia[32,33]	Awake patient ↓Recovery time ↓ peristalsis / bowel shrinkage Fewer drugs ↓ allergic /non allergic side effects avoided ↓ cost effective Problems of GA prevented	Carboperitoneum inadequacy Unsuitable for lengthy surgery Patient apprehension
General Anaesthesia[34,35]	Rapid onset Good analgesia Comprehensive airway control Good muscle relaxation Quiet surgical field Adequate carboperitoneum	↑ recovery time Drugs adverse effects Costly

Irrespective of the anaesthesia technique and monitoring methods applied, laparoscopic surgery should only be performed where equipment is immediately available for GA, exploratory laparotomy and resuscitation.

Airway

Tracheal intubation with a cuffed tracheal tube has been the gold standard for achieving a secured airway in patients undergoing gynaecologic laparoscopy. But for the problems of prolonged intubation (tracheal mucosal trauma, silent aspiration, vocal cord events, laryngeal oedema, etc.) and inadvertent displacement of tracheal tube (with inflation and deflation of carboperitoneum), tracheal intubation and PPV appears to be the airway method of choice.

The recent development of various modifications of LMA have enabled the anaesthesia physician to have an alternative airway during laparoscopic surgery. Routinely, use of c-LMA has become popular with the outpatients because of the ability to avoid sore throat and related laryngeal morbidity as seen with conventional tracheal intubation. PLMA is a modified LMA device which allows adequate PPV during laparoscopy and in addition it has a gastric drain tube which allows the gastric fluid to bypass the airway in case of regurgitation.[36] Moreover, one may pass a gastric tube through the drain tube to carry out gastric suctioning. However, enough experience with c-LMA is mandatory before PLMA can be tried.

COMPLICATIONS OF GYNECOLOGIC LAPAROSCOPY

The reported incidence of minor and major complications secondary to Gynaecologic laparoscopy ranges between 1-4 per cent and 0.3-2.8 per cent respectively. Generally, the complications are similar to any other laparoscopic intervention. Table 15.3 depicts possible complications that may arise out of Gynaecologic laparoscopic intervention.

CURRENT RESEARCH

Regional neuraxial anaesthesia has been in vogue for outpatient laparoscopy since 1978 when Burke[37] put forward a review of over one thousand cases undergoing laparoscopy. A renewed interest in regional anaesthesia technique arose when Vaghadia et al (1997) analysed the effects of selective spinal anaesthesia (SSA) during gynaecologic laparoscopy.[38] In the same year, Chilvers et al investigated the utility of low dose hypobaric lidocaine with fentanyl for outpatient gynaecologic laparoscopy cases.[39] These studies outlined the beneficial effects of SSA (no hypotension faster recovery) in outpatient gynaecologic laparoscopies, although postdural puncture headache remained a problem in some patients. Very recently, Lennox et al (2002)[40] compared the effects of SSA (lidocaine 10 mg + sufentanil 10 mg) with GA (desflurane–N$_2$O) and concluded that SSA patients had favorable impact on time to straight leg raise, ambulation, recovery domain (patients more awake and oriented at the end of surgery), and most importantly had significantly less postoperative pain.

Table 15.3: Complications

Complication	Pathophysiological	Prevention
Cardiac arrhythmias	Hypercarbia, acidemia	IAP < 12 mmHg Use of alternative insufflating gas, e.g. N$_2$O Use of 'Apneumic' techniques
Bradycardia	Vagal stimulus due to peritoneal stretching	Slow insufflation
Hypotension	Inappropriate vagal discharge in response to high IAP Volume depleted patients Pre-existing CV disease	Slow insufflation Preloading
Gastric reflux	Trendelenburg position Obesity Hiatal hernia Gastric outlet obstruction Gastroparesis	Aspiration prophylaxis Early airway security Aspiration with gastric tube Operate at lowest IAP Extubation after normalising patient position
Haemorrhage aorta IVC common iliac vessels	Surgical Trauma	Trocar / insufflation needle insertion with patient on horizontal position
Elevation of diaphragm	Basilar atelectasis V/Q mismatch R → L shunt	Frequent ventilatory adjustments Increase FiO$_2$ Bronchodilation
Trendelenburg position	Hypoventilation Regurgitation / Aspiration Bronchospasm Pneumonitis/ Pneumonia	Cuffed tracheal tube Bronchodilators Antibiotics
CO$_2$ – embolism	Intravascular placement of insufflation needle CO$_2$-macroemboli in central venous system	Ensure absence of blood from Needle before insufflation Operating with IAP < 20 mmHg Hemostasis Use of 'apneumic' laparoscopy

CONCUSSIONS

CLINICAL PEARLS

- Laparoscopy was initially started with minor gynaecological procedures conducted in young, healthy females.
- It has now extended to various major procedures: total abdominal hysterectomy and laparoscopic assited vaginal hysterectomy.
- Laparoscopy is often accompained with hysteroscopy which require fluid to be introduced into the uterine cavity.

REFERENCES

1. Stellato TA. The history of laparoscopic surgery. In: MacFadyen BV, Ponsky JL, eds. Operative Laparoscopy and Thoracoscopy. Philadelphia: Lippincott – Raven, 1996; 3-12.
2. Webb TD. Monitoring for laparoscopic surgery.Seminar Laparosc Surg 1994; 1: 223-27.
3. Marco AP, Yeo CJ, Rock P. Anesthesia for patients undergoing laparoscopic cholecystectomy. Anesthesiology 1990; 73: 1268-70.
4. Wittgen CM, Andrus CM, Fitzerland SD, et al. Analysis of hemodynamic and ventilatory effects of laparoscopic cholecystectomy. Arch Surg 1991; 126: 997-1001.
5. Pandit SK, Kothary SP, Pandit UA, Mathai MK. Comparison of fentanyl and butorphenol for outpatient anesthesia. Can J Anaesth 1987; 34: 130-34.
6. Skacel M, Sengupta P. Morbidity after day case laparoscopy : A comparison of two techniques of tracheal anaesthesia. Anaesthesia 1986; 41: 537-41.
7. Degrood PMRM, Harbers JBM, Egmond J, Crul JF. Anaesthesia for Laparoscopy: a comparison of five techniques including propofol, etomidate, thiopentone, and isoflurane. Anaesthesia 1987; 42: 815-23.
8. Eng back J, Ording H, Ostergaard D, Viby-Mogensen J. Edrophonium and neostigmine for reversal of the neuromuscular blocking effects of vecuronium. Acta Anaesthesiol Scand 1985: 29: 544-46.
9. Crily H, Mcleod K. Use of the laryngeal mask airway – a survey of Australian Anaesthetic Practice. Anaesth Intens Care 200; 28: 224.[abstract]
10. Brimacombe JR. The specialized LMAs 1989-2000. In Brimacombe JR (ed). Laryngeal mask Anesthesia, 2nd edn. Philadelphia: Saunders, 2005; 27-31.
11. Akthar TM, Shankar RK, Street MK. Is Guedels airway and facemask dead? Today's Anaesthetist 1994; 9: 56-58.
12. Dingley J, Asai T. Insertion methods of the laryngeal mask airway. A survey of current practice in Wales. Anaesthesia 1996; 51: 596-99.
13. Brain AIJ. The laryngeal mask – a new concept in airway management. Br J Anaesth 1983; 55: 801-5.
14. Matins AF, Cooper GM. Laparoscopy and laryngeal mask airway. Br J Anaesth 1994; 73: 121.
15. Lefert P, Visseaux H, Gabriel R, Palot M, Pire JC. Use of laryngeal mask airway for laparoscopy. Ann Fr Anesth Reanim 1993; 12: R231
16. Bapat P, Verghese C. Laryngeal mask airway and the incidence of regurgitation during gynecological laparoscopies. Anesth Analg 1997; 85: 139-43.
17. Brimacombe J, Berry A. Aspiration and the laryngeal mask airway. A survey of Australian Intensive care units. Anaesth Intens Care 1992; 20: 534-5.
18. Swann DG, Sipens H, Edwards SA, Chestnict RJ. Anaesthesia for Gynecological laparoscopy – a comparison between laryngeal mask airway and tracheal intubation. Anesthesia 1993; 48: 431-34.
19. Verghese C, Smith TGC, Young E. Prospective survey of use of the laryngeal mask airway in 2359 patients. Anaesthesia 1993; 48: 58-6.
20. Verghese C, Brimacombe J. Survey of laryngeal mask airway usage in 11910 patients; safety and efficacy for conventional and non-conventional usage. Anesth Analg 1996; 82: 129-33.
21. El Mikatti N, Luthra AD, Healy TEJ, Mortimer AJ. Gastric regurgitation during general anesthesia in different positions with the laryngeal mask airway. Anaesthesia 1995; 50: 1053-55.
22. Smith BE, Suchak M, Siggins D, Challands J. Rectus sheath block for diagnostic laparoscopy. Anaesthesia 1988; 43: 947-48.
23. Monk TG, Weldon BC. Anesthetic consideration for laparoscopic surgery. In: Clayman RV, McDougal EM, eds. Laparoscopic Urology. St. Louis : Quality Medical Publishing, 1993; 19-27.
24. Taylor E, Feinstein R, Soper N, White PF. Effect of nitrous oxide on surgical conditions during laparoscopic cholecystectomy. Anesthesiology 1991; 75: 541-43.
25. Lonie DS, Harper NJN. Nitrous oxide anaesthesia and vomiting : the effect of nitrous oxide anaesthesia on incidence of vomiting following Gynecological laparoscopy. Anaesthesia 1986; 41: 703-7.
26. Scarr M, Maltby JR, Jani K, Sutherland LR. Volume and acidity of residual gastric fluid after oral fluid ingestion before elective ambulatory surgery. Can Med Assoc J 1989; 141: 1151-4.
27. Maltby J, Beriault MT, Watson NC, Fick GH. Gastric distension and ventilation during laparoscopic cholecystectomy: LMA-classic vs tracheal intubation. Can J Anaesth 2000; 47(7): 622-6.

28. Gomar C, Fernandez C, Villalonga A, Nalda MA. Carbon dioxide embolism during laparoscopy and hysteroscopy. Ann Fr Anesth Reanim 1985; 4: 380-82.

29. Peterson JB, Hulka JF, Speilman FJ, Lee S, Marchbanks PA. Local versus general anesthesia for laparoscopic sterilisation: a randomised study. Obstet Gynecol 1987; 70: 903-8.

30. Penfido AJ. Gynecologic surgery under local anesthesia. Baltimore: Urban and Schwarzenberg 1986; 21.

31. Wheeless CR Jr. Anesthesia for diagnostic and operative laparoscopy. Fertil Steril 1971; 22: 690.

32. Aribarg A. Epidural analgesia for laparoscopy. J Obstet Gynecol Br Commonw 1973; 80: 567.

33. Bridenbaugh LD, Soderstrom RM: Lumbar epidural block for outpatient laparoscopy. J Reprod Med 1979; 23: 85.

34. Smith I, White PF. Anesthetic consideration for laparoscopic surgery, Semin Laparosc Surg 1994; 1: 198-206.

35. Andreas CH, Wittgen CM, Naunheim KS. Anaesthetic and physiologic changes during laparoscopy and thoracoscopy:the surgeons' view. Semin Laparosc Surg 1994; 1: 228-40.

36. Brimacombe J, Keller C, Bochler M, Puchringer F. Positive pressure ventilation with the ProSeal versus Classic laryngeal mask airway: a randomised, crossover study of healthy female patients. Anesth Analg 2001; 93:1351-3.

37. Burke RA. Spinal anesthesia for laparoscopy; a review of 1,063 cases. J Reprod Med 1978; 21: 59-61.

38. Vaghadia H, McLeod DH, Mitchell GWE, et al. Small-dose hypobaric lidocaine – fentanyl spinal anesthesia for short duration outpatient laparoscopy. A randomised comparison with conventional dose hyperbaric lidocaine. Anesth Analg 1997; 84: 59-64.

39. Chilvers CR, Vaghadia H, Mitchell GWE, Merrick PM. Small dose hypobaric lidocaine – fentanyl spinal anesthesia for short duration outpatient laparoscopy. Optimal fentanyl dose. Anesth Analg 1997; 84: 65-70.

40. Lennox PH, Vaghadia H, Henderson C, et al. Small dose selective spinal anesthesia for short-duration outpatient laparoscopy: recovery characteristics compared with desflurane anesthesia. Anesth Analg 2002; 94: 346-50.

CHAPTER 16

Laparoscopic Surgery in Pregnancy

INTRODUCTION

A few years back laparotomy was considered as the gold standard for all intra-abdominal surgeries in pregnant patients.[1]

Infact laparoscopic surgery was contraindicated in pregnancy due to the various pathophysiological changes of laparoscopy which would probably superimpose on the already existing changes associated with pregnancy. However with more technical advancement and expertise, laparoscopy has now become the technique of choice as compared to laparotomy in a pregnant patient due to various advantages associated with it. However, although laparoscopy has become a technique of choice, it is also fraught with various concerns due to various pathophysiological changes associated with carboperitoneum, raised intraabdominal pressure and patient positioning.

A few basic, but important, concerns which arise when dealing with a pregnant patient undergoing laparoscopic surgery are:

a. The maternal physiologic alterations associated with pregnancy
b. Factors unique to pregnancy and carboperitoneum that can affect uteroplacental blood flow
c. The overall effect of these influences on the well being of the fetus.
d. Surgical considerations
   – space
   – trocar insertion
   – manipulation

PHYSIOLOGICAL CHANGES (TABLE 16.1)

Physiological adaptations and changes occur early in pregnancy and continue throughout gestation, hormonal changes in the first trimester, mechanical effects of the gravid uterus in the second trimester and increasing metabolic demand throughout pregnancy. The systems that are uniquely affected by carboperitoneum and therefore important to address in the preparation of the gravida for laparoscopic surgery will be elaborated.

EFFECT OF CARBOPERITONEUM ON THE RESPIRATORY SYSTEM

There is an increase in oxygen demand and consumption during pregnancy. To provide this, the alveolar ventilation increases by 25 per cent by the 16th week of gestation to a maximum of 70 per cent at term. Due to this increased alveolar ventilation at term, maternal $PaCO_2$ is usually decreased from 35 to 32 mmHg. The pH remains unchanged as there is a compensatory metabolic alkalosis. It is important for an anaesthesiologist to become aware of this fact as maternal hyperventilation leads to hypocarbia (below 30 mmHg) which leads to uterine vasoconstriction, reduced cardiac output secondary to increased intrathoracic pressure and a leftward shift in the maternal oxygen dissociation curve impairing oxygen release from maternal blood to the foetus..

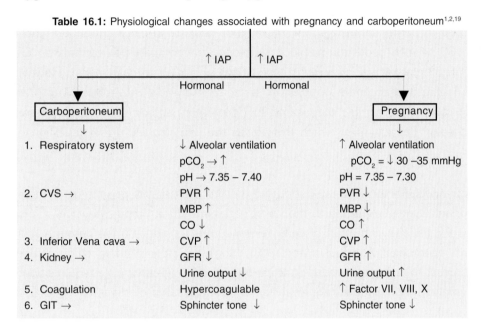

Table 16.1: Physiological changes associated with pregnancy and carboperitoneum[1,2,19]

	Carboperitoneum	Pregnancy
1. Respiratory system	↓ Alveolar ventilation $pCO_2 \rightarrow \uparrow$ pH → 7.35 – 7.40	↑ Alveolar ventilation $pCO_2 = \downarrow$ 30 –35 mmHg pH = 7.35 – 7.30
2. CVS →	PVR ↑ MBP ↑ CO ↓	PVR ↓ MBP ↓ CO ↑
3. Inferior Vena cava →	CVP ↑	CVP ↑
4. Kidney →	GFR ↓ Urine output ↓	GFR ↑ Urine output ↑
5. Coagulation	Hypercoagulable	↑ Factor VII, VIII, X
6. GIT →	Sphincter tone ↓	Sphincter tone ↓

There is a reduction in the functional residual capacity by about 20 per cent due to the gravid uterus pressing on the diaphragm. Due to the decrease in functional residual capacity which is the oxygen reserve of the lung, even brief periods of apnoea can cause desaturation. Apnoea lasting one minute has been found to reduce oxygen tension by 139 mmHg in parturients as compared to 58 mmHg in non pregnant patients.[4] Introduction of carboperitoneum in a pregnant patient further limits the diaphragm expansion thus leading to a further decrease in FRC, increase in V/Q mismatching, increase in arterio-alveolar gradient, decrease in thoracic cavity compliance and increase in plateau pleural pressure. Trendelenburg position further raises the diaphragm and increases the intrathoracic pressure and compounds the respiratory related physiological changes. Any increase in maternal $PaCO_2$ or decrease in PaO_2 can affect fetal well being.[13] Thus, the combination of pregnancy and carboperitoneum predisposes the parturient to hypoxemia and hypercarbia. Insufflation of CO_2 results in its absorption into the blood stream. Elimination of this CO_2 depends on an increase in minute ventilation, but mechanical hyperventilation can reduce uteroplacental perfusion. This has important clinical implications. Firstly, it is necessary to improve maternal oxygen reserve and neonatal outcome by adequate preoxygenation. Three minutes of preoxygenation or four vital capacity breaths within 30 seconds of induction satisfactorily increases maternal oxygenation. Secondly, it is essential to begin mask ventilation early rather than persist with intubation attempts.

CARDIOVASCULAR SYSTEM[7]

The cardiac output starts to increase as early as five weeks of gestation and increases upto 40 per cent above the non pregnant state by the end of second trimester. Mean arterial blood pressure falls due to the effect of progesterone on the vascular system. The gravid uterus presses on the inferior vena cava in the supine position resulting in hypotension and a reduction in cardiac output of 25-60 per cent (supine hypotension). Introduction of carboperitoneum, coupled with aortocaval compression further accentuates the hypotension.[6] The addition of reverse Trendelenburg position further produces a fall in blood pressure.[6] A combination of reverse Trendelenburg position, general anaesthesia and peritoneal insufflation decreases the cardiac index by as much as 50 per cent.[10] In studies involving pregnant maternal ewes maternal perfusion pressure decreased approximately 22 per cent in response to peritoneal insufflation with carbon dioxide to cause intraabdominal pressure of 20 mmHg resulting in a 60 per cent reduction in placental blood flow compared to controls[8,9,15] (Table 16.2). But there was no reduction of fetal perfusion pressure, blood flow, pH or blood gas tension. However extrapolating from human studies in the non pregnant population, it seems likely that intra-abdominal pressure above 20 mmHg or 15 mmHg can reduce cardiac output and blood pressure sufficiently to result in some decrease in uteroplacental blood flow.[8] The extent to which this affects the fetus awaits further investigation. [8]

RENAL SYSTEM[3,4,5,7]

The renal plasma flow and GFR increase rapidly during the first trimester of pregnancy, being elevated 50 per cent above non pregnant values by the fourth month of gestation. Urine output, however, does not reflect this increase. In non obstetric patients, the effect of carboperitoneum is to reduce urine output and this is attributed to the release of stress hormones, vasopressin and renin. However, there is no specific reference to this in an obstetric patient. The effect of carboperitoneum on urine output, although reversible requires adequate hydration preoperatively and careful surveillance intraoperatively to optimize renal blood flow[3,4,5] (Table 16.2).

COAGULATION

The pregnant woman becomes hypercoagulable as gestation progresses. Factors VII, VIII, X and fibrinogen are markedly increased.[5] Two of the factors in the Virchow's triad (hypercoaguability and venous stasis) are affected in laparoscopy; therefore, the hypercoaguable state of pregnancy along with the DVT susceptibility in laparoscopy, places the parturient at substantial risk of DVT during the raised IAP produced by carboperitoneum. Graded compression stockings, intermittent pneumatic compressions with or without prophylactic subcutaneous heparin at the onset of surgery should be the standard protocol.[24]

GASTROINTESTINAL SYSTEM[2,3,4,11]

The pregnant patient is at a high risk of silent gastric regurgitation and pulmonary aspiration due to effect of progesterone and mechanical consequences of the gravid uterus producing a change in the angulation of the gastroesophageal junction. Gastric stasis is also common phenomenon in pregnancy. The normal upper esophageal sphincter (UES) pressure is 38 cm of H_2O; while the normal lower esophageal sphincter (LES) pressure is 28 cm of H_2O with normal intra-gastric pressure (IGP) being 10 cm of H_2O. Therefore, the barrier pressure is around 18 cm of H_2O. In pregnancy there is disproportionate increase in both LES pressure (~35) and IGP (~34) as a result of which the effective barrier pressure is decreased. However in laparoscopic surgeries, creation of carboperitoneum increases the tone of the lower esophageal sphincter and thus increases the barrier pressure.

Table 16.2: Summary of the effect of carboperitoneum on pregnant patient

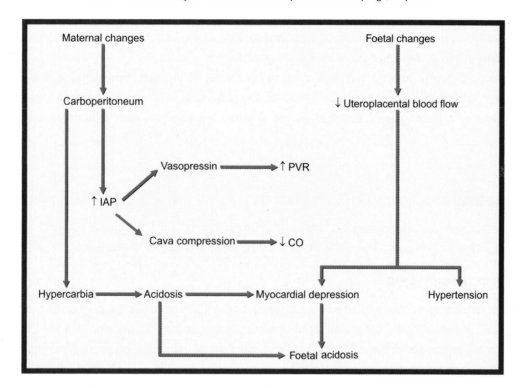

The hormone gastrin produced by the placenta raises the acid, chloride and enzyme content of the stomach and thus, makes gastric pH less than 2.5. All parturients must be considered at risk of pulmonary aspiration of acid material producing the acid aspiration syndrome of Mendelson. Thus all precautions must be taken to minimize gastric acidity preoperatively. Liberal use of a nasogastric tube to assure gastric emptying and careful patient positioning intraoperatively are additional measures to minimise this risk[5,6] (Table 16.1).

UTEROPLACENTAL BLOOD FLOW

Normal uterine blood flow at term is 600-700 ml per minute. Any decrease in maternal blood pressure due to supine hypotension syndrome or increased IAP (carboperitoneum) will further decrease uterine blood flow.[6,7] The introduction of carboperitoneum leads to activation of the renin angiotensin pathway which leads to increased uterine vascular resistance which further decreases the uteroplacental blood flow.

EFFECT OF CARBOPERITONEUM ON THE FETUS

The deleterious effects of carboperitoneum on human fetus have not been reported.[10,11,12,13] However the study (only study) by Amos et al[10] reported fetal deaths in four out of seven women after laparoscopic appendectomy and cholecystectomy (three during the first postoperative week and one four weeks postoperatively). However literature survey by Mazen Bisharah[24] et al have evaluated over 250 cases of laparoscopic cholecystectomy and appendectomy and have found no adverse effects on the fetus. The incidence of fetal congenital anomaly is less than two of 400 laparoscopies in pregnancy in study by Bisharah et al and they have concluded that it is unlikely that laparoscopy is the cause.[24]

Soriano[24] et al have reported the largest series of operative treatment of adrenal masses during pregnancy. Thirty nine patients had laparoscopy while 54 patients underwent a laparotomy. The laparoscopy was done in the first trimester of pregnancy. In the laparoscopic group, five women had miscarriage and two newborns had congenital malformation – hypospadias, cleft lip and palate.

In the laparotomy group, two miscarriages were encountered in the first trimester and one transposition of great vessels was found in the second trimester. These are the only congenital anomalies reported after laparoscopic surgery in pregnancy and they have concluded that whether surgery had any relation to these anomalies is unknown.

OTHER ISSUES

IMMUNOLOGICAL STATUS

Pregnancy is a mildly immunocompromised state stemming from decreased chemotaxis and adherence ability of polymorphonuclear leucocytes. Thus use of perioperative antibiotics is mandatory.

ALTERNATIVES TO CARBOPERITONEUM

Carbon dioxide is the gas commonly used to create carboperitoneum during laparoscopic surgeries. A new approach to laparoscopic surgery utilizes an apneumic approach, mainly the abdominal wall lift method. This avoids the effects of carbon dioxide insufflation and increased intra-abdominal pressure. Preliminary data suggest that the gasless laparoscopy confers fewer hemodynamic changes. Akira et al and Tanaka et al[1] compared laparotomy with gasless laparoscopy for ovarian cystectomy during pregnancy and they have reported that patients with gasless laparoscopy required lesser analgesics, less tocolytic agents and were ambulatory earlier. Further, this procedure could be done under epidural anaesthesia, the parturients remained spontaneously breathing and maintained a $PaCO_2$ near baseline throughout the procedure.[6,7] Gasless laparoscopic cholecystectomy in pregnancy has also been reported.[6,7,8]

USE OF ELECTROCAUTERY IN A PREGNANT PATIENT

Electrocautery creates heat and vaporizes intracellular fluid and burns proteins and other organic molecules causing thermal necrosis in adjacent tissues. This process creates smoke containing carbon monoxide, which during laparoscopy can accumulate in the abdomen if not properly evacuated. Carbon monoxide combines with hemoglobin to form carboxyhemoglobin and methemoglobin both of which compete with hemoglobin for oxygen and reduce the oxygen carrying capacity of red blood cells if allowed to accumulate during laparoscopy. Carbon monoxide may also be absorbed into the maternal circulation and can affect oxygen delivery to the fetus. Beebe et al[25] showed that although carbon monoxide is present in the abdominal gases five minutes after electrocautery is initiated, maternal blood levels of carboxyhaemoglobin were not elevated either during surgery or postoperatively and authors attribute this to diligent evacuation of intraabdominal smoke – meticulous attention to this detail is essential.

REMOVAL OF SPECIMEN IN LAPAROSCOPY

When appropriate, specimens (gall bladder, appendix, etc.) should be placed in an endoscopic bag before removal from the abdomen, specifically in patients with a dermoid cyst as an intraabdominal spillage may increase the risk of peritonitis postoperatively. If spillage occurs, then irrigation with large quantities of warm saline is mandatory.[15]

WHICH TRIMESTER IS SAFE FOR SURGERY (Table 16.3)

The second trimester is the optimal time to operate as organogenesis occurs in the first trimester and the susceptibility to induce premature labor and delivery in the third trimester.[6] Surgical procedures that do not involve uterine manipulation incur the lowest risk of preterm labour. The miscarriage rate is 5.6 per cent in the second trimester[24] compared with 12 per cent in the first trimester. The rate of preterm labor in the second trimester is very low. However instead of operating in the third trimester, in most cases an operative procedure can be delayed until the postpartum period. It is, therefore, prudent to evaluate uterine size and feasibility of the laparoscopic approach in providing adequate visibility of abdominal organs without undue uterine manipulation. With advancing gestation the ureter is also at great risk of injury; however, there is no consensus on the gestational age at which the uterus will limit laparoscopic access. Each case must be assessed individually and matched with the operators expertise and level of comfort.

TIME AND EXPOSURE

The duration of any surgical procedure in pregnancy should be limited to minimize the inherent risk of prolonged anaesthesia on the fetus and laparoscopy is no exception. If the experience of the surgeon is such that the procedure

Table 16.3: Surgical recommendations for management of the pregnant surgical patient

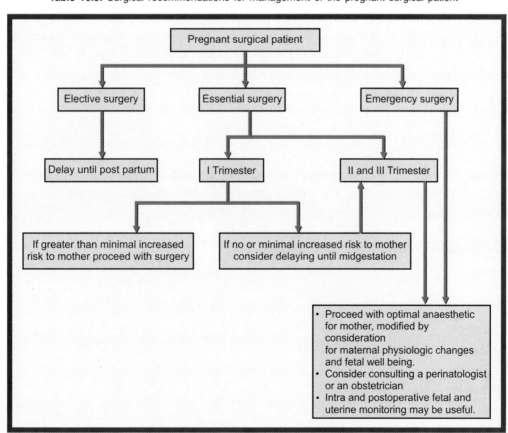

might take longer laparoscopically, it might be best to refer to a surgeon with more experience or perform the operation via laparotomy.[24]

ANESTHETIC DRUGS

The pharmacokinetic and pharmacodynamic profiles are altered in pregnancy, and drug administration must be titrated carefully to the desired effect. With the increase in blood volume, there is a greater volume of distribution, low albumin and increased $\alpha 1$ glycoprotein which may also alter free drug concentrations. MAC of inhalational anaesthetics is also reduced during pregnancy. The parturient is also sensitive to local anaesthetics. Careful titration of drugs is an important factor.

Nitrous oxide inactivates methionine synthetase, which in turn inhibits the synthesis of thymidine and DNA, inhibits cell division and potentially disrupts other biochemical pathways in methylation reactions. The concern is whether these known cellular effects of anesthetic agents are teratogenic, but to date, no clinical data link these cellular actions with teratogenic outcomes[5,6,7,8.]

Thiopentone (ultra short-acting barbiturates) is the induction agent of choice. It does cross the placenta very rapidly, however the fetal brain will not be exposed to high concentrations of barbiturate as the blood from the placenta first passes through the liver where most of it is cleared.

Propofol has still not been approved for obstetric anaesthesia and human studies are still debatable.

Muscle relaxants – being quarternary ammonium compounds cross the placenta in clinically insignificant amounts and therefore can be used safely in obstetric anaesthesia.

All opioids, can be used in pregnancy but in titrated doses as they all produce effective analgesia and some degree of respiratory depression, obtund reflexes and result in postural hypotension.

The use of liberal prophylactic tocolysis in these patients to prevent preterm labor is controversial as it is not without risk.

A baseline preoperative cervical examination with reservation of tocolysis for those at risk of preterm-labour (i.e. history of preterm labor), significant perioperative uterine activity and / or documented cervical change has been suggested.[2,3]

POSITIONING

During laparoscopy the position of the patient is altered several times to produce gravitational displacement of the viscera away from the surgical side. The Trendelenburg, reverse Trendelenburg, the left lateral tilt to avoid supine hypotension produce several haemodynamic and respiratory alterations.

MONITORING OF A PREGNANT PATIENT UNDERGOING LAPAROSCOPY

- Heart rate
- NIBP
- SpO_2
- $EtCO_2$
- Uterine contractions
- Fetal heart doppler
- Intra-abdominal pressure
- Airway pressure
- Urine output

Meticulous monitoring[11] of a pregnant patient is important as the surgery involves two lives instead of one. Monitoring of maternal heart rate, non invasive blood pressure and peripheral saturation of oxygen tension is important. Bhavani Shankar et al[6] states that there is little difference in the $PaCO_2$ and $EtCO_2$ levels (0.03 mmHg) and thus endtidal CO_2 is a good reflection of maternal $PaCO_2$ and is an essential monitor. They have also concluded that arterial blood gases monitoring during laparoscopy in pregnant patients with healthy lungs is not necessary. As with any surgical patient, adequate hydration, careful monitoring of urine output are of paramount importance. The SAGES guidelines clearly states that the intraabdominal pressure should be minimized to 8-12 mmHg and not allowed to exceed 15 mmHg. So a strict monitoring of the intraabdominal pressure is mandatory.

FOETAL MONITORING

Intermittent foetal heart rate auscultation to document foetal life[14] in the previable stage and continuous monitoring at viability with biophysical profile testing for nonreactive or nonreassuring tracings is essential to follow foetal well being. Rosen et al recommends the use of a sterile sleeve on a transabdominal ultrasound transducer and on a transesophageal echocardiography probe directly on the uterus if external abdominal ultrasound is not logically feasible. The decision to intervene for foetal distress should be made and prepared for in advance of the surgical procedure. There is no advantage of prophylactic tocolytic agents and they should be reserved for patients with documented uterine activity, cervical change and risk of preterm delivery.

Consultation with the neonatal team is integral in the planning of a possible emergent delivery and in informing the prospective parents of survivability at the gestational age in question.

Certain guidelines – should be routinely adopted to enhance operative safety. SAGES- guidelines for laparoscopic surgery during pregnancy are:[15]

1. Place the patient in the left lateral decubitus position as with open surgery to prevent uterine compression of the inferior vena cava. Minimising the degree of reverse Trendenlenburg position may also further reduce possible compression of the inferior vena cava.

2. An open Hasson technique for gaining access to the abdominal cavity is safer than a closed percutaneous technique as the potential for puncture of the uterus or intestine still exists, especially with increasing gestational age.

3. Maintain the intra-abdominal pressure as low as possible. A pressure less than 12-15 mmHg should be used until concerns about the effects of high intra-abdominal pressure on the fetus are answered.

4. Continuously monitor maternal $EtCO_2$ and maintain it between 25-30 mmHg by changing the minute ventilation. Promptly correcting any maternal acidosis is critical as the fetus is typically slightly more acidotic than the mother.

5. Use antiembolic devices to prevent deep venous thrombosis

6. Use continuous intraoperative fetal monitoring. If fetal distress is noted, release the carboperitoneum immediately.

7. If intraoperative cholangiography is to be performed, protect the fetus with a lead shield to protect it from radiation exposure.

8. Minimize operating time – several studies have demonstrated a direct relation between the duration of carboperitoneum and an increase in $PaCO_2$.

9. Tocolytic agents should not be administered prophylactically. If there is any evidence of uterine irritability then they have a role.

CONCLUSIONS

As with any intervention, the benefits must clearly outweigh the risks. In pregnancy, this is particularly important since we are dealing with two patients. Careful preoperative assessment and selection of cases likely to benefit from laparoscopic surgery is essential with the goal of optimising the health and well being of both the fetus and mother as the foremost concern.

Thus, one can safely conclude that laparoscopy is best reserved for anaesthesiologists and surgeons with extensive experience and expertise in performing these procedures in a carefully and wisely selected group of patients.

REFERENCES

1. Jonathan L. Benumof. Anaesthesia for minimally invasive surgery Laparoscopy, Thoracoscopy, Hysteroscopy. Anaesthesiol Clin N Am. 2001; 19(1).
2. Sol. M. Shnider and Gershon Levinson. Laparoscopic surgery during pregnancy. J Am Ass Gynaec Laparos 1999; 6: 229.
3. Sol. M. Shnider and Gershon Levinson. Anesthesia for Obstetrics. In : RD Miller (ed). Anesthesia, Churchill Livingstone; 4th Ed, Vol 2, pg 2031-77.
4. Rachel A. Farragher and Bhavani Shankar Kodali. Obstetric Anesthesia. In: Wylie and Churchill-Davidson's. 7th Ed, Chapter 57, pg 923-40.
5. Alan C. Santos, David A, O'Gorman and Mieczyslaw Feister. Obstetric Anesthesia. 4th Ed 2001 – Clinical Anaesthesia by Barash.
6. Bhavani Shankar K, Steinbrook R. Anaesthetic considerations for minimally invasive surgery. In Brooks DC (ed): Current Review of Minimally Invasive Surgery Ed 2, Philadelphia Current Medicine 1998;29-42.
7. Raul J. Rosenthal, Richard L. Friedman, Edivard H.Phillips eds. The Pathophysiology of carboperitoneum. Springer-Verlag Berlin Heidelberg 1998; Germany.
8. Hunter JG, Swanstrom I, Thoenburg K. Carbon dioxide carboperitoneum induces fetal acidosis in a pregnant ewe model. Surg Endos 1995;9:268-71.
9. Duncan PG, Pope WDB, Coher MM, et al. Fetal risk of anaesthesia and surgery during pregnancy. Anaesthesiology 1986; 64:790-94
10. Amos JP, Schor SJ, Norman PF, et al. Laparoscopic surgery during pregnancy. Am J Surg 1996;171:435-37.
11. Lachman E, Schienfeld A, Voss E, et al. Pregnancy and Laparoscopic surgery. J Am Assoc Gynaecol Laparoscopy 1999; 6:347-51.
12. Soper NJ, Hunter JG, Petric RH. Laparoscopic cholecystectomy during pregnancy. Surg Endos 1992;6:115-17.
13. Steinbrook RA, Brooks DC, Datta S. Laparoscopic cholecystectomy during pregnancy. Surg Endos 1996;10:511-15.
14. Kevin Stepp, Tommaso Falcone. Laparoscopy in the second trimester of pregnancy. Obst. & Gynaecol Clin N Am 2004; 31:485-96.
15. Guidelines for laparoscopic surgery during pregnancy. Surg. Endosc 1998;12:189-90.
16. Lyass S, Pikarsky A, Eisenberg VH, Elchalal U, Schenker JG Russman. Is Laparoscopic Appendectomy safe in pregnant women? Surg Endosc April 2001;15(4):377-9.
17. Rallins MD, Chan KJ and Price RR. Laparoscopy for appendicitis and cholelithiasis during pregnancy: a new standard of care. Surg Endosc Feb. 2004;18(2):237-41.
18. Kim WW, Chon JY, Chun SW, Jeon HM, Kim EK. Laparoscopic procedures during the third trimester of pregnancy. Surg Endos May 2000;14(5):501-3.
19. Lanzafame RJ. Laparoscopic cholecystectomy during pregnancy. Surg Oct. 1995;118(4):627-31.
20. Curet MJ, Allen D, Josloff RK, et al. Laparoscopy during pregnancy. Archives of Surg 1996;131:546-51.
21. Hardwick RH, Slade RR, Smith PA. Laparoscopic splenectomy in pregnancy. J Laparo Endos Adv Surg Tech 1999;9: 439-41.
22. Affleck DG, Handrahan DL, Figger MJ, et al. Laparoscopic Management of appendicitis and cholelithiasis during pregnancy. Am J Surg 1999;178:523-28.
23. Fetal response to carbon dioxide carboperitoneum in the pregnant ewe. Obstet Gynaec 1995;85:669-70.
24. Mazen Bisharah, Togas Tulandi. Laparoscopic surgery in pregnancy. Clinical Obstetrics and Gynaecology, 2003;46(1): 92-97.
25. Beebe DS, Svica H, Carlson N, Palahnuirk RJ et al. High levels of carbon monoxide are produced by electrocautery of tissue during laparoscopic cholecystectomy. Anesth Analg 1993;77:338-41.
26. Bhavani Shankar K, Steinbrook RA, Brooks David C, Datta Sanjay. Arterial to end tidal carbon dioxide pressure difference during laparoscopic surgery in pregnancy. Anesthesiology, 2000;93(2):370-73.

Anaesthesia for Laparoscopy in Paediatric Patients

CHAPTER 17

INTRODUCTION

The basic techniques of paediatric laparoscopy do not differ significantly from that of the adult patient. Laparoscopy has been in use since 1923 when it was first described by Kelling.Only in the last decade, however, has its use in the child become more popular. In addition to its enthusiastic utilization by general surgeons in adults, improvements in video technology and development of smaller endoscopic instruments have encouraged the application of laparoscopic techniques to paediatric problems. The availability of telescopes as small as 2 mm in diameter now permit applications even for neonates.

The documented benefits of shorter hospital stay, better recovery, improved cosmetic results and a markedly reduced incidence of postoperative pain, ileus and hernias have made laparoscopy an attractive option in children also.

Table 17.1: Laparoscopy: Advantages and disadvantage

Advantages	Disadvantage
1. Less pain, early recovery	Slow learning curve → more operative time
2. Small incision → small scar → good healing	
3. Less incidence of atelectactasis and pneumonitis	
4. Less incidence of postoperative small bowel slowing or malfunction	
5. Less duration of hospitalization → less stress to family	

An increasing number of pediatric surgical conditions are now amenable to minimally invasive techniques. It is nowadays being routinely performed in pediatric patients for therapeutic procedures like cholecystectomy, appendicectomy, esophageal fundoplication, gastrostomy, closure of bowel perforation and also as an important diagnostic tool for evaluation of undescended testis, intersex, acute abdomen and staging of abdominal carcinomas. With increasing experience in paediatric laparoscopy more sophisticated procedures such as colectomy, "pull-through" for Hirschsprung's disease,[1, 2] pyeloplasty, and treatment for vesico-ureteral reflux, gut malrotation and choledocal cysts are now possible (Fig. 17.1).

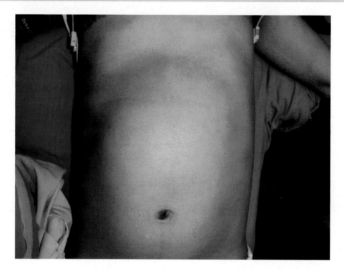

Fig. 17.1: Child with acute abdomen

Size and weight are no longer considered contraindications to laparoscopic approach. Judgment must, however, be carefully applied in instances of pre-existing coagulopathy and cardiorespiratory compromise (which might be exacerbated by carboperitoneum).

PAEDIATRIC LAPAROSCOPIC PROCEDURES

1. Laparoscopic exploration of contralateral hernia.
2. Laparoscopic repair of recurrent inguinal hernia.
3. Diagnostic laparoscopic exploration and orchidopexy for undescended testis.
4. Diagnostic laparoscopy in chronic and recurrent abdominal pain.
5. Pyloromyotomy.
6. Appendicectomy.
7. Nissen Fundoplication.
8. Laparoscopic appendicectomy for faecal incontinence.
9. Cholecystectomy and common bile duct exploration.
10. Splenectomy.
11. Excision of mesenteric cysts.
12. Division of Ladd's bands in Malrotation of small bowel.
13. Pull through surgery for Hirschsprung's disease.
14. Laparoscopic or lap assisted excision of Meckle's diverticulum.
15. Liver biopsy and operative cholangiogram in biliary atresia and other conditions.
16. Retroperitoneal lymph node sampling for diagnosis and staging of lymphoma.
17. Nephroureterectomy, ureterolithotomy and pyelolithotomy.
18. Oopherectomy, Oopheropexy, Ovarian biopsy, Excision of ovarian cyst.

Carbon dioxide (CO_2) has so far proved to be the ideal gas for insufflation and is being used almost universally[3] so much so that term pneumoperitoneum is now almost synonymous to carboperitoneum. Carbon dioxide is cheap, noncombustible and soluble with an Oswald's blood gas solubility coefficient of 0.48. Residual carboperitoneum after CO_2 exsufflation of is cleared more rapidly than that created by other gases, hence minimizing postoperative discomfort.

Several anaesthetic concerns are unique to laparoscopic procedures and they are more so in paediatric patients.[3] As in adults, the main trespasses to normal homeostasis during laparoscopy are patient positioning, insufflation of gas (CO_2) and raised intra-abdominal pressure.

PATHOPHYSIOLOGY OF CARBOPERITONEUM IN A CHILD

In children the small size of the abdomen restricts the volume of gas that can be used for insufflation as the stretch limit of the abdomen is easily exceeded. While adults may require 2.5 to 5 L, a 10 kg-child would need only about 0.9L.[4]

The pathophysiological changes in cardio-respiratory system appear very fast. Difficulty in maintaining adequate carboperitoneum during change of instruments at the ports results in time loss making procedures longer in children.[5] The already compromised therapeutic window for safe laparoscopy in children is further constricted by presence of comorbidities like anemia, sepsis and congenital heart disease. Large flows of cold CO_2 adds to hypothermia further depressing cardiorespiratory functions. Hence, for smaller and sicker, infants greater caution has to be exercised for laparoscopy (Fig. 17.2).

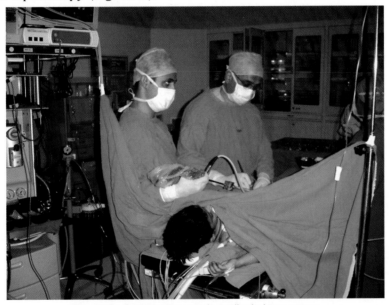

Fig. 17.2: Carboperitoneum in pediatric laparoscopy

INTRA-ABDOMINAL PRESSURE AND LAPAROSCOPY

EFFECTS ON HAEMODYNAMICS

As in adults the IAP (intraabdominal pressure) is the most important factor affecting the haemodynamics in paediatric laparoscopy. Carboperitoneum and resulting raised intra-abdominal pressure produce a fall in preload and rise in afterload with resultant fall in cardiac output. Hypercapnia can provoke sympathetic nervous system activity, leading to an increase in blood pressure, heart rate, myocardial contractility and arrhythmias. It also sensitizes the myocardium to catecholamines, particularly when volatile anaesthetics like halothane are being used.[6] Children with no cardiorespiratory disease tolerate these changes in preload and afterload better but in the presence of poor

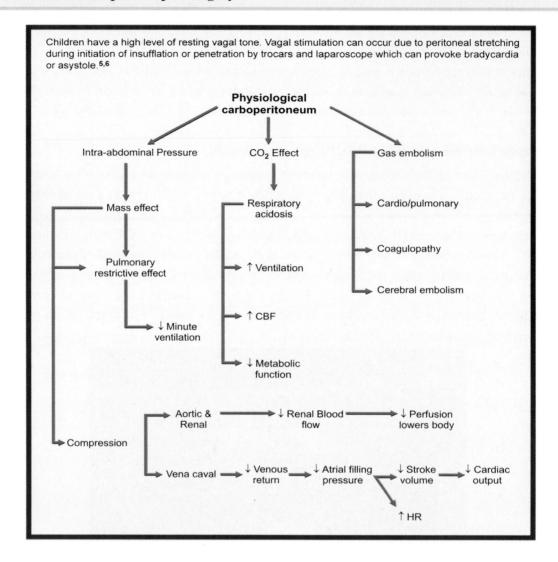

Children have a high level of resting vagal tone. Vagal stimulation can occur due to peritoneal stretching during initiation of insufflation or penetration by trocars and laparoscope which can provoke bradycardia or asystole.[5,6]

cardiorespiratory reserve, anaemia or hypovolaemia, haemodynamic instability can occur, especially during insufflation, positioning and volume loading.[6]

Technical details such as optimum intra-abdominal pressure as applied to children are still open to discussion. A compromise has to be reached between optimal surgical conditions, intra-abdominal pressure and haemodynamic effects.[7, 8]

Tobias JD et al studied the factors that determine haemodynamic changes after carboperitoneum, raised IAP and changes in patient position in children. They found that at IAP less than 15 mmHg venous return is augmented by compression of venous bed of viscera thereby increasing cardiac output whereas at IAP of more than 15 mmHg direct pressure on inferior vena cava (IVC) produces fall in the venous return and hence the cardiac output. In open surgeries the fall in cardiac output due to compression of IVC is compensated by collaterals but during carboperitoneum the collaterals are compressed as well thereby producing profound fall in blood pressure.[6,7]

Raised IAP may cause inferior vana caval (IVC) compression and arise in arterial blood pressure. Heart rate increases as a response to decreased ventricular stroke volume and cardiac output. Mechanical pressure on the kidney directly reduces urine output and the liver is underperfused. Animal studies (on newborn lambs) showed that at IAP of 25 mmHg there is 35 per cent reduction in renal, hepatic and intestinal blood flow.[9] As long as IAP is kept below 12 mmHg the pathophysiological changes are well tolerated. Cautious use of narcotics that depress respiration and medications that suppress cardiac function and circulatory homeostatic mechanisms is advised. Monitoring of cardio-respiratory functions should extend into 3-hour postoperative period. Anaesthesiologist must be cautious of exacerbation of gastro-oesophageal reflux as a consequence of raised IAP.

The adverse effects of carboperitoneum on the haemodynamics led to recommendations limiting IAP to 6 mmHg in infants because of the risk of re-opening of right-left shunts (foramen ovale) and to 12 mmHg in older children.[10]

Patient's position and duration of surgery further aggravate cardiovascular changes. ETCO$_2$ is not a reliable monitor of PaCO$_2$ in patients with congenital cyanotic heart disease (CCHD) undergoing laparoscopic procedures. Wulkan ML et al recommend close monitoring; including arterial blood gas measurements, and an experienced anaesthesia team to perform laparoscopic procedures in children with CCHD.[10-13]

EFFECTS ON RESPIRATORY SYSTEM

Controlled ventilation with modifications of minute volume is prudent. Minimal change in vital signs and ventilatory settings is seen even during brief procedures. The infant is a diaphragmatic breather. Increased IAP restricts diaphragmatic excursions and carboperitoneum results in rapid diffusion of carbon dioxide into the blood stream producing catastrophic effects on gas exchange. Correction of these abnormalities can be achieved by increasing the minute ventilation or by altering the balance of pressures across the diaphragm by placing the patient in Trendelenburg or reverse Trendelenburg position. These effects on a normal child may be minimal but may result in circulatory and respiratory insufficiency in a sick child. Raised IAP and carboperitoneum require careful monitoring of respiratory mechanics, minute ventilation, pulmonary compliance, arterial blood gases, pH and ETCO$_2$. Even though CO$_2$ uptake in paediatric patients is much more efficient as the absorptive area of peritoneum in relation to body weight is greater, hypercapnia develops when carboperitoneum lasts greater than 1 hour. The end-tidal CO$_2$ (EtCO$_2$), however can be restored to basal level by increasing the minute ventilation by 25-30 per cent.[4,11]

The magnitude of rise in EtCO$_2$ maybe to the extent that it prevents its correction by ventilatory adjustment. In such cases it is advisable to discontinue laparoscopy to allow CO$_2$ elimination and resume carboperitoneum thereafter at lower insufflation rate and pressure (Fig. 17.3).

Anaesthesia itself may result in hypoventilation, acidosis, atelectasis and decreased urine output.

Functional residual capacity (FRC) is low in children i.e. 10 per cent of Total lung capacity (TLC) and quickly falls below closing capacity under general anaesthesia (20%). When carboperitoneum ensues there is cephalad displacement of diaphragm, leading to small airway collapse, atelectasis, intrapulmonary shunting and hypoxemia. The result is ventilation–perfusion mismatch, which gets further aggravated in Trendelenburg position. The rise in peak airway pressure and fall in lung compliance returns to near normal levels after exsufflation much faster in children as compared to adults perhaps due to different chest wall configuration and greater thoracic distensibility.[11,12]

Intraoperatively arterial oxygen saturation can be improved by use of PEEP.[6] Much adjustment is required in minute ventilation because of use of uncuffed tubes and hence pressure cycled ventilators are preferred in

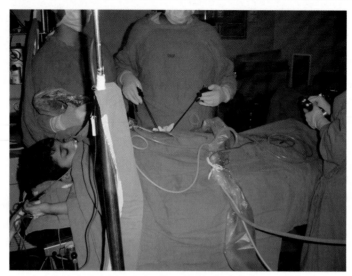

Fig. 17.3: Laparoscopy in progress

children so that there is leak around tracheal tubes is minimized, more so after carboperitoneum and Trendelenburg position.[5]

On exsufflation there is short-lived increase in EtCO$_2$, which may be related to an increase in venous return from the lower limbs after release of the abdominal pressure. The additional CO$_2$ load can persist into the postoperative period resulting in increased ventilatory requirement when the ability to increase ventilation is impaired by residual anaesthetic drugs and diaphragmatic dysfunction.[5]

Children undergoing laparoscopic Nissen fundoplication may have coexisting respiratory disease due to chronic aspiration of gastric contents. Due to interference with diaphragmatic function postoperative hypoxemia may persist and develop upto 3 hours after surgery. Raised IAP may allow escape of insufflating gases to gain access into tissue spaces and produce pneumothorax and pneumomediastinum. This surgery should be followed by chest radiograph.[4, 14]

These findings suggest that small children warrant close monitoring during laparoscopy and during the immediate postoperative period.

EFFECTS ON INTRACRANIAL PRESSURE

Laparoscopy produces elevation in intracranial pressure due to hypercapnia, increased SVR and head-down positioning and so it should not be performed in children with reduced intracranial compliance.IAP of 25 mmHg increases the intracranial pressures from a mean of 7.6 to 21.4 mmHg and produces a fall in cerebral perfusion pressure from 82 to 62 mmHg.In is inadvisable to perform laparoscopy in patients with reduced intracranial compliance.[15]

STRESS RESPONSE

The neuroendocrine axis is activated to same extent after laparoscopy as compared to open procedures in children. Blood levels of lactate, glucose and interleukin-6 after laparoscopy are similar to open procedures.[16]

ANAESTHETIC MANAGEMENT

Thorough preoperative evaluation is required as in any other major surgical procedure. Premedication is a matter of anesthesiologist's or institutional preference and adjusted according to underlying disease. It can vary from midazolam (oral), triclofos and opioids to ketamine. Metoclopramide (0.02mg/kg) and H_2 receptor blockers are advisable to prevent regurgitation and aspiration of gastric contents. Anaesthesia should be tailored according to severity of pre-existing disease and urgency of the procedure. A haemogram and urine analysis is required as routine preoperative investigations.

While some laparoscopic surgeries in adults can be performed under local or regional anaesthesia, general anaesthesia is recommended in all paediatric patients undergoing laparoscopy. Ventilation is controlled and may have to be increased to maintain normocapnia. If a Jackson-Rees modification of the Ayre's T-piece is used it may be necessary to increase the gas flows to maintain nonrebreathing however the closed circuit with sodalime absorber is a better choice in paediatric laeparoscopic procedures.[3]

Preloading with crystalloid 20-ml/kg fluid bolus is recommended to offset haemodynamic effects of carboperitoneum. Peripheral intravenous access should be adequate to permit rapid fluid resuscitation in face of accidental vascular injury during blind Veress needle insertion or during procedures like laparoscopic nephrectomy or splenectomy.[16] Venous access should preferably be secured above level of diaphragm as elevated IAP compresses the IVC (inferior venacava) and impairs access of drugs and fluids from legs into circulation. Some surgeons instill fluid laparoscopically to improve surgical field; this should be isotonic e.g. Ringer's lactate and allowance must be made for systemic absorption when calculating fluid maintenance.[17,18]

Either inhalational or intravenous induction of anaesthesia can be chosen. Sevoflurane or halothane in nitrous oxide and oxygen produce smooth inhalational induction but intravenous route should be preferred if intravenous access is already available. Agents that depress or sensitize myocardium to catecholamines e.g. halothane should be avoided, especially in patients with myocardial disease. Sevoflurane is safe and etomidate is better than propofol or barbiturates.[5] A rapid-sequence-induction with cricoid pressure as in adults is recommended for children requiring emergency exploration. Facemask or LMA has been used for laparoscopies of brief duration but tracheal intubation is recommended for long laparoscopic procedures (the details of use of LMA are discussed later in this chapter).[19,20]

Due to small abdominal capacity and constraints of intra-abdominal pressures Oxygen—air mixtures for maintenance are preferable to oxygen—nitrous oxide to prevent distention of bowel.[17,18] Nitrous oxide has been blamed to produce distention of bowel, postoperative nausea, vomiting and fatal venous gas embolism. Total intravenous technique may be used if there are concerns over myocardial depression by volatile anaesthetics.[18] After induction of anaesthesia a nasogastric tube is inserted to decompress the stomach and urinary catheter for bladder decompression prior to insertion of Veress needle.

Mandatory monitoring includes pulse oximetry, non-invasive blood pressure, ECG, capnography and temperature. Precordial or oesophageal stethoscope should be routinely used to allow continuous auscultation of breath and heart sounds, should endobronchial intubation occur following carboperitoneum and Trendelenburg position. Precordial doppler probe and transoesophageal echocardiography are very sensitive gadgets to detect embolized gas. In advanced centers transoesophageal echocardiography is being used in preference to CVP monitoring for assessing preload and myocardial contractility in children with heart disease. Children warrant the use of core temperature monitoring. Since several factors including high body surface area-to-mass ratio and little subcutaneous fat, less body hair, surgical exposure of the entire abdomen, insufflation of large volumes of cold, non-humidified CO_2 contribute to hypothermia. Heat loss can be combated with convective forced air-warmer, infrared radiant heater, a warming mattress, and heated and humified inspired gases.

Exhaled tidal volume should be measured to detect fall in pulmonary compliance that follows carboperitoneum, secondary to leak around the tracheal tube.

Complete deflation of carboperitoneum at the completion of surgery is advised to prevent irritation of diaphragm and consequent referred shoulder pain and also PONV.

Muscle relaxants and agents that release histamine (mivacurium, rapacuronium and morphine) should be avoided to prevent fall in cardiac output and preload. Multimodal analgesia with non-opioid analgesics and infiltration of local anesthetics at incision site reduces the need for postoperative analgesia.

Inflation and deflation should be gradual. IAP should never be allowed to exceed 15 mmHg. Arterial blood gases may be analysed to assess $PaCO_2$. Surgery should be preferably performed in supine position.

STATUS OF LMA IN LAPAROSCOPY

Despite concerns about aspiration, gastric distension and hypercapnia LMA has proved to be a very useful adjunct to anaesthesia in pediatric practice. Use of Trendelenburg position, increased IAP, surgeon pressing on abdominal wall and peritoneal stimulation are expected to increase the risk of regurgitation. Inflation of LMA cuff reflexly lowers the lower oesophageal sphincter tone.

If required it has been recommended that procedures be kept as brief as possible (<30 mt) and low IAP, but never in patients with cardiorespiratory disease even for brief procedures. The anaesthesiologist should be constantly vigilant to detect any dislodgement of LMA leading to gastric distention and underventilation. Epigastrium should be regularly auscultated to look for gas insufflation.[20, 21] A case of supercarbia (pCO_2 17.5 kPa) in a 4-month-old baby undergoing laparoscopic repair of inguinal hernia has been reported.[20-22]

ProSeal LMA (PLMA) is a recent introduction in paediatric anaesthesia practice. It is being increasingly used in adults for laparoscopic procedures. Paediatric PLMA has been shown to have higher oropharyngeal seal pressures as compared to classic LMA and may be used as an alternative to endotracheal tubes for laparoscopy. Recently the ProSeal has been successfully used for paediatric laparoscopy of brief duration.[23,24]

MANAGEMENT OF POSTOPERATIVE PAIN

Postoperative pain following laparoscopy is usually mild, however severity is related to the degree of distention, volume of residual gas after desufflation, excitation of phrenic nerve by residual CO_2 and by unusual position for some procedures. Shoulder pain is less common in pediatric patients.[18] Usually non-opioid analgesics in form of paracetamol are sufficient and are required for first 24 hours postoperatively. Use of local anaesthetics at trocar site and instillation into the peritoneum at the end of the procedure is beneficial. Rectus sheath block, epidural and caudal epidural have been shown to be better than opioids for adequate analgesia.[18]

MANAGEMENT OF PONV

PONV is common following laparoscopy. Factors contributing to it are bowel manipulation and peritoneal irritation. Ondansetron 100 µg/kg, dexamethasone 150 µg/kg and droperidol 25 µg/kg have been used as prophylactic antiemetics.[18] Ensuring complete deflation of carboperitoneum is a beneficial practice.

GASLESS LAPAROSCOPY

In this technique the abdominal wall is lifted to create an intra-abdominal space at atmospheric pressure and no gas is used. This is particularly useful in infants in whom even a small leak can reduce the working space. Valveless ports and instruments of differing calibers are used without the inconvenience of a variable pneumoperitoneum and the disadvantages of raised IAP. [25]

CONCLUSIONS

The anaesthetic management of children undergoing laparoscopy has to take into account surgical requirements as well as physiological changes due to carboperitoneum. The techniques of laparoscopic surgery can be used effectively in many diseases of children to decrease the morbidity associated with the traditional surgery. Laparoscopic techniques in general have slow learning curve and hence increases the operative time in the initial phase. Surgeons should be willing to convert to open procedure as and when the laparoscopic work becomes difficult. Experienced laparoscopic surgeons can perform many abdominal surgeries using laparoscopic or laparoscopic assisted techniques. Looking at the trends in all specialties laparoscopy appears to be the future of surgery.

CLINICAL PEARLS

1. Look for vagal stimulation at initiation of insufflation and penetration of trocars and laparoscope.
2. Restrict intra abdominal pressure to 10-12 mmHg and allow slow insufflation.
3. For procedures lasting greater than 1 hour, $EtCO_2$ can be restored to normal by increasing minute ventilation by 25-30 percent.
4. Use of closed circuit with sodalime absorption is preferable more so in procedures lasting more than an hour.
5. Strict maintenance of temperature and fluid balance.
6. Children with cyanotic heart disease need intra abdominal pressure between 6 and 10 mmHg and more intensive monitoring of haemodynamics including arterial blood gas analysis.
7. Intra-operative oxygenation can be improved by addition of PEEP.
8. Monitoring and supplemental oxygenation should extend into postoperative period.

REFERENCES

1. Georgeson KE: Minimally invasive pediatric surgery: Current status. Semin Pediatr Surg 1998;7:193.
2. Waldschmidt J, Schier F: Laparoscopic surgery in neonates and infants. Eur J Pediatr Surg 1991;1:145.
3. George A. Gregory, Pediatric Anaesthesia, Fourth Edition, pp 580-581 Churchill Livingstone.
4. Tobias JD, Holcomb GW: Anesthetic management for laparoscopic cholecystectomy in children with decreased myocardial function: Two case reports. J Pediatr Surg 1997;32:743.
5. McHoney M, Corizia L, Eaton S, Kiely EM et al. Carbon dioxide elimination during laparoscopy in children is age dependent.: J Pediatr Surg. 2003; 38(1): 105-10
6. Sfez M, Guerard A, Desruelle P: Cardiorespiratory changes during laparoscopic fun doplication in children. Paediatr Anaesth 1995;5:89.
7. Tobias JD: Anesthetic considerations for laparoscopy in children. Semin Laparosc Surg 1998;5:60.
8. Bannister C, Brosius K, Wulkan The effect of insufflation pressure on pulmonary mechanics in infants during laparoscopic surgical procedures. Paediatr Anaesth 2003;13:785-89.
9. P.Bozkurt, G.Kaya et al. The cardio respiratory effects of laparoscopic procedures in infants. Anaesthesia, 1999;54.831-34.
10. Wulkan ML, Vasudevan SA.Is end-tidal CO_2 an accurate measure of arterial CO_2 during laparoscopic procedures in children and neonates with cyanotic congenital heart disease? J.pediatr.Surg.2001; 36(8):1234-6

11. Manner T, Aantaa R, Alanen M: Lung compliance during laparoscopic surgery in paediatric patients. Paediatr Anaesth 1998;8:25.
12. Hsing CH, Hseu SS, Tsai SK, et al: The physiological effect of CO_2 pneumoperitoneum in pediatric laparoscopy.Acta Anaesthesiol Sin 1995;33:1.
13. Lynch FP, Ochi T, Sculty JM, et al.Cardiovascular effects of increased intra-abdominal pressure in newborn piglets.J Pediatr Surg 1974;9:621.
14. Tobias JD, Holcomb GW III, Brock JW III, et al: Cardiorespiratory changes in children during laparoscopy. J Pediatr Surg 1995;30:33.
15. BloomfieldGL, Ridings PC, Blocher CR, et al: Effects of increased intra-abdominal pressure upon intracranial and cerebral perfusion pressure before and after volume expansion .J Trauma 1996;40:936.
16. Bozkurt P, Kaya, Altintas Y, et al: Systemic stress response during operations for Acute abdominal pain performed via laparoscopy or laparotomy in children.Anaesthesia 55:5, 2000.
17. Walsh MT, Vetter TR: Anesthesia for pediatric laparoscopic cholecystectomy. J Clin Anesth 1992;4:406.
18. Pennant J H, Anesthesiology Clinics of North America, 2001; 19:1.69-88.
19. Tobias JD, Holcomb GW III, BrookJW, et al: General anesthesia by mask with spontaneous ventilation during brief laparoscopic inspection of the peritoneum in children.J Laparoendosc Surg 1994;4:379.
20. Tobias JD, Holcomb GW III, Rasmussen E, et al: General anesthesia using the laryngeal mask airway during brief, laparoscopic inspection of the peritoneum in children. J Laparoendosc Surg 1996;6:175.
21. Rabey PG, Murphy PI, Langton JA, et al: Effect of the laryngeal mask airway on lower oesophageal sphincter pressure in patients during general anaesthesia. Br J Anaesth 1992;69:346.
22. Lew YS, Thambi Dorai CR, Phyu PT. A case of supercarbia following pneumoperitoneum in an infant. Paediatr Anaesth 2005; 15 (4): 346-9.
23. Maltby JR, Beriault MT, Watson NC, et al: The LMA-ProSeal ™ is an effective alternative to tracheal intubation for laparoscopic cholecystectomy: Can J Anesth. 2002;49:857.
24. Sinha A, Sharma B, Sood J. ProSeal™ in paediatric laparoscopy. Accepted for publication in Paediatric Anaesthesia (20th Sept. 2006).
25. Luks FL, Peers KHE, Deprest JA, et al: Gasless laparoscopy in infants, the rabbit model. Pediatr Surg 1995;30:1206.

CHAPTER 18

Anaesthetic Considerations in Urologic Laparoscopic Surgery

INTRODUCTION

Surgeons strive to perform procedures that are less invasive and cause less patient morbidity while remaining technically and therapeutically sound. Based on these aspirations, laparoscopy is a significant advancement. Advantages of laparoscopic surgery include the following:

- Decreased pain
- Decreased hospital stay
- Decreased convalescence
- Decreased wound infections
- Improved cosmesis
- Decreased pulmonary complications

Laparoscopy, the concept of closed inspection of intra-abdominal organs took root through the primitive efforts of Ott in 1901 when he introduced a speculum through a small abdominal incision. The credit for a true endoscopic examination that paved the way to laparoscopy goes to George Kelling who reported his views of abdominal viscera after filling a dog's abdomen with air and inserting a Nitze cystoscope. Over the next 75 years, several innovations like improved optics, electrical light source and specially designed laparoscopic instruments gave a boost to the minimally invasive or laparoscopic surgery. The advent and success of laparoscopic cholecystectomy led to a surge of interest in laparoscopic procedures, especially in the field of urology.

Initially great enthusiasm for learning laparoscopy was generated by the successful demonstration of laparoscopic pelvic lymph node dissection by Schuessler and co-workers.[1] A survey, after couple of years, showed that 86 per cent of urologists actually performed laparoscopy after one year of formal training.[2] Subsequent survey at the same institution revealed that only 53.6 per cent respondents had performed laparoscopy after 5 years of formal training.[3] Decreased patient interest, increased costs, higher complication rates, decreased institutional support, decreased indications and increased operative time were the cited reasons for waning use of laparoscopic urologic procedures. Possibly the real reason behind this decline is the inherent difficulty, compounded by the fact that, in the field of urology, there is no single procedure akin to laparoscopic cholecystectomy to sustain skill and interest.

Encouragingly, there are selected laparoscopic centres committed to the pursuit of excellence where caseload per year for the interested laparoscopic urologist has actually increased. In 1991 Winfield listed more than 20 potential, but not tried, urologic laparoscopy procedures and by 1995 Gill and co-workers reported on 26 procedures that had been performed clinically or in the laboratory.[4,5]

Cortesi et al in 1976 reported the first use of laparoscopy for urologic surgery in an 18-year-old male student with bilateral undescended nonpalpable testes.[6] Although diagnostic laparoscopy in urology became more widespread, therapeutic procedures were not used until Clayman et al completed the first radical laparoscopic nephrectomy in 1990.[7] Therapeutic urological laparoscopic procedures for both benign and malignant disease have since become commonplace and have ever-expanding applications to internal genitourinary pathology.

Cardiovascular changes, mechanical consequences of pneumoperitoneum, neurohormonal responses, systemic absorption of carbon dioxide and physiological changes associated with patient positioning are the major points for consideration during laparoscopic urology surgery. Most of these effects are very well studied and documented, mainly in context to the pneumoperitoneum created for laparoscopic cholecystectomy and this surgery is used as a theoretical template for abdominal laparoscopy. Alterations in the dynamics other than the cholecystectomy model may play significant role in urological laparoscopic procedures. These include, organ specific issues, handling of the genitourinary system, difference in positioning and co-morbid conditions specific to this class of patients. While general and systemic effects of CO_2 insufflation have been discussed elsewhere in the book; effects pertaining to retroperitoneal insufflation of CO_2 are discussed here with comparative references to intraperitoneal CO_2 insufflation.

LAPAROSCOPIC APPROACHES IN UROLOGY SURGERY

For any laparoscopic surgery, the first requirement is reaching the lesion. Multiple factors decide the approach to the surgical site: the diseased organ, site and size of the lesion, the procedure planned and the experience of the surgeon. Insufflation of carbon dioxide as a means of creating adequate working space uses either intra-peritoneal (pneumoperitoneum) or extraperitoneal (pneumoretroperitoneum) routes for accessing urologic organs. The two routes of carbon dioxide insufflation lead to different haemodynamic and gas exchange effects.

PATIENT POSITIONING DURING UROLOGICAL LAPAROSCOPY

The position of the patient during laparoscopic surgery varies according to the procedure to be done and the type of approach used in that procedure.[8] Various positions according to the type of approach are:
- Transperitoneal – anterior approach – supine with Trendelenburg position
- Transperitoneal – lateral – complete flank position (kidney position)
- Extraperitoneal – lateral – complete flank position
- Extraperitoneal – posterior – prone position
- Transperitoneal – pelvic surgery – supine with Trendelenburg position (head-down)
- Extraperitoneal – pelvic surgery – supine with Trendelenburg position

PHYSIOLOGICAL CHANGES PERTAINING TO POSITIONING OF PATIENT

Most of the urological laparoscopic procedures are carried out in lateral decubitus renal position with Trendelenburg position.

THE LATERAL DECUBITUS (THE KIDNEY POSITION) POSITION

The lateral decubitus position (kidney position) and the kidney rest is commonly used during renal surgery, laparoscopic or otherwise. In a simple lateral position, patient is made to lie on the side that is not to be operated (Fig. 18.1). Care should be taken while positioning the patient in lateral decubitus position. Without the head pillow, neck gets acutely flexed causing the brachial plexus of upper side to stretch excessively, while the shoulder gets compressed by the weight of the patient leading to narrowing of axillary space, thereby, compressing axillary contents.

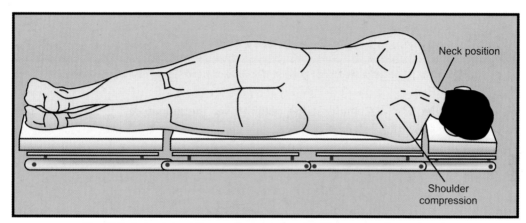

Fig. 18.1: Lateral decubitus position showing shoulder compression and neck extension because of poor support to these structures

A proper lateral decubitus can be achieved by placing head rest of adequate height so that the cervical spine remains in a horizontal position (Fig. 18.2). Addition of shoulder rest will decrease the pressure on the axillary contents.

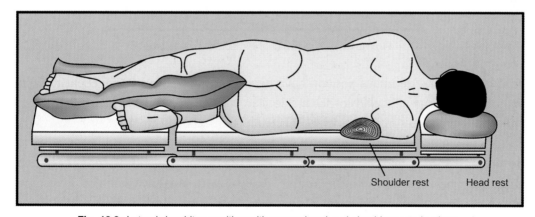

Fig. 18.2: Lateral decubitus position with proper head and shoulder rests in place

There are profound changes in cardiovascular, respiratory and musculoskeletal systems in lateral decubitus and lateral decubitus with the kidney rest (Fig. 18.3) positions. The addition of lateral angulation caused by elevating the kidney rest until the up-side flank is taut, imposes severe skeletal stresses and ventilatory restrictions.

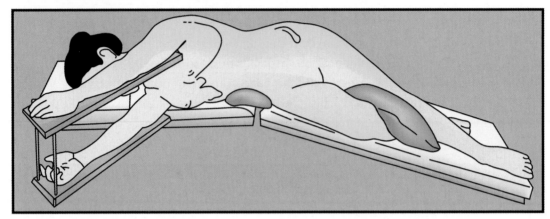

Fig. 18.3: Right lateral decubitus position with jackknife and kidney rest augmentation

The debate regarding the best placement of the patient over the kidney rest is a continuing process. Flock and Clup advocated a posture (Fig. 18.4) that allows the kidney rest to strike just above the iliac crest[9].

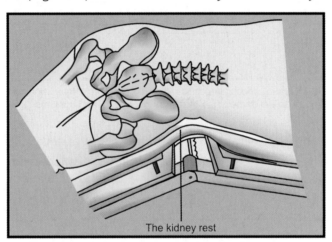

The kidney rest

Fig. 18.4: The kidney rest is just above the iliac crest

All variations of the lateral decubitus position have been shown to decrease vital capacity.[10] Elevation of the kidney rest into the soft tissue cephalad to down-side iliac crest compresses the flank and restricts descent of the ipsilateral hemidiaphragm, as in Figure 18.4. This flank encroachment in the right lateral decubitus position might directly compress the vena cava and impede venous return.

Smith et al recommended positioning the twelfth rib over the kidney rest (Fig. 18.5). In this position, negligible or minimal compression of vena cava does not reduce venous return but down-side ribs get compressed causing marked reduction in diaphragmatic movement of the ipsilateral hemidiaphragm.

Grayhack and Graham[11] recommended that the kidney rest be placed directly under the iliac crest (Fig. 18.6). This position offers the least interference with the functions of the down-side lung and diaphragm.[12]

Supporting hip straps for the lateral decubitus position can also be a source of sciatic nerve damage to the up-side hip if the straps are pulled too tight. Straps should not be placed over the femoral head because of the possibility of the aseptic necrosis from a compression of the vessels that cross the hip joint to supply the femoral head. Correctly placed straps are shown in Figures 18.7A and 18.7B.

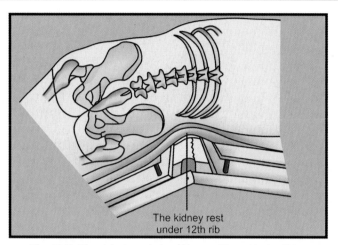

Fig. 18.5: The right lateral decubitus position with the kidney rest under the twelfth rib

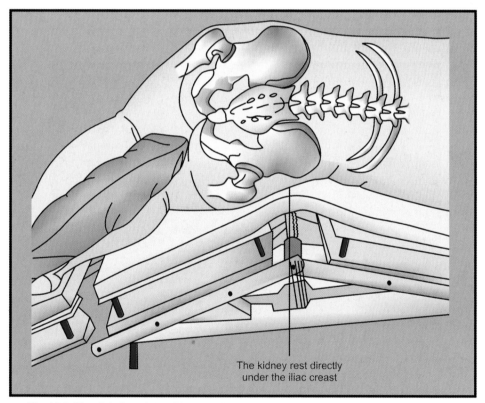

Fig. 18.6: The right lateral decubitus position with the kidney rest directly under the iliac crest

Very few workers have paid attention to cardiovascular changes during kidney position in healthy subjects undergoing renal surgery. In a study, conducted by M Yokoyama et al 2000[13], haemodynamic effects of the lateral decubitus position with kidney rest during anaesthesia were evaluated. They demonstrated significant reduction in mean arterial, right atrial, pulmonary artery mean and wedge pressures. There was significant increase in systemic vascular resistance index with no change in pulmonary vascular resistance index.

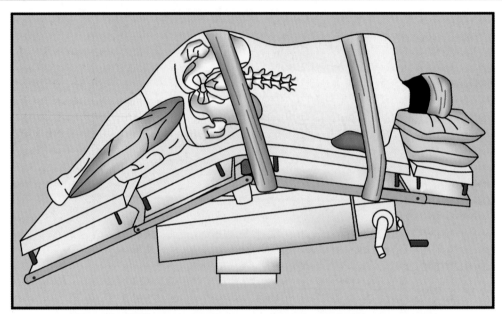

Fig. 18.7A: Properly placed hip and shoulder straps

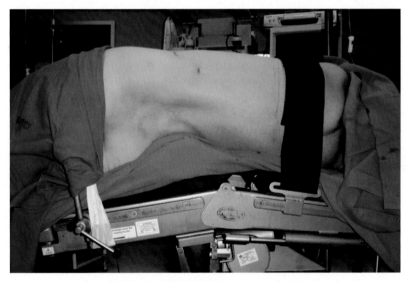

Fig. 18.7B: Properly placed hip and shoulder straps

Cardiovascular collapse is possible when the anaesthetised patient is turned from the supine to the lateral decubitus position, especially after lateral flexion. Sudden postural changes are tolerated poorly in the anaesthetised patient. General anaesthesia depresses the carotid and aortic baroreceptors so that they can no longer effectively compensate for cardiovascular instability produced by altered body posture. In addition, the lateral decubitus position shifts the mediastinum down and rotates the heart on its axis. Such changes can interfere with venous return and reduce cardiac output. Other mechanisms responsible for decreased cardiac output is reduced venous return as the heart is placed at a hydrostatic level above the lower extremities. In addition, the kidney rest and flexion of trunk compress great vessels in the abdomen and alter the venous return. The reduction in venous return is reflected by decreased right atrial pressure (RAP) and pulmonary capillary pressure (PCWP) during the institution of kidney position.

Eggers and associates demonstrated that marked reduction in arterial pressure occurred with almost all lateral positions during anaesthesia compared with the supine position.[14] The lowest mean arterial blood pressure was noted in those patients placed in the right lateral decubitus and right lateral decubitus jackknife positions. The left lateral decubitus position produced little changes in blood pressure compared with supine. Addition of the kidney rest and jackknife position to the lateral decubitus position, further, exaggerates impairment of venous return. Kidney rest constitutes a source of vena caval occlusion. The right lateral decubitus position appears to place the patient at greater risk for vena caval constriction with kidney rest than does the left lateral decubitus, possibly because of the proximity of the vessel to the right flank. Application of positive end-expiratory pressure may cause inferior venal caval constriction in patients in the left lateral decubitus position.[15]

In case of hypotension due to positional change, the position should be reverted back to supine and repositioning tried more cautiously with adjustments in the kidney rest. Volume expansion or vasoactive drug therapy are two alternatives to treat the reduced cardiac output state. Transfusion of excessive fluid as the primary measure to combat hypotension, may lead to cardiac decompensation when the patient is returned to the supine position at the end of the surgery.[16,17]

Formation of atelectatic areas in the dependant portions of the lung is a well-recognised and documented fact.[18] Atelectasis in each lung may also be affected by change of position from supine to the lateral decubitus position. The single most important effect of posture on ventilation is simple mechanical interference with chest movement limiting expansion of the lung.[19] While atelectasis usually develops in the dependant areas during both transperitoneal and retroperitoneal approaches in urological surgery, the nondependant lung can also get affected by the pressure exerted by the insufflating gas.

THE TRENDELENBURG POSITION

The Trendelenburg position is the other most commonly employed position during laparoscopic urological surgery to get an optimised access to pelvic organs. This can vary from minimum head-down tilt (10 to 20 degrees) to steep head-down tilt (30 to 45 degrees). Laparoscopy for pelvic surgery introduces three major physiological alterations.[20]

1. Trendelenburg position: usually with a 30° head-down tilt to allow better visualisation of the pelvic viscera. This can cause cardiovascular and gas exchange impairments.
2. CO_2 pneumoperitoneum: this further increases abdominal pressure and exaggerates the ventilation/ perfusion mismatch due to the Trendelenburg position.
3. CO_2 absorption: the combination of hypercarbia and alveolar hypoventilation can lead to cardiac arrhythmias and even cardiac arrest.

The other variant of the Trendelenburg position, used commonly in the laparoscopic pelvic surgery, is hyperlordotic position. When an awake patient is maintained in head-down tilt, a series of events commonly occur with varying speed of onset. The individual becomes anxious and restless, often develops a pounding vascular headache, becomes dyspneic, may develop a stuffy nose, gradually becomes less cooperative and often tries to sit up to escape the head-low posture. All these symptoms relate to vascular congestion in the form of raised jugular venous pressure, vascular overload in the superior caval circuit, pulmonary vascular congestion, disrupted ventilation due to interference with diaphragmatic excursion and impaired cerebral circulation.[21]

Changes in arterial blood pressure seen just after a patient is tilted head down is caused by baroreceptor activity with following events:

1. A rapid movement of blood from lower extremities to the central circulation to the extent of 1000 ml.
2. This initial increase in central blood volume is pumped from the heart as an increase in cardiac output, raising hydrostatic pressure in the arch of aorta and in the carotid sinuses at the bifurcation of the carotid arteries.
3. Reflex generalised vasodilatation and a decreased stroke volume leading to a reduced cardiac output and decreased perfusion of vital organs.
4. Cerebral circulation is impaired because of increased cerebral venous pressure and postural migration of cerebrospinal fluid which increases hydrostatic pressure of intracranial CSF. These impede cerebral blood flow and additively contribute to stagnant cerebral hypoxia.[22,23]

Kubal and co-workers[24] observed a significant increase in myocardial oxygen consumption and CVP in patients with coronary artery disease, occasionally leading to ST segment changes on the electrocardiogram while performing central line cannulation in the Trendelenburg position. Incidence of malignant dysrhythmias increases significantly when positioned with head down tilt during pulmonary artery catheterisation in coronary artery disease.[25]

Haemodynamically stable patients tolerate mild to moderate head-down tilt well but patients with coronary artery disease have marked tendency to develop congestive heart failure when placed in head-down position.[26] Therefore, during preanaesthetic evaluation the effect of desired degree of head-down tilt can be assessed. If the patient complains of dyspnoea, or if the position results in decrease in blood pressure, an alternative posture should be sought for the operation.

The Trendelenburg position along with lithotomy, can cause severe perfusion problems in the lower extremities[27] (Fig. 18.8). In a similar fashion, a rise in the mean arterial pressure at the circle of Willis is difficult to justify especially in patients with cerebrovascular pathology and prolonged surgery.

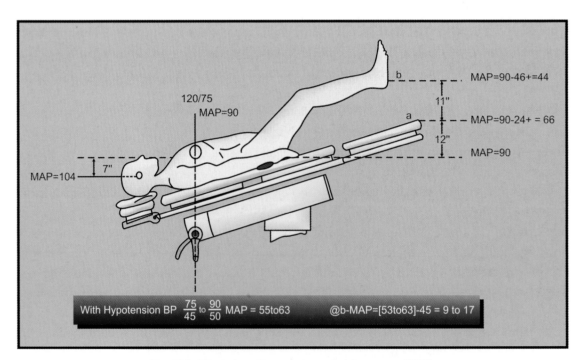

Fig. 18.8: Effect of position on mean arterial pressure (MAP)
at various sites in relation to the heart[28]

During laparoscopic surgery, abdominal distension produced by insufflation of CO_2 into the peritoneal cavity is combined with some degree of head-down tilt to provide working room for the surgeon amid abdominopelvic viscera that are displaced cephalad to varying degrees (Fig. 18.9).

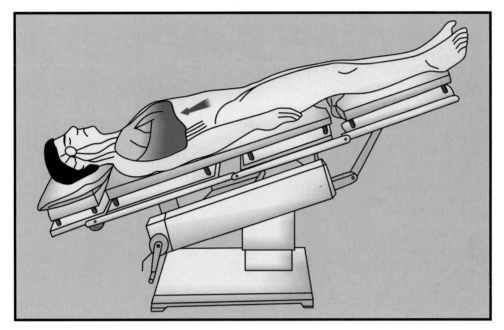

Fig. 18.9: Visceral forces acting on the diaphragm during head-down tilt and the resultant effect

Johannsen and associates reported a reduction of stroke index and cardiac index by 42 per cent at the time of maximum haemodynamic stress.[29] Total peripheral vascular resistance increased by 50 to 100 per cent while there was no significant change in the pulse rate and mean arterial pressure.

There are various effects on the respiratory system by virtue of various positions used during the surgery. The lung and chest wall impedance to inflation increases during mechanical ventilation with head-down tilt and increased intra-abdominal pressure.[30] This requires higher alveolar pressures for lung inflation, which can add to the risk of barotrauma. The increase in chest wall impedance increases intrathoracic pressure during positive pressure lung inflation and has possible inhibitory effect on cardiac output. There is decrease in pulmonary compliance due to increased pulmonary blood volume and gravitational force on the mediastinal structures and the diaphragm.

The other aspect, during the Trendelenburg position, is to keep the patient stable on the mattress of the operating table. With increasing degree of head-down tilt, there remains a possibility of patient to slip from the table. Various types of restraints have been described. Hewer in 1953 described a non-slip mattress (Fig. 18.10) for patients in the Trendelenburg position up to 30° head-down tilt.[31]

Use of wrist or shoulder braces to sustain head-down tilt threatens to pull (wrist) or push (shoulder) the mobile shoulder mechanism caudad, closing the retroclavicular space by moving the clavicle onto the first rib (Fig. 18.11).

The retroclavicular neurovascular bundle of subclavian vessels and brachial plexus can get stretched or compressed by closure of retroclavicular space. At risk is perfusion of the extremity with potential for a compartment syndrome and abnormal neural function with dysesthesias or anaesthesia of the extremity. Placing the shoulder braces medially against the root of the neck (Fig. 18.12) can directly compress vessels that emerge from the thoracic outlet as well as nerves that exit the cervical foramina and adjacent soft tissue.

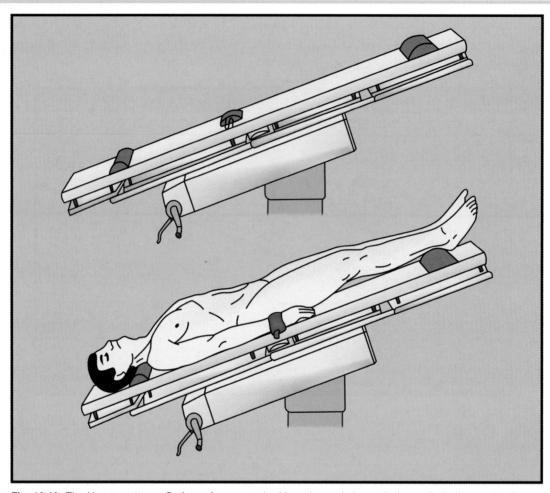

Fig. 18.10: The Hewer mattress. Surface of corrugated rubber plus pads beneath the neck, lumbosacral spine and ankles retain patient in head-down tilt without use of shoulder braces and restrictive straps

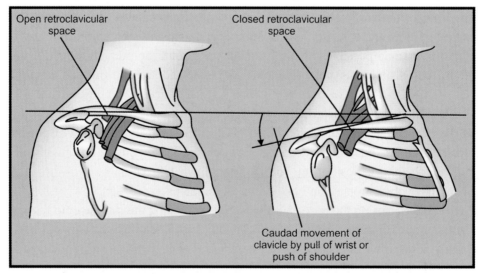

Fig. 18.11: Retroclavicular space and position of the clavicle in relation to the first rib

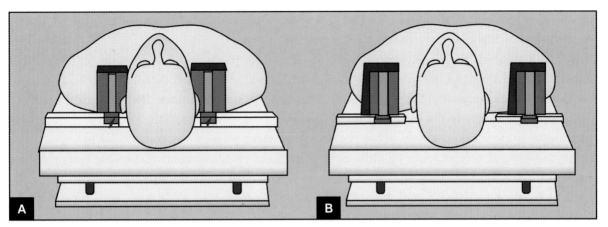

Figs 18.12: A: Shoulder braces placed at the root of the neck, B: shoulder braces placed laterally over the cap of the shoulder joint

The traditional advice about the safest location for shoulder braces has been that they should be situated laterally over the cap of the shoulder. But even then the risk of retroclavicular space closure remains. Heavier patients and steeper tilt accentuate the possibility of the structural damage from wristlets and shoulder braces. When the head-down posture is no longer needed at the end of the surgical procedure, greater care is required to return the patient to horizontal position. A sudden return to the horizontal position may unmask the inadequate volume replacement and provoke hypotension by adding vascular capacitance of the lower limbs because of the delayed response of the compensatory vasomotor system that is depressed by anaesthesia. If leg holders had been used to elevate the lower extremities, the legs should be brought together, straightened slowly and lowered simultaneously.

HYPERLORDOTIC POSITION

This position is a variant of the Trendelenburg position, where hyper-extension of spine is achieved by putting the patient on operation table in a reverse jackknife position (Fig. 18.13).

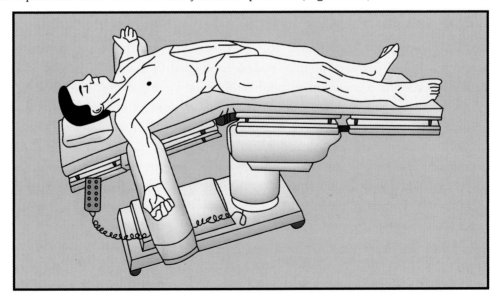

Fig. 18.13: The hyperlordotic position for transabdominal access to the ventral pelvis and retropubic space

Despite its ability to improve transabdominal access to pelvic organs, several aspects of the hyperlordotic position have the potential of being a major insult for the patient.

1. Arching the lumbar spine excessively can seriously stress the joints and ligaments of the angulated area. Postoperative backache can be anticipated, particularly in elderly patients with an arthritic spine.
2. The arched spine elongates and flattens the major vessels on its ventral surface. Reduced caliber of the vessels in this position can impede the blood flow. Consequently, changes in pressure in collateral circulation may affect intraspinal perfusion, causing either congestion or ischaemia of the contents of the spinal cord.
3. Placement of the legs at level lower than the atrium promotes venous stasis in distensible vessels of the lower extremities.

Increased intraspinal pressure secondary to compression of the inferior vena cava by the hyperlordotic position is implicated as a possible cause of lumbar canal stenosis.[32]

PHYSIOLOGICAL EFFECTS PERTAINING TO CO_2 INSUFFLATION

CARDIOVASCULAR EFFECTS

The effects of carbon dioxide during pneumoperitoneum for gynaecological endoscopic surgery were determined in the early 1970s.[33,34] Several experimental and clinical studies have addressed the physiologically complex haemodynamic effects of CO_2 insufflation including mechanical (increased intra-abdominal pressure) and pharmacological consequences and cardiovascular effects. The interaction of several patient and surgical factors contribute to the alterations in cardiovascular function. These include intra-abdominal pressure (IAP), patient position, CO_2 absorption, ventilatory strategy, surgical technique, surgical site, the nature and duration of the procedure. Haemodynamic alterations caused by pneumoperitoneum and retropneumoperitoneum are also influenced by the patient's intravascular volume, preexisting cardiopulmonary status, neurohormonal factors, patient's medications and the anaesthetic agents used.

There is absorption of CO_2 during pneumoperitoneum or pneumoretroperitoneum in the systemic circulation. Under normal circumstances, mild hyperventilation maintains normocarbia and no significant cardiovascular effects are encountered. However, moderate to severe hypercarbia (50 to 70 mmHg) has a direct myocardial depressant and vasodilatory effect.

Very few studies have been conducted to assess cardiovascular and respiratory effects of pneumoretroperitoneum. One of the experimental studies conducted by Reiner M Giebler et al[35], has shown different cardiovascular effects during pneumoperitoneum and pneumoretroperitoneum in supine animals. Central venous and iliac venous pressure increase significantly under both pneumoperitoneum and pneumo-retroperitoneum. There is an increase in pressure gradient along the inferior caval vein during CO_2 insufflation in the peritoneum and retroperitoneum, but this gradient is significantly greater during peritoneal rather than retroperitoneal insufflation. This can be explained in terms of the area of inferior vena cava (IVC) exposed to the pressure increases created by intraperitoneal CO_2 insufflation in comparison to the area exposed during retroperitoneal insufflation. Pooling of blood in the thoracic compartment by compression of abdominal vasculature produces a rise in central venous pressure. The additional factor contributing to an increase in central venous pressure (CVP) is displacement of the diaphragm in a cephalad direction resulting in an increase in intrathoracic pressure.

The cardiovascular effects of pneumoretroperitoneum are influenced greatly by the position of the patient, volume loading and type of population studied.[36] There is an increase in cardiac output during CO_2 insufflation in normovolaemic patients in both pneumoperitoneum and pneumoretroperitoneum during the initial phase of insufflation. This can be explained by the fact that there is increased blood volume displacement during increased intra-abdominal pressure. In contrast, there is less translocation of blood in the central pool during increases in retroperitoneal pressure.

There is an insufflation mediated increase in aortic systolic and diastolic pressures.[37] Both diastolic and systolic aortic pressures tend to return towards baseline after 15-30 minutes of CO_2 insufflation but do not reach baseline readings. The magnitude of systemic haemodynamic changes are significantly less as compared to the changes during pneumoperitoneum. The transient increase in aortic pressure is possibly caused by increased peripheral vascular resistance due to compression of splanchnic vasculature.

RESPIRATORY EFFECTS

During retroperitoneoscopic procedures, the majority of pulmonary effects are the result of CO_2 insufflation rather than pressure changes in the retroperitoneal space. The effects of retroperitoneal insufflation of CO_2 are less well known than intraperitoneal insufflation. Animal studies are scarce and their results differ or even contradict one other. There are studies indicating increased as well as decreased carbon dioxide absorption during extraperitoneal CO_2 insufflation.[35,38,39] Various factors have been attributed to both the contradicting conditions. Guillonneau B 1995, reported effect on the arterial CO_2 pressure similar to those seen in intraperitoneal laparoscopy, while performing retroperitoneoscopy in goats.[40] A study conducted by Baird JE 1999 on pigs, showed that $PaCO_2$ was directly related to insufflation pressure and time to return to baseline was less with retropneumoperitoneum than with pneumoperitoneum.[41]

In medical practice, different investigators have made different observations with regard to CO_2 absorption and elimination. It is observed that the magnitude of CO_2 elimination and end-tidal CO_2 ($EtCO_2$) change was significantly different while studying intraperitoneal and extraperitoneal CO_2 insufflation.[42] They observed that retroperitoneal insufflation of CO_2 during pelviscopy was associated with a higher rate of elimination of CO_2 from the lungs. Values for $etCO_2$ and V_eCO_2 measured 45 minutes after cessation of CO_2 insufflation were still higher than preinsufflation values.

While during intraperitoneal insufflation a plateau is reached after 15-20 minutes, no plateau is observed for $EtCO_2$ and V_eCO_2 during extraperitoneal insufflation.[42] One or both of the following factors can explain this. First, extraperitoneal insufflation may require more time to reach a steady state due to the nature of the exchange area in contact with CO_2. Second, there may be a continual recruitment of more gas-exchange area caused by the continued dissection of extraperitoneal space. The other probable contributory factor is subcutaneous emphysema, which is created by CO_2 insufflation of the retroperitoneal compartment.[38] It was suggested that direct intravascular uptake of CO_2 may be facilitated by disruption of the microvasculature and lymphatic channels during the development of an extraperitoneal cavity.[43]

In 1999 Ng CS reported equivalent CO_2 elimination for either transperitoneal or retroperitoneal approach in renal and adrenal surgery.[44] In retrospect, it was realised that during transperitoneal urological laparoscopic surgery, the line of Toldt is incised and the retroperitoneum is entered within first thirty minutes of surgery. During the next three to four hours of procedure, surgical dissection and mobilisation are performed largely at the retroperitoneal organs, adipose tissue and fascial planes. Thus, during more than 75 per cent of the surgical intervention, the retroperitoneal cavity is exposed to CO_2 and participates in resorption. This is in contrast to the intraperitoneal approach for any other surgery where the retroperitoneum is not entered at all, thus giving rise to equivalent elimination of CO_2 during intraperitoneal and extraperitoneal CO_2 insufflation techniques.

Persistence of acidosis and hypercapnia despite the cessation of insufflation is a well known phenomenon where the retroperitoneum has been involved, which can be partly explained by the existence of CO_2 in the subcutaneous emphysema which persists in the postoperative period.[42]

Absorption of a gas from a closed cavity depends on its diffusability and the perfusion of the walls of that cavity. Rate of insufflation of gas does not influence the absorption into the circulation. Carbon dioxide absorption cannot be measured directly. Carbon dioxide elimination, which is easier to estimate, gives a fairly accurate estimate of CO_2 absorption. CO_2 elimination is the sum of CO_2 production and CO_2 absorption at steady state and can be calculated by the following equation:

$$VCO_2 = \frac{EtCO_2 \times TV \times RR}{(P_B - P_{H_2O}) \times Wt}$$

(VCO_2; carbon dioxide elimination (ml/kg/minute), $EtCO_2$; end-tidal carbon dioxide, TV; tidal volume, RR; respiratory rate, P_B; barometric pressure, P_{H_2O}; partial pressure of water vapour, Wt; weight in kilogram)

From a practical point of view, the increase in CO_2 load is not a problem if controlled ventilation is instituted. Excessive values of $EtCO_2$ may be avoided by increasing minute ventilation. Cessation of controlled ventilation should be considered only after the return of $EtCO_2$ to physiologic values. However, if the surgical procedure is performed during regional anaesthesia, or if tracheal extubation occurs soon after CO_2 insufflation, patients will have to increase alveolar ventilation and work of breathing to keep arterial PCO_2 within normal range. This imposed CO_2 load must be considered in patients with restricted ventilatory reserves or receiving sedative drugs during regional anaesthesia.

RENAL EFFECTS

In 1923, Thorington and Schmidt observed that urine output improved following paracentesis in a patient with malignant ascites.[45] They subsequently demonstrated in an animal study that animals became oliguric at an IAP of 15-30 mmHg and anuric when it exceeded 30 mmHg.

During increased intra-abdominal pressure, renal cortical and medullary blood flow, glomerular filtration, creatinine clearance and urine production decrease. There is an increase in plasma renin and antidiuretic hormone release due to handling of the kidney.[13,46] The adverse effects of increased IAP on renal haemodynamics are due to changes in cardiac output and a direct effect on renal blood flow. It has been demonstrated in animal studies that renal perfusion deficit with increased IAP persists despite normal or even supra-normal values of cardiac output.[47]

Decreased urine output with ureteral compression, because of increased IAP, has been discounted by various studies that utilised ureteric stents to counter the mechanical compression of ureters. Ureteric stents failed to resolve the impaired renal function. Local compression effects on renal parenchyma, decreased cardiac output and impaired venous return are identifiable factors that lead to renal haemodynamic changes. Among them, local compression appears to be the most important factor. Local compression has persistent influence on the renal tissue perfusion for fairly longer periods. There is reversal of the renal tissue perfusion changes towards normal once the pressure is released. In some animals studied for these changes, tissue perfusion increased temporarily after the release of pressure. This may be due to transient hyperperfusion phenomenon that has been reported in various organs, including the kidney.[48] Superficial cortical arteries are particularly sensitive to sympathetic activity because of their rich innervation and a high blood flow rate as compared to other regions of the kidney.[49] Variation in the cortical blood flow may not be applicable to the human kidney. The human kidney, which is located in the retroperitoneal space, is in close contact with a number of overlying structures. Human peritoneum and renal capsule are tougher, and the perinephric fat is more abundant in humans than the studied animals. Nevertheless, before results of such clinical studies are available, a cautious approach is recommended.

Mechanical compression of renal cortex may lead to parenchymal ischaemia leading to so called 'renal compartment syndrome'. Increase in renal venous pressure may increase renal vascular resistance by mechanically obstructing renal venous outflow and leading to a secondary decrease in renal artery blood flow. Increased sympathetic activity from raised IAP or from hypercarbia may lead to renal vasoconstriction. Increase in IAP causes elevation of plasma antidiuretic hormone (ADH) presumably mediated by activation of central baroreceptors. There is evidence of increased plasma renin and aldosterone activities that respond to volume loading.

Oxidative stress is thought to be another component of CO_2 pneumoretroperitoneum induced kidney injury. The most likely causes of ROS (reactive oxygen species) production as a consequence of CO_2 pneumoretroperitoneum are an inflammatory reaction due to tissue trauma, ischaemia and reperfusion as a result of increased abdominal pressure and diaphragmatic dysfunction. Reactive oxygen species (ROS) and related molecules have shown to have toxic renal effects with contributory roles in the development of glomerular as well as tubulointerstitial damage, acute and chronic renal failure.[50,51]

CEREBROVASCULAR EFFECTS

Positioning during bladder and prostate surgery poses an additional stress on the cerebral circulation. Acute elevations in IAP produce an immediate increase in intracranial pressure (ICP), more so when increased IAP is associated with a head-down tilt. Various mechanisms have been postulated for the sudden rise in ICP, like mechanical venous effects mediated by cranial displacement of the diaphragm with inferior vena cava obstruction and increased intra-thoracic pressure and the subsequent sudden onset of decreased venous drainage from the central nervous system. Other factors include hypercarbia and reflex cerebrovascular vasodilatation. Because of the head-down position, there is an increase in cardiac output by virtue of the increased venous return. This increase in central blood volume is sensed by baroreceptors which lead to a reflex decrease in the systemic vascular resistance (SVR) to compensate for increased blood flow velocity. Therefore, during CO_2 insufflation along with a head-down position the brain may not be protected from an increased blood flow.

Increase in the ICP is multifactorial in origin. Acute elevation of IAP leads to a cranial displacement of the diaphragm thereby compressing the IVC and increasing intrathoracic pressure as well as venous pressure below the diaphragm. The increase in intrathoracic pressure increases the filling pressure of the right atrium, which is reflected in the superior vena cava. This causes an increase in cerebral venous circulation contributing to an increased ICP. Increases in the venous pressure above and below the diaphragm leads to increased venous pressure in the sagittal sinus in the CNS and arachnoid villi in the spinal cord resulting in decreased CSF absorption and a rise in ICP. Further, there is sufficient evidence in literature supporting the direct effect of an elevated $PaCO_2$ on ICP.[52-54]

There are few reports on the effect of CO_2 insufflation on the cerebral vascular system in the Trendelenberg position. Abe K found a positive correlation between $PaCO_2$ and middle cerebral artery blood flow velocity (MCABFV) in their patients.[55] Rosenthal et al 1998, did a large animal study to determine the probable cause of increased ICP with variables like increased IAP, increased or decreased $PaCO_2$, arterial blood pressure and CVP above and below the diaphragm.[56] They found that while increased IAP directly increased ICP other variables contributed significantly to it.

Therefore, laparoscopy with peritoneal or extraperitoneal CO_2 insufflation should be considered as a relative contraindication in patients with suspected or documented intracranial injuries or space occupying lesions.

TEMPERATURE CHANGES

Hypothermia has been defined as core temperature below $36°c$ and results from influence of general anaesthesia.[57] In addition to hypothermia caused by general anaesthesia, gas insufflation contributes to body cooling. This is due to the creation of a large surface area by the circulating insufflating gas filling the abdominal cavity, thereby, leading to heat loss by conduction and convection. Another factor that plays a role in lowering the body temperature is the temperature of the gas itself. Gas which is supplied from the high pressure cylinders, gets cooled when released into the abdominal cavity since there is loss of heat due to sudden expansion of gas. The higher the flow rate of gas, the larger the heat loss and the greater the fall in gas temperature. In procedures where higher flow rates are required patient temperature falls to a greater extent. Temperature monitoring is therefore recommended in laparoscopic procedures of long duration.

VENOUS THROMBOEMBOLISM

Deep vein thrombosis (DVT) is a common risk in medicine. DVT and venous thromboembolism (VTE) is a significant postoperative complication in urological surgery and more so in laparoscopic procedures. The majority of available data comes from the field of general surgery.[58, 59] For all indications and for all ages, reported incidence of DVT is 50 per 100,000 patients. DVT rarely occurs in age below 20 years, but the incidence increases with age. The incidence of DVT, in patients over 70 years of age, is 200 per 100,000.[60] The incidence reported for VTE and fatal pulmonary embolism (PE) in patients who received some form of prophylaxis against VTE is 0.03 and 0.02 per cent respectively.[58] Patel et al reported an incidence of as high as 55 per cent in patients who underwent laparoscopic cholecystectomy without prophylaxis.[59] In urological laparoscopic procedures, postoperative VTE has been reported in 0.13 to 1.3 per cent.[61,62]

During laparoscopic surgery, decreased venous return from lower limbs, decreased venous peak flow rate in femoral veins, increased femoral venous pressure and reduced venous pulsatility contribute to development of VTE. These conditions arise due to pneumoperitoneum or retropneumoperitoneum used during laparoscopic urological surgery. Other important contributing factor is venodilatation in lower limbs because of venous stasis, this in turn leads to intimal tears exposing thrombogenic subendothelial collagen.

DVT and VTE is an important preventable complication that puts patients at risk of pulmonary embolism (PE), recurrent VTE and post thrombotic syndrome.[63] The prevention of VTE in the postoperative period represents a medical topic of high clinical interest. The appropriate use of prophylaxis is based on the knowledge of specific risk factors for VTE (Table 18.1). The risk factors depend on the type of surgery, presence of clinical risk factors and the presence of acquired or congenital thrombophylic disorders. The highest risk of VTE occurs with orthopaedic surgery, whereas, risk decreases to 50 per cent in case of general surgery. Urologic laparoscopic surgery carries the minimum risk of VTE as per data available in the literature. Among many clinical risk factors, age over 40 years, previous VTE, obesity, varices and estrogen use are especially relevant for surgical patients.

During the last few years, the approach to the problem has become increasingly evidence-based and some relevant medical professional societies worldwide have formulated recommendations and clinical practice guidelines.

Table 18.1: Risk factors associated wth higher incidence of VTE[64, 65]

Risk Factor	Incidence
Chronic respiratory failure	53.4%
Age > 75 years	50.3%
Chronic heart failure	32.0%
Varicose veins	25.0%
Obesity	20.1%
Cancer	14.3%
History of venous thromboembolism	9.4%
Hormone therapy	2.0%
Two or more risk factors	66.5%

According to the incidence of DVT among surgical patients, 4 levels of risk emerged (Table 18.2) and appropriate preventive strategies were developed for each.

Table 18.2: Thromboembolic risk stratification for surgery patients

Low risk	Uncomplicated surgery in patients aged <40 years with minimal immobility postoperatively and no risk factor
Moderate risk	Any surgery in patients aged 40-60 years, major surgery in patients <40 years and no risk factors
High risk	Surgery in patients aged >60 years, major surgery in patients aged 40-60 years with 1 or more risk factors
Very high risk	Major surgery in patients aged >40 years with previous VTE, cancer or known hypercoagulable state, major orthopedic surgery, elective neurosurgery, multiple trauma or acute spinal cord injury

METHODS OF PROPHYLAXIS

While some of the methods proved modestly effective (e.g. aspirin), until recently the use of heparins appeared to provide the maximal risk reduction. Means of VTE prophylaxis include pharmacologic agents such as fractionated heparin (FH) and unfractionated heparin, and mechanical methods, including lower extremity sequential compression devices (SCD) and elastic stockings.

Aspirin is shown to decrease incidence of VTE by 22 percent. Low-dose unfractionated heparin (LDUH) and low molecular weight heparin (LMWH) are the most effective therapies in the prevention of VTE providing a 68 to 72 percent of risk reduction.[66,67]

LMWH and LDUH appear to be equally effective in preventing DVT in general surgery patients.

As for their side effects, some studies have reported significantly fewer wound haematomas and bleeding complications with LMWH,[66-68] while other well-designed trials have shown that LMWH causes more bleeding than LDUH.[69,70] The discrepant findings appear to be related to dosage; there is a clear dose-response effect of LMWH on bleeding complications and probably also on the efficacy of the prophylaxis. The incidence of hemorrhage after the use of LMWH is related to dosage; higher doses of LMWH >3400 IU is associated with more bleeding complications as compared to LDUH.[71]

In contrast, lower doses of LMWH (< 3400 anti-Xa units daily) are equivalent to LDUH in preventing VTE in moderate risk patients and have a lower rate of bleeding complications.[72]

Mechanical prophylaxis with sequential compression devices, also called intermittent pneumatic compression (IPC), is an attractive form of VTE prophylaxis owing to lack of bleeding risk and proven efficacy.[73] These devices have been suggested to have haemodynamic action (increase of blood flow velocity) and to stimulate endogenous fibrinolytic activity via the production of tissue-type plasminogen activator by the vascular endothelium, which might contribute to their antithrombotic properties.[74] Intermittent pneumatic compression (IPC) showed an increased risk reduction of 88 percent.[75,76] IPCs are probably more effective than graduated compression stockings or LDUH in patients at moderate to high risk.[77,78]

PREVENTIVE STRATEGIES

Different patient risk groups (Table 18.2) have to be treated with different strategies. While in low-risk patients no specific prophylaxis is needed, high-risk patients benefit from a combination of heparins (LMWH or LDUH) and IPC or ES (Table 18.3).

Table 18.3: Evidence-based use of antithrombotic prophylaxis in general surgery[79]

Low risk	Early mobilization
	Low dose unfractionated heparin (LDUH) 5000 IU 12 hourly starting 2 hours before surgery
	or
	Low molecular weight heparin LMWH (<3400 anti-Xa IU daily.
Moderate risk	Compression elastic stockings (ES)
	or
	Intermittent pneumatic compression (IPC)
	LMWH (>3400 anti-Xa IU daily.
High risk	LDUH 5000 IU 8 hourly starting 2 hours before surgery plus ES
	or
	IPC if anticoagulation contraindicated
	Perioperative warfarin (INR = 2-3.
Very high risk	LMWH (>3400 anti-Xa IU daily) + ES

SELECTION OF PATIENT

Patient selection is an important consideration before any surgical procedure to optimize outcome. Hypercarbia and increased abdominal pressure from pneumoperitoneum or pneumoretroperitoneum coupled with patient's posture during urologic laparoscopic surgery can cause significant cardiovascular, respiratory and neurological effects. Various reports are available indicating safe laparoscopic procedures in patients belonging to Goldman class III and IV or American Society of Anesthesiologists class III.[80,81] Although healthy patients usually tolerate hypercarbia associated with CO_2 insufflation, patients with pre-existing cardiorespiratory disease do not and an intraoperative arterial blood gas monitoring or $EtCO_2$ monitoring is required in such patients.

Obesity is another area where conflicting reports are available regarding morbidity in relation to laparoscopic surgery. Scribner and Kuo separately reported safety of laparoscopic surgery in obesity and found obesity not a significant predictor of laparoscopic success.[82, 83] Mendoza et al reported a 22 per cent intraoperative and 26 per cent postoperative complication rate in obese patients in a multi-institutional review of 125 cases and concluded that obesity does place the patient at increased risk when undergoing laparoscopic surgery.[84] A detailed discussion on the subject is cited elsewhere in this book.

Previous abdominal surgery has also been considered a relative contraindication to laparoscopic surgery. In a review of 700 cases by Parsons et al, 15 per cent patients had a history of earlier surgery at the same anatomic region as their urologic surgery and 33 per cent had a history of abdominal surgery at other anatomic sites. There were no significant differences in operative blood loss, rate of conversion to open surgery or rate of operative complications among these three groups. However, a review of 190 cases of transperitoneal laparoscopic renal or adrenal procedures by Seifman et al, found significantly higher operative and major complication rates in patients with previous abdominal operations.[85] Although the data are confounding, patients with prior surgery or comorbidities should be counseled before surgery about their possible increased risks.[85,86]

SPECIFIC APPLICATIONS

Virtually all benign conditions have been impacted by laparoscopic surgery. Depending on the severity of the procedure and skill of endourologist, urological laparoscopic procedures can be classified as under:

Classification of urological laparoscopic producers

Easy procedures:
Orchiopexy
Orchiectomy
Varicocelectomy
Diagnostic laparoscopy

Moderately difficult procedures:
Cystectomy
Renal biopsy
Peritoneal lymph node dissection
Ureterolysis
Lymphocele drainage
Renal cyst decortication
Partial cystectomy
Bladder neck suspension

Difficult procedures:
Donor nephrectomy
Adrenalectomy
Partial nephrectomy
Simple nephrectomy
Radical nephrectomy
Nephroureterectomy
Pyeloplasty
Ureterectomy
Radical prostatectomy
Bladder augmentation
Pelvic lymphadenectomy
Retroperitoneal lymphadenectomy
Promontofixation for uterovaginal prolapse

LAPAROSCOPIC ADRENALECOMY

Since the work of Gagner et al in 1992 laparoscopic adrenalectomy has become the standard of care for benign adrenal lesions.[87] The small size of the adrenal gland, the benign nature of most adrenal tumours and difficulty of gaining access to the organ by open surgical means make laparoscopic approach particularly suitable for adrenalectomy. Laparoscopic adrenalectomy is appropriate for both functional and non-functional benign adrenal tumours.

Surgery is performed in modified flank (kidney) position (Fig. 18.14). Patient is put in lateral position with affected adrenal side up. The shoulders are dropped back by 30°. It is not necessary to flex table because the pneumoperitoneum will provide adequate working space. Table flexion has been implicated as a factor for neuromuscular injury during laparoscopic renal and adrenal surgery.[88]

The decreased morbidity and excellent patient satisfaction afforded by needlescopic technique prompted Gill and associates to explore the possibility of outpatient adrenalectomy.[89] They performed needlescopic adrenalectomies in 14 patients on outpatient basis. These patients fulfilled all of the following preoperative and perioperative inclusion criteria: informed consent, age 70 years or less, BMI < or = 40 kg/m², adrenal tumour less than 5 cm, no pheochromocytoma, the laparoscopic procedure is uncomplicated and finished by noon, perioperative haemodynamic stability and postoperative pain control with oral analgesics.

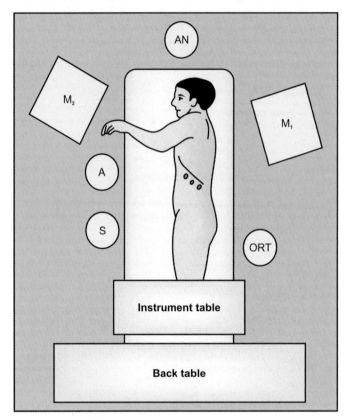

Fig. 18.14: Operating room layout for left transperitoneal laparoscopic adrenalectomy. (S, surgeon; A, assistant; AN, anaesthesiologist; ORT, operating room technician; M₁, primary video monitor; M₂, optional second video monitor)

LAPAROSCOPIC SURGERY FOR PHEOCHROMOCYTOMA

Surgery for pheochromocytoma carries specific risks not known with other adrenal tumours. Life-threatening hypertension or hypotension may occur during surgery. Pheochromocytomas may develop not only in the adrenals but also in extra-adrenal sites, therefore, careful preoperative evaluation is of outmost importance. Preoperative preparation of the patient with pheochromocytoma includes blockade of α-adrenergic receptors to preclude intraoperative hypertension. An additional β-blockade may be required to treat cardiac dysrhythmias. Phenoxybenzamine is the most commonly used a-adrenegic blocking agent.[90] A completely different approach to preoperative preparation has been described with the use of calcium-channel blockers.[91]

Intraoperative manipulation of the tumour may induce excessive catecholamine excretion, resulting in life-threatening hypertensive crisis. Because of lack of catecholamines following removal of the tumour, hypotensive crises may occur as well. It has been speculated that the pneumoperitoneum may induce hypertensive crisis owing to hypercapnia or the positive pressure. This coupled with handling of tumour, may increase the catecholamine levels more than those seen during open surgery. Various other investigators have shown that the amount of catecholamine secreted during laparoscopic surgery is lower than with open surgery.[92] Low IAP (8-10 mmHg) has shown to produce fewer haemodynamic changes and less catecholamine release during adrenalectomy.[93]

Balanced anaesthesia is the procedure of choice with continuous arterial blood pressure and central venous pressure monitoring. Pulmonary artery catheterisation may be considered in high-risk patients. Hypertensive crisis is treated with sodium nitroprusside, nitroglycerine, labetalol, esmolol and magnesium sulphate on a patient-specific basis.

LAPAROSCOPIC DONOR NEPHRECTOMY

As the waiting list of patients for cadaveric renal allografts grows longer, living related donation has become an increasingly popular option. Introduction of laparoscopic donor nephrectomy programme, has substantially reduced the donor morbidity and increased number of living donor volunteers. Laparoscopically procured kidneys have been shown to provide equivalent recipient outcomes and donor safety when compared with the traditional open surgical technique.[94-96] Laparoscopic donor nephrectomies have been shown to reduce postoperative pain, shorten hospital stay, allow faster return to work and improve cosmetic results.[94,95,97] With the introduction of laparoscopic donor nephrectomy, the number of donations has increased possibly decreasing disincentives to donations.[98]

Briefly, the laparoscopic donor nephrectomy technique includes induction of endotracheal general anaesthesia, insertion of nasogastric tube and Foley catheter. Patient is placed in modified lateral decubitus position at 45° and the torso is allowed to rotate posteriorly to allow exposure to the lower midline. Surgery is carried out through three port or four port options after pneumoperitoneum with carbon dioxide. After careful and complete dissection, the kidney is removed through a paraumbilical incision large enough to remove the kidney. The renal bed and trocar sites are inspected for bleeding and carbon dioxide is evacuated.

Postoperative recovery data from several series comparing laparoscopic donor nephrectomy with open donor nephrectomy are summarised in Table 18.4.

Table 18.4: Postoperative recovery data

| | Ratner et al[100] | | Ratner et al[101] | | Odland et al[102] | | Flowers et al[99] | |
	LDN	ODN	LDN	ODN	LDN	ODN	LDN	ODN
Number	20	19	25	37	26	30	70	65
PO intake resumed (days)	0.8	2.5					1.7	3.2
LOS (days)	3.1	5.7	2.9	5.5	2.7	3.8	2.2	4.5
Analgesic usage	34*	124*	4.2**	11.8**	1.0#	2.5#	1.2#	2.5#
Driving (weeks)			1.9	3.2			1.6	4.5
Full activity (weeks)	2.2	4.2			1.4	3.6		
Returned to work (weeks)	3.9	6.4	4.4	6.3	2.7	5.3	2.3	7.4

LDN, laparoscopic donor nephrectomy; ODN, open donor nephrectomy; LOS, length of stay
*mg parenteral morphine sulphate used
**days of prescription analgesic used
days of parenteral analgesic used

These results show that laparoscopic donor nephrectomy is associated with low morbidity and has eliminated many of the disincentives to live donor nephrectomy. Since the inception of the laparoscopic donor nephrectomy programme, Ratner and co-workers have reported more than a 100 percent increase in live donor transplants.[103]

LAPAROSCOPIC RADICAL PROSTATECTOMY

Laparoscopic radical prostatectomy was first performed by Schuessler and colleagues in 1991 who published their experience of nine cases in 1997.[104] The objective of laparoscopic radical prostatectomy is to allow more precise operative procedure in addition to reduce perioperative morbidity. The quality of surgery is improved by a better visualisation of the operative site owing to the optical magnification and the manoeuverability of the laparoscope. In addition to the improved postoperative course, laparoscopic radical prostatectomy allows better preservation of periprostatic vascular, muscular and neurovascular structures.

The operation is performed under general anaesthesia with the patient in supine position with head-down tilt. Thoracic wrap with elastic adhesive tape is more suitable and comfortable for the patient than shoulder supports because of the risk of postoperative shoulder pain by compression on the shoulders. The arms are kept by the side of the patient to avoid brachial plexus injury by exaggerated abduction at the shoulder joint for a prolonged period. The legs are positioned in flexion-abduction on foam support with the buttocks at the end of the operating table.

Perioperatively, an antithrombotic regimen is an essential element because of three risk factors: cancer surgery, pelvic surgery and a laparoscopic procedure. Specific complications associated with this procedure include haemorrhage from the dorsal venous complex, epigastric arterial injury, rectal injury, peritonitis and bladder or ureteric injury leading to urinary leak.[105]

URINARY INCONTINENCE

Urinary incontinence is the involuntary loss of urine and is estimated to affect females predominantly. In females, the normal continence mechanism consists of an intrinsic coapting ability of proximal urethra, a critical functional urethral length, the ability of the pelvic floor to increase urethral pressure at the time of stress and the proper anatomic location of this sphincteric unit. Stress incontinence results from the loss of the normal supporting backboard effect of the levator muscles and the urethral pelvic ligaments on the bladder neck and the proximal urethra. Surgical correction of stress incontinence include securing the anterior vaginal wall with its overlying endopelvic fascia to a strong ligamentous or bony structure anterosuperiorly, in such a manner that the bladder neck and proximal urethra are elevated and secured in a retropubic position.

Laparoscopic bladder neck suspension, the procedure involved, was first described by Vancaillie et al.[106] This procedure is performed using either extraperitoneal or transperitoneal approach. The main concerns for the anaesthesiologists remain the position of the patient, Trendelenburg position with slight lithotomy and adequate relaxation for better retropubic access.

ANAESTHESIA

Careful choice of anaesthetic technique must be tailored to the type of surgery. General anaesthesia using balanced anaesthesia technique including inhalational agents, intravenous induction agents and a variety of muscle relaxants have been reported. The use of more rapid and short-acting volatile anaesthetics such as desflurane and sevoflurane along with ultrashort-acting opioid analgesic such as remifentanil has allowed the anaesthesiologist to achieve a recovery profile that facilitates fast tracking after general anaesthesia. Sevoflurane, desflurane and continuous infusion of propofol represents the maintenance agents of choice. Moreover, propofol does have the advantage of producing less postoperative nausea and vomiting (PONV).[107, 108]

The use of an auditory evoked potential or Bispectral Index monitor to titrate the volatile anaesthetic, in comparison to standard monitoring practices, leads to significant reduction in the anaesthetic requirement, resulting in a shorter stay in post anaesthesia care unit and an improved quality of patient's recovery.[109]

The ultrashort-acting opioid remifentanil, which is rapidly hydrolysed by circulating and tissue nonspecific estrases, has been shown to provide better control of perioperative haemodynamic responses compared with alfentanil.[110] Moreover, doses of remifentanil required to attenuate cardiovascular responses can be used without the risk of postoperative respiratory depression and delayed recovery, however, postoperative analgesia should be considered. Preemptive analgesic techniques using nonopioids such as acetaminophen, nonsteroidal anti-inflammatory drugs, a_2-agonists and N-methyl D-aspartate antagonists proved to be of benefit in multimodal analgesia where rapid recovery was the aim.[111]

Nitrous oxide, the oldest anaesthetic agent, is commonly used to provide perioperative analgesia and to reduce the requirements for inhaled or intravenous anaesthetics. Its contribution towards postoperative nausea and vomiting is still controversial. There is apparently no clinical advantage in omitting nitrous oxide and benefits from its elimination must be balanced against a greater risk of awareness. Earlier anaesthetic techniques described for laparoscopic cholecystectomy avoided nitrous oxide. Further studies have confirmed similar surgical conditions regardless of whether nitrous oxide was used or not, questioning its contraindication during laparoscopic surgery. However, omission of nitrous oxide improves surgical conditions for intestinal and colonic surgery by avoiding the possible nitrous oxide diffusion into the bowel lumen. During urologic laparoscopic surgery, particularly in renal surgery, the use of nitrous oxide is avoided for the same reason. Because of the limited space available for dissection during laparoscopic nephrectomy, the dilated gut may further limit the access to the kidney and increase the risk of bowel injury as well.

Succinylcholine was commonly as muscle relaxant of choice for short laparoscopic procedures, but it was associated with a high incidence of postoperative muscle pains. There is a considerable choice in short-acting nondepolarising neuromuscular blocking agents these days, but none of them are quite as short acting as succinylcholine. In urological laparoscopic procedures shorter duration of muscle relaxants is not an issue, but postoperative muscle pains even with intubating dose of succinylcholine is definitely an issue when considered along with the postoperative pain because of long duration of unusual posture. However, it is desirable to use repeated doses of short-acting agents during short surgical procedures rather than occasional doses of longer-acting drugs. Reversal of residual muscle paralysis by neostigmine at the end of surgery is reported to be associated with PONV, for the same reason some anaesthesilogists do not reverse their patients.[112] There are other studies where increased incidence of PONV after reversal of neuromuscular block is not reported.[113] In prolonged surgical procedures, as in urological laparoscopy, there should not be any concern regarding duration of neuromuscular blockade. For smooth conduct of anaesthesia and adequate relaxation an infusion of neuromuscular blocking drug is desirable along with the use of neuromuscular block monitor to titrate the dose of relaxant drug.

General anaesthesia with endotracheal intubation and controlled ventilation remains the best choice for urological laparoscopic surgery. A correctly placed classical LMA or a ProSeal LMA is as effective as an endotracheal tube for positive pressure ventilation without clinically important gastric distension.[114] However, it should be restricted to short laparoscopic procedures performed using low IAP and small degrees of tilt. In the kidney position, pneumoperitoneum is associated with decreased thoracopulmonary compliance resulting in airway pressures exceeding 20 cmH$_2$O. Since the LMA cannot guarantee an effective airway seal above this pressure, its use for controlled ventilation in this position is limited.

During pneumoperitoneum, controlled ventilation must be adjusted to maintain EtCO$_2$ at approximately 35 mmHg, requiring usually an increase in minute ventilation by 15 to 25 per cent. In patients with chronic obstructive airway disease and in patients with a history of spontaneous pneumothorax or bullous emphysema, an increase in respiratory rate rather than tidal volume is preferable to avoid increased alveolar inflation and reduce the risk of pneumothorax. Because of the potential for reflex increase in vagal tone during laparoscopy, atropine should be administered before the induction of anaesthesia or should be available for injection if necessary.

MONITORING

Appropriate anaesthetic techniques with proper monitoring to detect and reduce complications must be used to ensure optimal anaesthesia care. Electrocardiogram, noninvasive blood pressure monitor, $EtCO_2$ concentration monitor, pulse oximetry, peripheral nerve stimulation and temperature monitor should be used routinely. Invasive arterial blood pressure monitoring, blood gas analysis and urine output monitoring should be considered for haemodynamically unstable patients and in prolonged surgical procedures.

Adequacy of ventilation during laparoscopic surgery is most commonly assessed by $EtCO_2$ monitoring as a noninvasive substitute for $PaCO_2$ (partial pressure of carbon dioxide in arterial blood). A careful consideration should be taken for the gradient between $PaCO_2$ and $EtCO_2$ because $EtCO_2$ may differ considerably from $PaCO_2$ because of ventilation/perfusion (V/Q) mismatch in patients with cardiopulmonary compromise or ASA III-IV patients. Direct estimation of $PaCO_2$ by arterial blood gas analysis may become necessary in patients with compromised cardiopulmonary dysfunction as the gradient between $EtCO_2$ and $PaCO_2$ increases to become unpredictable. Therefore, a radial artery cannulation for continuous blood pressure monitoring and frequent arterial blood gas analysis should be considered in patients with preoperative cardiopulmonary disease and in situations where intraoperative hypoxaemia, high airway pressures or elevated $EtCO_2$ are encountered.[115]

An airway pressure monitor, present on the ventilator of anaesthesia machine, is routinely used during intermittent positive pressure ventilation. An activated high airway pressure alarm can aid detection of excessive elevation in IAP.[115] The use of a Bispectral Index monitor, a possible monitor of depth of anaesthesia, can help to reduce the occurrence of awareness. It can further assist in titrate intravenous and inhalation agents to fasten emergence and improved recovery.[116-118]

CLINICAL PEARLS

1. Laparoscopic urological procedures are gaining popularity due to the well documented benefits.
2. General anaesthesia with endotracheal intubation and controlled ventilation is recommended.
3. Meticulous monitoring essential since the procedures involve intraperitoneal and extraperitoneal insufflation of CO_2.

REFERENCES

1. Schuessler WW, Vancaillie TG, Reich H, et al: Transperitoneal endosurgical lymphadenectomy in patients with localised prostate cancer. J Urol 1991;145:988.
2. See WA, Cooper CS, Fisher RJ. Urological laparoscopic practice patterns 1 year after formal training. J Urol 1994;151:1595.
3. Colegrove PM, Winfield HN, Donovan JF, et al. Laparoscopic practice patterns among urologists 5 years after formal training. J Urol 1999;161:881.
4. Winfield HN, Donovan JF, See WA, et al. Urological laparoscopic surgery. J Urol 1991;146:941.
5. Gill IS, Clayman RV, McDougall EM. Advances in urological laparoscopy. J Urol 1995;154:1274.
6. Cortesi N, Ferrari P, Zambardae A, Baldini A, Morano FP. Diagnosis of bilateral abdominal cryptorchidism by Laparoscopy. Endoscopy 1976;8:33.
7. Clayman RV, Kavoussi LR, Soper NJ, Dierks SM, Darcy MD, et al. Laparoscopic nephrectomy: initial case report. J Urol 1991; 146:278.

8. Abdelmaksoud A et al. Laparoscopic approaches in urology. BJU International 2005; 95: 244.

9. Flocks RH, Culp D. Surgical urology. Chicago Year Book Medical Publishers, 1967.

10. Horswell JL. Anesthetic techniques for thoracoscopy. Ann Thorac Surg 1993; 56: 624.

11. Grayhack JT, Graham J. Renal surgery. In Glenn JF (ed.): Urologic Surgery. Hagerstown, MD, Harper & Row, 1975.

12. Kroppa KA. Unusual positions in urology: Surgical aspects. In Martin JT (ed.): Positioning in Anaesthesia and Surgery. Philadelphia, WB Saunders, 1987.

13. Yokoyama M, Ueda W, Hirakawa M. Haemodynamic effects of the lateral decubitus position and kidney rest lateral decubitus position during anaesthesia. Br J Anaesth 2000; 84: 753.

14. Eggers GNW, DeGroot WJ, Tanner CR, et al. Hemodynamic changes associated with various surgical positions. JAMA 1963; 185: 1.

15. Fessler HE, Brower RG, Shapiro EP, et al. Effects of positive end-expiratory pressure and body position on pressure in the thoracic great veins. Am Rev Respir Dis 1993; 148: 1657.

16. Baraka A, Moghrabi R, Yazigi A. Unilateral pulmonary edema/ atelectasis in the lateral decubitus position. Anaesthesia 1987; 42: 171

17. Snoy FG, Woodside JR. Unilateral pulmonary edema (down-lung syndrome) following urological operation. J urol 1984; 132: 776

18. Klingstedt C, Hedenstierna G, Lundquist H, et al. The influence of body position and differential ventilation on lung dimentions and atelectasis formation in anesthetized man. Acta Anaesthesiol Scand 1990; 34: 315.

19. Meyhoff HH, Hess J, Olesen KP. Pulmonary atelectasis following upper urinary tract surgery on parients in the 25 and 45 degree jack-knife position. Scand J Urol Nephrol 1980; 14: 107.

20. Calverly RK, Jenkins LC. The anaesthetic management of pelvic laparoscopy. Can Anaesth Soc J, 1973; 20: 679.

21. Wilkins RW, Bradley SE, Friedland CK. The acute circulatory effects in the head-down position (negative G) in normal man, with a note on some measures designed to relieve cranial congestion in this position. J Clin Invest 1950; 29: 940.

22. Little DM Jr. Posture and anesthesia. Can Anaesth Soc J 1960; 7: 2.

23. Abel FL, Pierce JH, Guntheroth WG. Baroreceptor influence on postural changes in blood pressure and carotid blood flow. Am J Physiol 1963; 205: 360.

24. Kubal K, Komatsu T, Sanchala V, et al. Trendelenburg position used during venous cannulation increases myocardial oxygen demand. Anesth Analg 1984; 63: 239.

25. Keusch DJ, Winters S, Thys DM. The patient's position influences the incidence of dysrhythmias during pulmonary artery catheterization. Anesthesiology 1989; 70: 582.

26. Dripps RD. Anesthesia. In Rhoads JE, Allen JG, Harkins HN, Moyer CA, (eds.): Surgery: Principles and Practice, 4th ed. Philadelphia, JB Lippincott, 1970.

27. Enderby GEH. Postural ischaemia and blood pressure. Lancet 1954; 1: 185

28. Martin JT. Compartment syndromes: Concepts and perspectives for the anesthesiologist. Anesth Analg 1992; 75: 275.

29. Johannsen G, Andersen M, Juhl B. The effect of general anaesthesia on the haemodynamic events during laparoscopy with CO_2 insufflation. Acta Anaesthesiol Scand 1989; 33: 132.

30. Fahy BG, Barnas G, Nagle S, et al. Effect of Trendelenburg and reverse Trendelenburg posture on lung and chest wall mechanics. Anesthesiology 1995; 83: A1224.

31. Hewer CL. Latest pattern of non-slip mattress. Anaesthesia 1953; 8: 198.

32. AmoiridsG,Wohrle JC, Langkofel M, et al. Spinal cord infarctionafter surgery in a patient in the hyperlordotic position. Anesthesiology 1996; 84: 228.

33. Hodgson C, McClelland RMA, Newton JR. Some effects of the peritoneal insufflation of carbon dioxide at Laparoscopy. Anaesthesia 1970;25: 382.

34. Seed RF, Shakespeare TF, Muldoon MJ. Carbon dioxide homeostasis during anaesthesia for lapaoscopy. Anaesthesia 1970;25:223.

35. Giebler RM, Kabatnik M, Stegen BH, Scherer RU, Thomas M, Peters J. Retroperitoneal and intraperitoneal CO_2 insufflation have markedly different cardiovascular effects. Journal of Surgical Research 1997; 68: 153.

36. Odeberg S, Ljungqvist O, Svenberg T, Gannedahl P, Backdahl M, von Rosen A, Sollevi A. Haemodynamic effects of pneumoperitoneum and the influence of posture during anaesthesia for laparoscopic surgery. Acta Anaesthesiol Scand 1994; 38: 276.

37. Chiu AW, Chang LS, Birkett DH, et al. The impact of pneumoperitoneum, pneumoretroperitoneum, and gasless laparoscopy on the systemic and renal hemodynamics. J Am Coll Surg 1995; 181: 397.

38. Wolf JS Jr.,Monk TG, McDougall EM, McClennan BL, Clayman RV. The extraperitoneal approach and subcutaneous emphysema are associated with greater absorption of carbon dioxide during laparoscopic renal surgery. J Urol 1995; 154: 959.

39. Christopher S, Gill IS, Sung GT, Whalley DG, Graham R, Schweizer D. Retropritoneoscopic surgery is not associated with increased carbon dioxide absorption. J Urol 1999; 162: 1268.

40. Guillonneau B, Wetzel O, Lepage JY, Vallancian G, Buzelin JM. Retroperitoneal laparoscopic nephrectomyanimal and human anatomic studies. J Endourol 1995;9:487.

41. Baird JE, Granger R, Klein R, Warriner CB, Phang PT. The effects of retroperitoneal carbon dioxide insufflation on hemodynamics and arterial carbon dioxide. Am J Surg 1999;177:164.

42. Mullet CE, Viale JP, Sagnard PE, et al. Pulmonary CO_2 elimination during surgical procedures using intra- or extraperitoneal CO_2 insufflation. Anesth Analg 1993; 76: 622.

43. Gascock JM, Winfield HN, Lund GO, Donovan JF, Ping ST, Griffiths DL. Carbon dioxide homeostasis during transperitoneal or extraperitoneal laparoscopic pelvic lymphadenactomy: a real-time inraoperative comparison. J Endourol 1996; 10: 319.

44. Ng CS, Gill IS, Sung GT, Whalley DG, Graham R, Schweizer D. Retroperitoneoscopic surgery is not associated with increased carbon dioxide absorption. J Urol 1999;162:1268.

45. Thorington JM, Schmidt CF. A study of urinary output and blood pressure changes resulting in experimental ascites. Am J Med Sci 1923; 165: 880.

46. Leonard IE, Cunningham AJ. Anaesthetic considerations for laparoscopic cholecystectomy. Clin Anaesthesiol 2002; 89: 535.

47. Harmon PK, Kron I, McLochlan HD, et al. Elevated intra-abdominal pressure and renal function. Ann Surg 1982; 196: 594.

48. Lennon G, Ryan PC, Gaffney EF, et al. Changes in regional renal perfusion following ischemia/ reperfusion injury to the rat kidney. Urol Res 1991; 19: 259.

49. Spelman FA, Oberg PA, Astley C. Localized neural control of blood flow in the renal cortex of the anaesthetized baboon. Acta Physiol Scand 1986; 127: 437.

50. Sies H. Oxidative stress oxidants and antioxidants. Exp Physiol 1997; 82: 291.

51. Andreoli SP. Reactive oxygen molecules, oxidant injury and renal disease. Pediatr Nephrol 1991; 5: 733.

52. Schob OM, Allen DC, Benzel E, et al. A comparison of the patho-physiologic effects of carbon dioxide, nitrous oxide and helium pneumoperitoneum on intracranial pressure. Am J Surg 1996; 172: 248.

53. Hargeaves DM. Hypercapnia and raised cerebrospinal fluid pressure. Anesthesia 1990; 45: 7.

54. Fujii Y, Tanaka H, Tsurukoa S, et al. Middle cerebral artery blood flow velocity increases during laparoscopic cholecystectomy. Anesth Analg 1994; 78: 80.

55. Abe K et al. Middle cerebral artery blood flow velocity during laparoscopic surgery in head-down position. Surg Laparosc Endosc 1998; 8: 1.

56. Rosenthal et al. Effects of hyperventilation and hypoventilation on $PaCO_2$ and intracranial pressure during acute elevations of intraabdominal pressure with CO_2 pneumoperitoneum: large animal observations. J Am Coll Surg 1998; 187: 32.

57. Morris RH, Ktunar A. The effect of warming blankets on maintenance of body temperature of the anesthetized, paralysed adult patient. Anesthesiology 1972; 36: 408.

58. Lindberg F, Bergqvist D, Rasmussen I. Incidence of thromboembolic complications after laparoscopic cholecystectomy: review of the literature. Surg Laparosc Endosc 1997; 7: 324.

59. Patel MI, Hardman DT, Nicholls D, Fisher CM, Appleberg M. The incidence of deep vein thrombosis after laparoscopic cholecystectomy. Med J Aust 1996; 164: 652.

60. Fowkes FJ, Price JF, Fowkes FG. Incidence of diagnosed deep vein thrombosis in general population: systematic review. Eur J Vasc Andovasc Surg 2003; 25: 1.

61. Kavoussi LR, Sosa E, Chandhoke P, Chodak G, Clayman RV, Hadley HR et al. Complications of laparoscopic pelvic lymph node dissection. J Urol 1993; 149: 322.

62. Cadeddu JA, Wolf JS Jr, Nakada S, Chen R, Shalhav A, Bishoff JT, et al. Complications of laparoscopic procedures after concentrated training in urological laparoscopy. J Urol 2001; 166: 2109.

63. Prandoni P, Lensing A W, Cogo A, Cuppini S, Carta M, et al: The long-term clinical course of acute deep venous thrombosis. Ann Intern Med 1996; 125: 1.

64. Samama MM. An epidemiologic study of risk factors for deep vein thrombosis in medical outpatients. The Sirius Study. Arch Intern Med 2000; 160: 3415.

65. Heit JA, Silverstein MD, Mohr DN, et al. Risk factors for deep vein thrombosis and pulmonary embolism. Arch Intern Med 2000; 160: 809.

66. Kakkar VV, Cohen AT, Edmonson RA, et al. Low molecular weight versus standard heparin for prevention of VTE after major abdominal surgery. Lancet 1993; 341: 259.

67. Nurmohamed MT, Verhaeghe R, Hass S, et al. A comparative trial of a low molecular weight heparin (enoxaparin) versus standard heparin for the prophylaxis of postoperative deep vein thrombosis in general surgery. Am J Surg 1995; 169: 567.

68. Kakkar VV, Boeckl O, Boneu B, et al. Efficacy and safety of a low-molecular-weight heparin and standard heparin for prophylaxis of postoperative venous thromboembolism: European multicenter trial. World J Surg 1997; 21: 2.

69. Bergqvist D, Matzsch T, Burmark US, et al. Low molecular weight heparin given the evening before surgery compared with conventional low-dose heparin in prevention of thrombosis. Br J Surg 1988; 75: 888.

70. Etchells E, McLeod RS, Geerts W, et al. Economic analysis of low-dose heparin vs the low-molecular-weight heparin enoxaparin for prevention of venous thromboembolism after colorectal surgery. Arch Intern Med 1999; 159: 1221.

71. Koch A, Bouges S, Ziegler S, et al. Low molecular weight heparin and unfractionated heparin in thrombosis prophylaxis after major surgical intervention: update of previous meta-analysis. Br J Surg 1997; 84: 750.

72. Mismetti P, Laporte S, Darmon JY, et al. Meta-analysis of low molecular weight heparin in the prevention of venous thromboembolism in general surgery. Br J Surg 2001; 88: 913.

73. Hull RD, Pineo GF. Intermittent pneumatic compression for the prevention of venous thromboembolism. Chest 1996; 109: 6.

74. Christen Y, Wutschert R, Weimer D, et al. Effects of intermittent pneumatic compression on venous haemodynamics and fibrinolytic activity. Blood Coagul Fibrinolysis 1997; 8(3): 185.

75. Butson ARC. Intermittent pneumatic calf compression for prevention of deep venous thrombosis in general abdominal surgery. Am J Surg 1981; 142: 525.

76. Hills NH, Pflug JJ, Jeyasingh K, et al. Prevention of deep vein thrombosis by intermittent pneumatic compression of calf. BMJ 1972; 1: 131.

77. Vanek VW. Meta-analysis of effectiveness of intermittent pneumatic compression devices with a comparison of thigh-high to knee-high sleeves. Am Surg 1998; 64: 1050.

78. Agu O, Hamilton G, Baker D. Graduated compression stockings in the prevention of venous thromboenbolism. Br J Surg 1999; 86: 992.

79. Turpie AG, Chin BS, Lip GY. ABC of antithrombotic therapy: venous thromboembolism: pathophysiology, clinical features, and prevention. BMJ 2002; 325: 887.

80. Sharma KC, Kabinogg G, Ducheine Y, Tierney J, Brandstetter RD. Laparoscopic surgery and its potential for medical complications. Heart Lung 1997;26:52.

81. Carroll BJ, Chandra M, Phillips EH, Margulies DR. Laparoscopic cholecystectomy in critically ill cardiac patients. Am Surg 1993; 59: 783.

82. Scribner Jr. DR, Walker JL, Johnson GA, McMeekin DS, Gold MA, Mannel RS. Laparoscopic pelvic and paraaortic lymph node dissection in the obese. Gynecol Oncol 2002; 84: 426.

83. Kuo PC, Plotkin JS, Stevens S, Cribbs A, Johnson LB. Outcomes of laparoscopic donor nephrectomy in obese patients. Transplantation 2000; 69: 180.

84. Mendoza D, Newman RC, Albala D, Cohen MS, Tewari A, Lingeman J, et al. Laparoscopic complications in markedly obese urologic patients. (a multi-institutional review) Urology 1996; 48: 562.

85. Seifman BD, Dunn RL, Wolf JS Jr. Transperitoneal laparoscopy into the previously operated abdomen: effect on operative time, length of stay and complications. J Urol 2003; 169: 36.

86. Parsons JK, Jarrett TJ, Chow GK, Kavoussi LR. The effect of previous abdominal surgery on urological laparoscopy. J Urol 2002; 168: 2387.

87. Gagner M, Lacroix A, Bolte E. Laparoscopic adrenalectomy in Cushing's syndrome and pheochromocytoma [letter]. N Engl J Med 1992; 327: 1033.

88. Wolf JS Jr, Marcovich R, GillIS, et al. Survey of neuromuscular injuries to the patient and surgeon during urologic laparoscopic surgery. J Endourol 1999; 13(Suppl 1): A 144.

89. Gill IS, Hobart MG, Schweizer D, et al. Outpatient adrenalectomy. J Urol 2000; 163: 717.

90. Hull CJ. Pheochromocytoma: Diagnosis, preoperative preparation and anesthetic management. Br J Anaesth 1986; 58: 1452.

91. Ulchaker JC, Goldfarb DA, Bravo EL, et al. Successful outcomes in pheochromocytoma surgery in modern era. J Urol 1999; 161: 764.

92. Fernandez-Cruz L, Taura P, Saenz A, et al. Laparoscopic approach to pheochromocytoma: Hemodynamic changes and catecholamine secretion. World J Surg 1996; 20: 762.

93. Sood J, Jayaraman L, Kumra VP, et al. Laparoscopic approach to pheochromocytoma: Is a lower intraabdominal pressure helpful? Anesth Analg 2006; 102: 637.

94. Jacobs SC, Cho E, Dunkin BJ. Laparoscopic donor nephrectomy: current role in renal allograft procurement. Urology 2000; 55: 807.

95. Fabrizio MD, Ratner LE, Montgomery RA, et al. Laparoscopic live donor nephrectomy. Urol Clin North Am 1999; 26: 247.

96. Brown SL, Bichl TR, Rawlins MC, et al. Laparoscopic live donor nephrectomy: a comparison with the conventional open approach. J Urol 2001; 165: 766.

97. Leventhal JR, Deeik RK, Joehl RJ, et al. Laparoscopic live donor nephrectomy – is it safe? Transplantation 2000; 70: 602.

98. Schweitzer EJ, Wilson J, Jacobs S, et al. Increased rates of donation with laparoscopic donor nephrectomy. Ann Surg 2000; 232: 392.

99. Flowers JL, Jacobs S, Cho E, et al. Comparison of open and laparoscopic live donor nephrectomy. Ann Surg 1997; 226: 483.

100. Ratner LE, Kavoussi LR, Saroka M, et al. Laparoscopic assisted live donor nephrectomy – a comparison with open approach. Transplantation 1997; 63: 229.

101. Ratner LE, Kavoussi LR, Schulam PG, et al. Comparison of laparoscopic live donor nephrectomy versus the standard open approach. Transplant Proc 1997; 29, 138.

102. Odland MD, Ney AL, Jacobs DM, et al. Initial experience with laparoscopic live donor nephrectomy. Surgery 1999; 126: 603,

103. Ratner LE, Montgomery RA, Kavoussi LR. Laparoscopic live donor nephrectomy: The four year John Hopkins University experience. Nephrol Dial Transplant 1999; 14: 2090.

104. Schuessler W, Schulam P, Clayman R, et al. Laparoscopic radical prostatectomy: Initial short-term experience. Urology 1997; 50: 854.

105. Guillonneau B, Rozet F, Barret E, et al. Laparoscopic radical prostatectomy: Assessment after 240 procedures. Urol Clin North Am 2001; 28: 189.

106. Vancaillie TG, Schuessler W. Laparoscopic bladder neck suspension. J Laparoendosc Surg 1991; 1: 169.

107. Eriksson H, Korttila K. Recovery profile after desflurane with or without ondansetron compared with propofol in patients undergoing outpatient gynecological laparoscopy. Anesth Analg 1996; 82: 533.

108. Reader JC, Mjaland O, Aasbo V, et al. Desflurane versus propofol maintenance for outpatient laparoscopic cholecystectomy. Acta Anaesthesiol Scand 1998; 42: 106.

109. Recart A, Gasanova I, White PF, et al. The effect of cerebral monitoring on recovery after general anesthesia: a comparison of the auditory evoked potential and Bispectral Index devices with standard clinical practice. Anesth Analg 2003; 97: 1667.

110. Philip BK, Scuderi PE, Chung F, et al. Remifentanil compared with alfentanil for ambulatory surgery using total intravenous anesthesia. Anesth Analg 1997; 84: 515.

111. Power I, Barratt S. Analgesic agents for the postoperative period. Nonopioids. Surg Clin North Am 1999; 79: 275.

112. Ding Y, Fredman B, White PF. Use of mivacurium during laparoscopic surgery: effect of reversal drugs on postoperative recovery. Anesth Analg 1994; 78: 450.

113. Hovorka J, Korttila K, Nelskyla K, et al. Reversal of neuromuscular blockade with neostigmine has no effect on the incidence or severity of postoperative nausea and vomiting. Anesth Analg 1997; 85: 1359.

114. Maltby JR, Beriault MT, Watson NC, et al. Classic and LMA-ProSeal are effective alternatives to endotracheal intubation for gynecological laparoscopy. Can J Anaesth 2003; 50: 71.

115. Neudecker J, Sauerland S, Neugebauer E, et al. The European Association for Endoscopic Surgery clinical practice guideline on the pneumoperitoneum for laparoscopic surgery. Surg Endosc 2002; 16: 1121.

116. Gan TJ, Glass PS, Windsor A, et al. Bispectral index monitoring allows faster emergence and improved recovery from propofol, alfentanil, and nitrous oxide anesthesia. Anesthesiology 1997; 87: 808.

117. Song D, Joshi GP, White PF. Titration of volatile anesthetics using Bispectral Index facilitates recovery after ambulatory anesthesia. Anesthesiology 1997; 87: 842.

118. White PF, Ma H, Tang J, et al. Does the use of electroencephalographic Bispectral Index or auditory evoked potential index monitoring facilitates recovery after desflurane anesthesia in the ambulatory setting? Anesthesiology 2004; 100: 811.

CHAPTER 19

Complications in Laparoscopic Surgery

INTRODUCTION

The advantages of laparoscopic approach for surgical procedures are quite well known now. This has led to performing more extensive procedures in older and sicker patients with significant co-existing cardiopulmonary disease. However these procedures have new potentially life threatening complications that are not traditionally seen with the conventional open approach. Awareness of these potential complications and knowledge of their management should reduce morbidity and mortality thus improving patient care and safety.

INCIDENCE

The incidence of laparoscopic complications is 1.1 to 5.2 per cent in minor procedures and 2.5 to 6 per cent in major ones.[1] The incidence of anaesthesia related complications is remarkably low-probably due to better monitoring facilities.

CLASSIFICATION

It can be divided into intraoperative and postoperative.

A. Intraoperative

1. Anaesthesia related
2. Laparoscopy related
   a. *Introduction of pneumoperitoneum*
      - Cardiovascular
        - Arrhythmias
            Vasovagal
            Brady arrhythmias
            Tachy arrhythmias.
        - Hypotension
            Cardiac arrest.

> – Hypertension.
>
> – Respiratory
>> – Hypercarbia.
>> – Gas embolism
>
> – Due to extravasation of gas
>> – Subcutaneous emphysema
>> – Pneumothorax
>> – Pneumomediastinum.

b. *Insertion of Trocars*
  - Similar to above
  - Injury to the organs
    - Stomach, liver, spleen
    - Urinary bladder.
  - Injury to the vessels.

c. *Positioning of Patient*
  - Nerve injuries
  - Endobronchial intubation

d. *Thermal Injuries*

B. Postoperative

1. Pain
2. Nausea and vomiting
3. Deep vein thrombosis
4. Infections
5. Spread of malignancy.

C. Specific – due to the surgery involved.

ANAESTHESIA RELATED

The problems related to anaesthesia like difficult intubation, hypoxemia etc. are not discussed here since with better perioperative management and monitoring, the anaesthesia related problems are very low.

Due to Introduction of Pneumoperitoneum

The first step in laparoscopy after anaesthesia is the introduction of Veress needle. This is a blind procedure and therefore can cause various complications.

Cardiovascular

Bradyarrhythmias: The introduction of gas in the abdomen produces a peritoneal stretch, which results in vagal stimulation leading to bradyarrhythmias. This can be accentuated if patient is on β-blockers. Anaesthetic drugs like fentanyl citrate, sufentanil, morphine along with the inhalational agent sevoflurane potentiate these bradyarrhythmias. Incidence of these arrhythmias has been reported to be 30 per cent in a study of forty nine patients.[1,2] The treatment of these bradyarrhythmias is atropine. Desufflation of the abdomen has to be done if the bradyarrhythmias do not improve with the conventional treatment.

Tachyarrhythmias: Lighter planes of anaesthesia and hypercarbia due to some cause can also precipitate tachyarrhythmias. Paroxysmal atrial tachycardia, ventricular tachycardia and ventricular fibrillation are rare complications, which have been reported during laparoscopic adrenalectomy.[1] Treatment is the conventional treatment of specific arrhythmias with xylocard and amiodarone. Failure to respond to medications warrants desufflation of abdomen.

Hypotension: The effect of the anaesthetic induction agents like thiopentone and inhalational agents like sevoflurane along with the decreased volume status of the patient coupled with a sudden inflation of abdomen with carbon dioxide compressing the inferior vena cava are causative agents for hypotension during anaesthesia. Adequate hydration of the patient and gradual carboperitoneum can prevent this complication. A sudden blood loss due to injury to the major vessels can also cause hypotension and should be dealt with accordingly.

Hypertension: Lighter planes of anaesthesia and hypercarbia are the two common causes of hypertension during laparoscopic surgery. Handling of the tumour during laparoscopic adrenalectomy can also precipitate hypertension. Management includes increasing the depth of anaesthesia with propofol, inhalation agents like sevoflurane, addition of opioids and use of calcium channel blockers and beta-blockers.

Respiratory Complications

The induction of pneumoperitoneum causes a cephalad shift of the diaphragm,[3,4] reduction of FRC, basal atelectasis leading to hypoventilation, V/Q mismatch, hypoxemia and hypercarbia. Management is by increasing tidal volume and respiratory rate and adjusting the minute ventilation to maintain normocarbia.

Gas embolism: One of the most dreaded complication in laparoscopic surgery is gas embolism. It is a rare but potentially lethal complication and thus early diagnosis and prompt management is paramount in enhancing the chances for patient survival. Most commonly embolic episodes occur during creation of pneumoperitoneum and can occur through a tear in a vessel in the abdominal wall or on the peritoneum. A large amount of carbon dioxide must enter the vessels rapidly (>1L/min) before significant embolism can occur.[5-13]

The embolism may lodge in the right atrium or ventricle to form a gas lock. This gas lock may impair venous return and obstruct right ventricular outflow, resulting in sudden cardiovascular collapse. Alternatively, the embolus may disperse and enter the pulmonary circulation resulting in acute pulmonary hypertension and right heart failure. One of the earliest diagnostic sign may be a transient increase in end tidal carbon dioxide.[5-13]

The diagnostic signs include sudden hypotension, tachycardia, arrhythmias, and cyanosis. A characteristic millwheel murmur can be heard on auscultation. Treatment of gas embolism consists of immediate cessation of CO_2 insufflation and release of pneumoperitoneum. 100 per cent oxygen should be administered. The patient should be turned to the left lateral decubitus with a head down position to allow the gas to rise into the apex of the right ventricle and prevent entry into the pulmonary artery. In addition to aggressive cardiopulmonary resuscitation, including management of arrhythmias, a central venous catheter placement will enable to aspirate gas. Hyperbaric oxygen and cardiopulmonary bypass have also been used to successfully treat gas embolism.[5-13]

Subcutaneous emphysema (Figs 19.1 and 19.2): During laparoscopy the first step which is introduction of Veress needle into the peritoneal cavity is a blind procedure. Subcutaneous emphysema may result from positioning of the Veress needle in the subcutaneous tissue during insufflation or unrecognized retraction of the tip of the primary insufflating trocar into the subcutaneous tissue. Diagnosis is made by the presence of crepitus in the

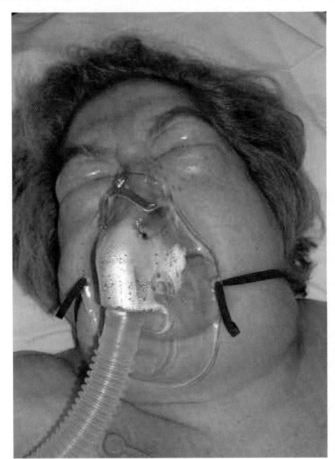

Fig. 19.1: Severe surgical emphysema

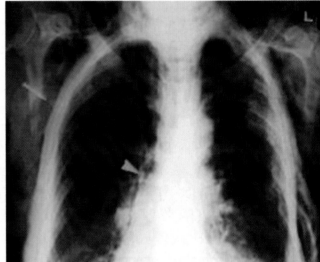

Fig. 19.2: Surgical emphysema

abdominal wall and an abrupt increase in the $EtCO_2$. Although the condition is usually mild and limited to the abdominal wall, it can become extensive, and may involve the extremities, the neck and the mediastinum. Spontaneous resolution of the subcutaneous emphysema results over few hours.[14-16] However continue positive pressure ventilation till the $EtCO_2$ levels are restored to normal. An ABG analysis is recommended. This complication can be prevented with the proper positioning of the insufflation needle. A variety of tests such as aspiration or saline placement in the Veress needle help. If at any time, the surgeon feels that the needle is not located intraperitoneally, it should be withdrawn and reinserted.

Pneumothorax (Figs 19.3)[17-22]

The development of pneumothorax and pneumomediastinum during laparoscopic surgery may arise from various mechanisms. The embryonic remnants constitute potential channels of communication between the peritoneal cavity and the pleural and pericardial sacs which can open when intraperitoneal pressure increases.[25] The defects in the diaphragm or weak points in the aortic and oesophageal hiatus, pleural tears during laparoscopic surgical procedures at the level of the gastro-oesophageal junction (fundoplication), other causes like rupture of emphysematous bullae due to increased airway pressures due to the carboperitoneum should be kept in mind. The opening of the pleuroperitoneal ducts result mainly in right sided pneumothorax while it is left sided during laparoscopic fundoplication.

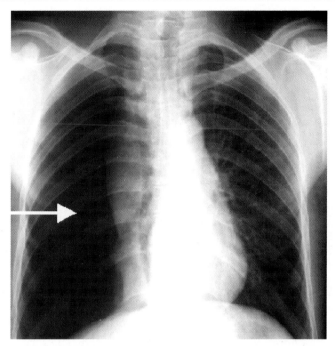

Fig. 19.3: Pneumothorax

The diagnosis of capnothorax is by decreased thoracopulmonary compliance, increased peak airway pressure, and a sudden increase in $EtCO_2$. There will be decreased breath sounds on auscultation of that hemithorax.

Management: As carbon dioxide is rapidly absorbed, there will probably be no need of any intervention. Usually spontaneous resolution occurs within 30-60 minutes after insufflation. Guidelines are to administer 100 per cent oxygen, discontinue N_2O, and adjustment of ventilatory settings. Treatment is according to the severity of cardiopulmonary compromise. Minimal compromise—treat conservatively with close observation. In case of moderate to severe compromise an intercostal drainage is recommended.

Pneumomediastinum and Pneumopericardium[17-22]

The above findings are also manifested due to the causes mentioned above. The management of pneumomediastimum and pneumopericardium depends on the severity of associated cardiopulmonary dysfunction. Desufflation of abdomen is usually adequate to treat these patients.

Trocar Injuries

The damage caused by sharp trocar penetration is usually more serious than injury from a Veress needle. Most often injury is created by the primary trocar because of its blind insertion.

Injury to Stomach and Bowel[4,23]

When a primary trocar inserted with closed technique penetrates the bowel, the diagnosis of bowel injury is made when the surgeon visualizes a mucosal lining after the insertion of laparoscope. The other ways of recognizing gastric entry by the trocar are increased intra-abdominal pressure in the beginning of pneumoperitoneum, asymetric distension of peritoneal cavity or sometimes by aspiration of gastric particulate matter through the lumen of the needle. Entry into the large bowel causes a feculent odour. Usually these complications occur in patients with previous abdominal surgeries. These injuries can be generally eliminated with the liberal use of an oral/nasogastric tube.

Injury to the Urinary Bladder[4]

These injuries can occur during surgeries like laparoscopic hysterectomy. Previous abdominal surgery and certain congenital anomalies of the lower urinary tract increase the chances of bladder injury. Prevention of these injuries is by decompression of the bladder by placement of a Foley's indwelling catheter.

Vascular Injuries[24,25]

The most dangerous haemorrhagic complications of needle entry are from injury to the great vessels, including the aorta and vena cava, common iliac vessels and their branches, internal and external iliac arteries and veins.

Most often the problem manifests in profound hypotension with or without the appearance of a significant volume of blood in the peritoneal cavity. Frequently bleeding is contained in the retroperitoneal space, which delays the diagnosis.

In major vessel injury, management is the treatment of the shock, replacement with blood and blood products. Immediate laparotomy may be required to repair the injured big vessels. The most commonly injured abdominal wall vessels are the inferior epigastric vessels during laparoscopic hernia repair. Haemorrhage has been reported during laparoscopic cholecystectomy due to injury to the cystic or hepatic artery. Sometimes concealed bleeding can occur in the postoperative period which can be diagnosed by the onset of hypotension in the recovery room.

Neurologic Injuries[1,3,4]

Peripheral neurological injury is usually related to the inappropriate positioning of the patient or to the pressure exerted by the surgeons or assistants inadvertently in the anaesthetised patient.

The incidence of brachial plexus injuries can be reduced by avoiding hyperabduction at the shoulder joint, and also by placing the arms by the side of the patient in an adducted position. Incidence of sciatic nerve and perineal nerve injuries have been reported during lithotomy position. Most injuries to peripheral nerves recover spontaneously.[1,4]

Thermal Injuries[26,27]

These injuries are most common due to the extensive use of cautery during laparoscopic surgeries. The extent of thermal injury will depend on the power of electric current used, the area and the duration of application.

Thermal injury to organs such as bowel may occur due to the leakage of current from the shaft of the instrument. The injury may range from minor blanching of the serosa to frank perforation. If blanching is significant, laparotomy is recommended and the excision of the damaged tissue required as failure to do so may result in ischaemic necrosis at the site of the burn. A high index of suspicion should be there in a patient complaining of vague abdominal symptoms, discomfort, anorexia and sometimes fever. A faecal fistula may not form within 48-72 hours. Urgent laparotomy, repair of the bowel, colostomy and drainage of the peritoneum is the treatment of choice.[1,4,23]

Deep Vein Thrombosis and Pulmonary Embolism

Pneumoperitoneum unites all three elements of Virchow's triad i.e, venous stasis of the lower limbs, microendothelial injury due to venodilatation and hypercoagulability. Certain features that increase the risk of deep vein thrombosis is due to a longer duration of procedure as compared to an open procedure. The increased intra-abdominal pressure causes a reduction in the femoral venous flow, thus contributing to the stasis of blood in the lower extremities. The decrease in venous flow is further aggravated by the reverse Trendelenburg position.

Prophylaxis should be done in all obese patients, patients with expected prolonged duration of surgery, surgery in the pelvis and pregnant patients and surgeries in which steep reverse Trendelenburg position is required. Low molecular weight heparins and application of sequential compression devices in the intraoperative period and early ambulation reduce the incidence of deep vein thrombosis.[1,4,13]

POSTOPERATIVE COMPLICATIONS

Pain

Shoulder tip pain is one of the common postoperative discomfort associated with laparoscopic surgeries. The carbon dioxide gas is converted to carbonic acid when it is in solution with body fluids. This acid is irritant to the peritoneum. Diaphragmatic peritoneal irritation produces pain which is referred to the shoulder by the phrenic nerve. The treatment consists of removal of all the gas at the end of surgery and local anaesthetic instillation in the subdiaphragmatic space.[1]

Multimodal analgesia using NSAIDs, local anaesthetic infiltration into the port sites and if required opioid analgesics can be used to alleviate the pain following laparoscopic surgeries.

Nausea and Vomiting

This complication is extremely common after laparoscopic surgery. Some of the causal factors are peritoneal gas insufflation, bowel manipulation and pelvic surgery. Wide range of antiemetics like 5HT3 antagonists like ondansetron, dolasetron and granisetron are quite effective. Other antiemetics used include metoclopramide, decadron and even accupressure at PC6 point are adequate.[1,3,4]

Infection

Wound and peritoneal infections can occur in elderly, obese, diabetic or immuno-compromised patient.[4]

Dissemination of Malignancy

A rare complication is dissemination of malignancy at the trocar insertion site. Seeding along the tracks of an instrument have been reported with primary cancers of the colon, stomach and ovary.[4]

CONCLUSIONS

A systematic approach and a good intraoperative monitoring can easily decrease the incidence of complications. Most episodes of altered cardiovascular haemodynamics during laparoscopy are self-limited. Most of the haemodynamic complications settle with desufflation of the abdomen.

CLINICAL PEARLS

Main keys to avoid complications are:

1. Gradual insufflation of abdomen.
2. Strict monitoring of intra-abdominal pressure, haemodynamics and ventilatory parameters.
3. An alert and experienced anaesthesiologist and laparoscopic surgeon are the main keys to avoid complications in any laparoscopic procedure.

REFERENCES

1. Girish Joshi. Anesthetic complications in laparoscopic surgery. Anaesthesiol Clin North America 2001; 19: 89-105.
2. Benitez P OR, Serra E, Jara L, Buzzi JC. Heart arrest caused by CO_2 embolism during a laparoscopic cholecystectomy. Rev Esp Anestesiol Reanim 2003; 50(6): 295-8.
3. Chir PT, Gin T, Oh TE. Anesthesia for laparoscopic general surgery. AIC 1993; 21(2): 163-71.
4. Crist DW, Gadacz TR. Complications of laparoscopic surgery. Surgical Clinics of N Am 1993;73(2): 265-89.
5. Wahba RW, Tessler MJ, Kleinman SJ. Acute ventilatory complications during laparoscopic upper abdominal surgery. Can J Anesth. 1996; 43: 77-83.
6. Imasogie N, Crago R, Leyland NA, Chung F, et al. Probable gas embolism during operative hysteroscopy caused by products of combustion. Can J Anesth 2002; 49(10): 1044-7.
7. Fatal gas embolism caused by over pressurization during laparoscopic use of argon enhanced coagulation. Hazard Health Devices 1994.; 23(6): 257-9.
8. Ishryama T, Hanagota K, Kashimoto S, Kumazawa T, et al. Pulmonary carbon dioxide embolism during laparoscopic cholecystectomy. Letters to the editor, Can J Anesth 2003; 50(2): 319-20.
9. Derouin M, Couture P, Boudreault D, Grard D, et al. Detection of gas embolism by transesophageal echocardiography during laparoscopic cholecystectomy. Anesth Analg 1996; 82: 119-24.
10. Councilman LM, Gonzales, Jolene D, McAllister, et al. A probable CO_2 embolus during laparoscopic cholecystectomy. Can J Anesth 2003; 50(3):311-5.
11. Scoletta P, Morsiani E, Ferroci G, Maniscalco P, et al. Carbon dioxide embolization: Is it a complication of laparoscopic cholecystectomy? Monerva Chic 2003; 58: 313-20.
12. Pendevillie P, Boufroukh D, Aunac S, Donnez J, et al. Perioperative desaturation during gynaecological laparoscopy-hysteroscopy. Ann Fr Anesth Reanim 2003; 22: 553-6.
13. Zacharoules, Dimitris, Kakkar, Ajay K. Venous thromboembolism in laparoscopic surgery current opinion. Pulmonary Medicine 2003; 9(5): 356-61.
14. Murdock CM, Walff AJ, Geem TV. Risk factors for hypercarbia, subcutaneous emphysema, pneumothorax and pneumomediastinum during laparoscopy. Obstet Gynae 2000 May; 95(5): 1.
15. Lo CH, Tratter D, Grassberg P. Unusual complications of laparoscopic totally entraperitoneal inguinal hernia repair. ANZ J Surgery 2005 Oct.; 75(10): 917-9.
16. Abreu SC, Sharp DS, Ramani AP, Steinberg AP, et al. Thoracic complications during urological laparoscopy. J Urol 2004; 171(4): 1415-5.
17. Shiraki K, Hamada M, Sugimoto K, Ito T, et al. Pneumothorax after diagnostic laparoscopy. J Urol 2004; 171(3): 1256-9.
18. Kusaka J, Goto K, Yamamoto S, Hasegarva A, et al. Pneumothorax during retroperitoneoscopic nephrectomy – a case report. Masui 2004; 53(12): 1411-3.
19. Karaviannakis AJ, Anagnostoulis S, Michailidis K, Vogratzaki T, et al. Spontaneous resolution of massive right sided pneumothorax occuring during laparoscopic cholecystectomy. Surg Laparos Endos Percutan Tech 2005; 15(2): 100-3.
20. Bartelmaos T, Blane R, De Claviere G, Benhamou D. Delayed pneumomediastinum and pneumothorax complicating laparoscopic extraperitoneal inguinal hernia repair. J Clin Anesth 2005; 17(3): 209-12.
21. Richard HM, Stancato-Pasik, Salky, Mendelson. Pneumothorax and pneumomediastinum after laparoscopic surgery. Clin Imaging 1997; 21(5): 337-9.
22. Waterman BJ, Robinson BC, Snow BW, Carturight PC, et al. Pneumothorax in pediatric patients after urological laparoscopic surgery: experience with four patients. ANZ J Surg 2005; 75(10): 917-9.

23. Shen CC, Wu MP, Lu CH, Hung YC, Lin H, et al. Small intestine injury in laparoscopic assisted vaginal hysterectomy. J Am Assoc Gynaecol Laparos 2003; 10(3): 350-5.
24. Mases, Anna, Montes, Antonio, et al. Injury to the abdominal aorta during laparoscopic surgery: an unusual presentation. Hepatogastroenterology 2002; 49(46): 1033-5.
25. Larobinam, Nattle P-complete evidence regarding major vascular injuries during laparoscopic access. Surg Laparosc Endos Percut Tech 2005; 15(3)-119-23.
26. Emam TA, Cuschiaria A. How safe is high power ultrasonic dissection? Ann Surg 2003; 237(2): 186-91.
27. Soro M, Garcia-Perez ML, Ferrandis R, Aguilar G, et al. Closed system anaesthesia for laparoscopic surgery: Is there a risk for carbon monoxide intoxication. Eur J Anaesthesiol 2004; 21(6): 483-8.

Anaesthetic Management for Laparoscopic Bariatric Surgery

INTRODUCTION

Obesity, derived from the latin word *'obesus'* which means 'fattened by eating', is a major health problem and has reached epidemic proportions in the western countries. The prevalence of obesity in the USA in the 18-29 years age group has increased from 12 per cent in 1991 to 18.9 per cent in 1999.[1]

According to the National Institutes of Health in America, obesity is a major health problem with clearly established health implications, including an increased risk of coronary artery disease, hypertension, hyperlipidemia, diabetes mellitus, gall bladder disease, degenerative joint disease, obstructive sleep apnoea, socio-economic and psychosocial impairment. Evidence continues to accumulate that obesity is associated with increasing morbidity and mortality.

Bariatric (comes from the Greek word 'weight treatment') and is the only surgery which provides significant and sustained weight loss option for the morbidly obese patients. With advancing surgical technology and success, anaesthesiologists are now faced with the reality of having to care for this high-risk population with increasing frequency. Since laparoscopic approach to surgical procedures is now very popular, laparoscopic bariatric surgery now presents a fairly new frontier in anaesthesiology.

WHO IS TERMED "OBESE"?

The Federal guidelines for obesity[2] state three important parameters to assess 'overweight'. These include (1) BMI (2) waist circumference and waist hip ratio and (3) patient's risk factors for diseases and conditions associated with obesity. They also state that a patient's waist circumference, which is strongly associated with abdominal fat, is an independent predictor of disease risk. The World Health Organisation has endorsed the body mass index as a measure of obesity.

Overweight - BMI in the range 25 to 29.9 kg/m^2

Obesity - BMI greater than 30 kg/m^2

Morbid obesity- BMI greater than 35 kg/m^2

Waist circumference exceeding 102 cm (40 inches) in men and 89 cm (35 inches) in women, waist hip ratio greater than 0.9 in men and 0.85 in women indicates an increased risk in individuals with a BMI of 25 to 34.9 kg/m^2.

In patients having a metabolic syndrome; the criteria are – atleast three or more of the following must be present:

Waist circumference > 102 cm (men), > 88 cm (women)

Serum triglycerides $\geq$ 150 mg/dL

High-density lipoprotein cholesterol < 40 mg/dL (men), < 50 mg/dL (women)

Systolic blood pressure $\geq$ 130 mmHg and/or diastolic $\geq$ 85 mmHg or on treatment for hypertension

Fasting serum glucose $\geq$ 110 mg/dL or on treatment for diabetes

ELIGIBILITY OR INDICATIONS FOR BARIATRIC PROCEDURES?

The indicators for surgical treatment of severe obesity as outlined in the 1996 National Institutes of Health consensus conference include: [3]

a. Absolute BMI > 40 kg/m^2 or BMI > 35 kg/m^2 in combination with life threatening cardiopulmonary problems or severe *diabetes mellitus.*

The patients seeking surgical weight loss must however have:

i. Proven attempts at medically supervised weight loss

ii. Documentation of loss of less than 5 or 10 per cent excess body weight or weight gain after atleast six months of diet modification, exercise and medical therapy, and

iii. Non-improvement in comorbid conditions during this period.

BARIATRIC SURGERY PROCEDURES [2]

The various bariatric surgery procedures available are classified as malabsorptive or restrictive.

Malabsorptive procedures include:

i. Jejunoileal bypass

ii. Biliopancreatic bypass

Restrictive procedures include:

i. Vertical banded gastroplasty

ii. Gastric banding (adjustable) AGB

iii. Endoscopic bioenteric intragastric balloon

Laparoscopic bariatric surgery was first introduced in 1994.[4] At our institution laparoscopic adjustable gastric banding (LAGB) and endoscopic placement of bioenteric intragastric balloon are the procedures done to treat morbid obesity.

From an anaesthesiologist's point of view, preoperative evaluation and optimization, intraoperative management and post-operative care represent a clinical challenge that may determine the success of the surgical procedure, the development of complications and the final prognosis of the patient undergoing bariatric surgery.

The main trespasses to normal homeostasis in laparoscopy are – patient positioning, insufflation of CO_2 to produce carboperitoneum and an increased intraabdominal pressure. It is important for the anaesthesiologist and surgeon to understand the fundamental differences between laparoscopic versus open surgery and the possible adverse consequences of carboperitoneum in the morbidly obese patient.

The physiological aspects of carboperitoneum include:

i. Systemic absorption of CO_2

ii. Haemodynamic and physiological alterations in all organs

PHYSIOLOGICAL CHANGES

EFFECTS OF CARBON DIOXIDE ABSORPTION DURING CARBOPERITONEUM

Pneumoperitoneum with carbon dioxide has been used in clinical practice since 1980s. It results in systemic absorption of CO_2 with alteration of acid base balance. CO_2 absorbed across the peritoneum is normally eliminated through the lungs because of its high aqueous solubility and diffusibility. In a study of laparoscopy[4] versus gastric bypass (GBP), VCO_2 levels were reported to increase from 20 ml/min to 26 ml/min at two and a half hours, which represents a 30 per cent increase in CO_2 load but VCO_2 was unchanged in patients who underwent open gastric bypass. If intra-operative ventilation is impaired, CO_2 absorption can result in hypercarbia and acidosis. Hypercapnia can cause cardiac arrhythmias, vasoconstriction of pulmonary vessels and a mixed response in cardiac function. Close monitoring of end tidal CO_2 is therefore essential. Tan et al[5] estimated that the volume of CO_2 absorbed from peritoneal cavity in non-obese patients ranged from 38 to 42 ml/min during laparoscopy, which represents a 30 per cent increase in the CO_2 load. Demiraluk et al[6] reported an increase of $PaCO_2$ from 34 mm Hg at baseline to 42 mm Hg after abdominal insufflation in patients undergoing laparoscopic adjustable gastric banding (LAGB). In a study of laparoscopic *versus* open gastric bypass, $EtCO_2$ levels were found to increase by 14 per cent from baseline (from 32 to 42 mmHg).[4] So appropriate ventilatory changes should be performed to eliminate the increased CO_2 load and prevent systemic acidosis. Dumont et al[7] reported that the minute ventilation was increased by 21 per cent to limit the rise in $EtCO_2$ in patients undergoing laparoscopic gastroplasty. In a study by Nguyen,[4] the VCO_2 levels increased from 20 ml/min to 26 ml/min at two and half hours in patients undergoing laparoscopic gastric bypass which represented a 30 per cent increase in CO_2 load, while the VCO_2 remained unchanged in patients who underwent open gastric bypass. The ventilatory adjustments were made by increasing the respiratory rate by 25 per cent and minute ventilation by 21 per cent to counteract the increase in CO_2 load and prevent intra-operative acidosis in patients who underwent laparoscopic bypass. As the elimination of CO_2 load is through the lungs, the total volume of exhaled CO_2 (VCO_2) during carboperitoneum is therefore an indirect method to quantify the amount of CO_2 absorbed during laparoscopy.[4,5,6]

EFFECT OF INCREASED IAP DURING CARBOPERITONEUM

The normal IAP of non-obese individuals is 5 mmHg or less. In contrast, the morbidly obese patients have a chronically elevated IAP at 9 to 10 mmHg.[8,9] Carboperitoneum results in a state of acutely elevated intra-abdominal pressure. Similar to non-obese subjects, the IAP during laparoscopy is set at 15 mm Hg to provide adequate visualisation and exposure of the operative field. However, studies clearly report that laparoscopy is well tolerated provided the intraabdominal pressure is maintained less than 15 mmHg.[4,6,9]

PATHOPHYSIOLOGY OF THE RESPIRATORY SYSTEM[10]

Obese individuals have increased oxygen consumption and carbon dioxide production as a result of the metabolic activity of the excess fat and the increased workload on supportive tissues. The body attempts to meet these increased demands by increasing, both cardiac output and alveolar ventilation.

Mass loading by accumulated fat on the chest wall and abdominal components of the chest wall results in alterations in both the static and dynamic performance of the respiratory system. The chest wall compliance is decreased. The expiratory reserve volume and functional residual capacity are reduced, so that tidal ventilation may fall within the range of closing capacity with ensuing ventilation perfusion abnormalities

(V/Q) leading to hypoxaemia. The dependent zones of the lung may be effectively closed throughout the respiratory cycle and the inspired gas becomes more distributed to the upper zones of the lungs leading to ventilation perfusion mismatch. Any kind of procedure which increases the subdiaphragmatic pressure such as the lithotomy or Trendelenburg position may be hazardous to the patient because of a further decrease in FRC and lung compliance leading to hypoxemia.

The increased pulmonary blood volume is also responsible for the decrease in lung compliance. This increased pulmonary blood volume is part of an overall increase in blood volume, as more volume is required to perfuse the additional body tissue in the form of fat. Polycythemia from chronic hypoxemia is also part of this increased total blood volume.

Obesity hypoventilation (Pickwickian)[11] syndrome affects approximately 5 to 10 per cent of the morbidly obese. It consists of extreme obesity, somnolence, cardiomegaly, polycythemia, hypoxemia, hypercarbia and eventually right ventricular failure. Alveolar hypoventilation which is independent of intrinsic lung disease is the main ventilatory impairment. OSA (obstructive sleep apnoea) affects 5 per cent of the morbidly obese population and is characterised by frequent episodes of apnoea / hypopnoea during sleep, snoring and day time sleepiness. Respiratory acidosis occurs in OSA. The long term sequlae is alteration in control of breathing leading to central apnoeic events.

Airway in patients with OSA is characterised by increased fat deposition in the pharynx resulting in decreased patency of pharynx. Any relaxation of the upper airway muscles will lead to collapse of the soft walled pharynx between uvula and epiglottis. So tracheal intubation and extubation decisions have to be properly planned and executed.[11]

EFFECT OF CARBOPERITONEUM ON THE RESPIRATORY SYSTEM (TABLES 20.1 AND 20.2)

The introduction of CO_2 into the abdominal cavity pushes the diaphragm, decreases FRC and lung compliance, and increases the peak airway pressure. Without ventilatory adjustments peak inspiratory pressures (PIP) can increase by 17 to 109 per cent during laparoscopy.[4] Dumont et al[7] reported an increase in airway pressure by 17 per cent. To limit the rise in peak inspiratory pressure ventilatory adjustment is commonly performed by decreasing the tidal volume.[6,7] Though carboperitoneum alters the respiratory mechanics, Sprung[14] reported no significant changes in the physiological dead space to tidal volume ratio or A-a gradient in patients undergoing lap gastric banding. Demiroluk et al[6] reported no significant differences in PaO_2 levels in morbidly obese patients undergoing laparoscopy.

Table 20.1: Effect of carboperitoneum on respiratory system

Respiratory mechanics:	
Peak inspiratory pressure	increased
Respiratory compliance	decreased
Ventilatory changes:	
Respiratory rate	increased
Tidal volume	decreased
Minute ventilation	increased
Physiological dead space to tidal volume ratio	unchanged
Alveolar arterial oxygen gradient	unchanged

Table 20.2: Effect of carboperitoneum on acid-base balance

ABG		
	$PaCO_2$	increased
	PaO_2	unchanged
	Bicarbonate	decreased
	Base excess	decreased
	pH	decreased
CO_2 Elimination:		
	Total volume of Exhaled CO_2 (VCO_2)	increased

HAEMODYNAMIC CHANGES AND CARDIOVASCULAR CHANGES[12]

Cardiovascular and derived haemodynamic variables dominate the pathophysiology of obesity. Morbidly obese patients have increased preload, afterload, right and left pulmonary artery pressure. Cardiac output rises about 0.1 L/min for each 1 kg addition in weight. Stroke volume is elevated because total blood volume increases to perfuse the added body weight.

EFFECT OF CARBOPERITONEUM ON THE CARDIOVASCULAR SYSTEM (TABLE 20.3)

Abdominal insufflation has been shown to increase mean arterial pressure and heart rate. In a study of morbidly obese patients, heart rate and MAP increased during both laparoscopy and open procedures.[2] Fried et al[12] have reported that the heart rate increase is more pronounced in obese individuals.

A few studies have examined the effects of carboperitoneum on cardiac function in the morbidly obese.[12] Fried et al compared the cardiac function of six morbidly obese patients and six normal body weight subjects. There was 12 per cent increase in cardiac output after carboperitoneum in morbidly obese patients.[13] Nguyen,[13] however, reported a decrease in cardiac output and stroke volume upon abdominal insufflation by 6 and 8 per cent of baseline values respectively. The mechanisms for reduction in cardiac output after abdominal insufflation include an increase in afterload due to raised SVR and decrease in preload by impeding venous return. Declan Fleming et al[14] have reported that SVR increased by 25 per cent of baseline after abdominal insufflation and decreased with desufflation. Nguyen[13] has reported an increase of SVR in laparoscopic gastric bypass by 34 per cent of baseline upon insufflation which returned to baseline within 1.5 hours after initiation of carboperitoneum. The timing for the increase in SVR correlates with the reduction in cardiac output and stroke volume.

Hypovolemia decreases the preload and cardiac output. Thus a euvolemic preoperative status is very important to minimise cardiac depression associated with carboperitoneum. Measurement of cardiac filling pressure, an accurate method of estimation of intravascular volume may be falsely elevated during carboperitoneum.[13] Nguyen et al[13] in their study have reported a significantly higher CVP and pulmonary artery pressure in laparoscopic gastric banding as compared to open gastric banding.

Table 20.3: Effect of carboperitoneum on haemodynamics

Heart rate	increased
MAP	increased
Cardiac output unchanged/	decreased
Stroke volume	decreased
SVR	increased
Mean pulmonary artery pressure	increased
PAWP	unchanged
CVP	increased

HEPATIC FUNCTION DURING LAPAROSCOPY (TABLE 20.4)

The mechanisms for alteration of post-operative hepatic function include direct operative trauma to the liver, general anaesthesia and reduction of portal venous flow during carboperitoneum which may lead to hepatic hypoperfusion and acute hepatocyte injury.[15,16] Jakimowics et al[15] reported a 53 per cent reduction in portal blood flow with abdominal insufflation to 14 mmHg.

Transient elevation of hepatic transaminases levels have been reported after laparoscopy and open gastric banding.[15,16] The transminases levels after laparoscopic gastric banding have been shown to increase by sixfold, peaking at 24 hours postoperatively and returning to baseline by third postoperative day. Although there was an increase in transminase levels after laparoscopic gastric banding, it was only transient and subsided by the third postoperative day.[15,16]

Therefore, carboperitoneum in the morbidly obese patient is considered safe in patients with normal baseline liver function. However, further studies are required to evaluate the safety of carboperitoneum in morbidly obese patients.

Table 20.4: Effect of carboperitoneum on hepatic function

Portal venous flow	decreased
Aspartate transferase	increased
Alamine phospatase	increased
Alkaline phosphatase	decreased
Albumin	decreased
Total bilirubin	decreased
Gamma GT	unchanged

CARBOPERITONEUM AND RENAL CHANGES (TABLE 20.5)

Increased intraabdominal pressure during laparoscopy has been shown to alter renal function. A reduction in urine output has been well documented during laparoscopic operations.[17,18]

Studies on morbidly obese subjects have also shown that intraoperative urine output decreased immediately after initiation of carboperitoneum during laparoscopic gastric banding and remained 31 to 64 per cent lower than during open gastric banding.[17,18] However, no significant changes in blood urea nitrogen or serum creatinine were observed in the postoperative period after laparoscopic adjustable gastric banding. Additionally, creatinine clearance in patients who underwent laparoscopic gastric banding was in the normal range, both, on the first and second postoperative day.[17,18]

Table 20.5: Carboperitoneum and renal function

Intraoperative urine output	decreased
ADH levels	increased
Aldosterone levels	increased
Plasma renin activity	increased
Postoperative renal function:	
BUN	decreased
S.Creatinine	decreased
Creatinine clearance	unchanged

CARBOPERITONEUM AND VENOUS STASIS (TABLE 20.6)

Morbid obesity is a major independent risk factor for sudden death from acute postoperative pulmonary embolism.[1,3,4,20]

The true incidence of DVT after laparoscopic operations compared with open operations is unknown. The factors contributing to DVT (according to the Virchow's triad) during laparoscopy is venous stasis and hypercoagulability.[4,19,20]

The increased intraabdominal pressure and reverse Trendelenburg position during laparoscopy have been shown to promote venous stasis. Other risk factors include high fatty acid levels, hypercholesterolemia and diabetes. In addition, morbidly obese patients demonstrate accelerated fibrin formation, fibrinogen- platelet interaction and platelet function. The increased IAP has a direct compressive effect on the inferior vena cava and iliac veins with a consequent decreased venous flow in the lower extremities.[4,19,20]

Development of venous stasis during laparoscopy in morbidly obese patients has been observed. Increased IAP during laparoscopic gastric banding results in reduced peak femoral systolic velocity by 43 per cent and increase in the femoral cross-sectional area by 52 per cent.[4,19,20]

Nguyen[19] reported that by combining carboperitoneum with reverse Trendelenburg position, peak femoral systolic velocity decreased to 57 per cent of baseline values.

The use of sequential compression devices (SCD) during laparoscopic gastric banding[20] has been only partially effective in augmenting the femoral peak systolic velocity, and the ineffectiveness is attributed to the larger calves and thighs of these individuals. The use of antithrombotics along with sequential compression devices (Fig. 20.1) is therefore important to decrease the incidence of DVT in morbidly obese patients.[4,19,20] An inferior vena cava filter may be considered in the preoperative period.[19,20]

Table 20.6: Carboperitoneum and femoral venous flow

Femoral peak systolic velocity	decreased
Femoral cross-sectional area	increased

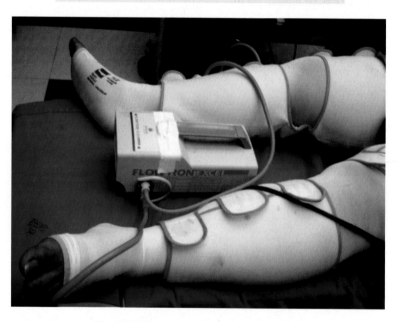

Fig. 20.1: Sequentional compression device

PREOPERATIVE EVALUATION

During the preoperative evaluation, attention should focus on issues unique to the obese patient, particularly cardiorespiratory status and airway. These patients suffer from hidden anxiety, especially if they have had unpleasant experiences with anaesthesia in the past. The planned procedure, i.e. general anaesthesia, including any anticipated complications or difficulties with performing the anaesthetic procedure, especially airway, the need for postoperative ventilation and the plans to minimize or avoid such problems should be discussed in detail with the patient. The regime for postoperative analgesia, the necessity of early postoperative ambulation and postoperative physiotherapy to reduce postoperative complications should be explained.

CARDIOVASCULAR SYSTEM [21-23]

Obese patients should be thoroughly evaluated for systemic hypertension, pulmonary hypertension, signs of right and/or left ventricular failure and ischaemic heart disease. A positive cardiac history may suggest the need for a cardiology consultation and a detailed planning for intra- and post-operative cardiovascular monitoring and care. Signs of cardiac failure such as raised jugular venous pressure, added heart sounds, pulmonary crackles, hepatomegaly and peripheral edema may be difficult to elicit in obese patients. ECG, chest radiography and echocardiography should be done and any adverse findings should be optimized with the help of a cardiologist. ECG may be of low voltage due to the excess fat on the chest wall. Transesophageal echocardiogram may be required in some cases. Sites for peripheral and central venous access and for arterial cannulation should be evaluated during preoperative assessment. [11,21-24]

RESPIRATORY SYSTEM

Assessment should seek to elicit signs and symptoms of respiratory disease including central or obstructive sleep apnoea, upper or lower airway obstruction and history of bronchospastic disease (common in obese smokers). Sleep studies are considered essential as part of the preoperative screening. [11, 21-24]

When obstructive sleep apnoea is identified, patients are immediately instructed to commence using appliances and positive airway pressure devices when sleeping. They should also bring their devices to the hospital for use postoperatively in the recovery room.

Regardless of the result of sleep studies, all obstructive sleep apnoea patients should be treated with prudence. Extreme caution is the rule when administering any pre- or post-operative medications that may have a depressant effect on respiratory function. Thus, the goal of intraoperative management should always be a rapid return to a fully alert, cooperative state in which the patient can protect the airway and maintain patency. [11, 21-24]

Bronchodilators, chest physiotherapy and consultation with a pulmonary physician may be necessary. He should be familiarised with the equipment for incentive spirometry. [11, 21]

GASTROINTESTINAL SYSTEM

Obese patients have delayed gastric emptying often combined with a low pH (<2.5) of gastric juice. [10,24] This combination together with increased intraabdominal pressure and increased incidence of hiatus hernia increase the risk of gastric content aspiration and subsequent pneumonitis. Therefore, these patients should always be considered as non fasting, even in elective surgery and due precautions should be taken. Before induction of anaesthesia, gastric aspiration must be considered and a slight antiTrendelenburg position should be used during induction. [27] The incidence of liver disease is greater in obese population, mainly fatty change and gallstones. [1,2]

ENDOCRINE SYSTEMS

Glucose tolerance is frequently impaired in morbidly obese patients. [24] This is reflected in a high prevalence of type II or maturity onset *diabetes mellitus*. Insulin is required to control postoperative glucose concentration, which is increased secondary to the catabolic response to surgery; otherwise, the patient is susceptible to wound infection and an increased risk of myocardial infarction. Hypothyroidism is frequently present in morbidly obese patients.

ANTIOBESITY AND OTHER CONCURRENT MEDICATIONS

During the preoperative visit,[2,24,38] a history of the patient's medications should be elicited to avoid adverse drug interactions, and very importantly, a history of appetite suppressants and other antiobesity medications should be sought.[2] Appetite suppressants such as fenfluramine combined with phenteramine can cause various complications in the perioperative period.[2,24,38] Fenfluramine has a catecholamine depleting effect so that indirect acting vasopressors will be ineffective during hypotension, necessitating the use of direct acting vasopressors. It also delays gastric emptying time for solids and potentiates the effects of insulin in diabetic patients and increases the risk of hypoglycaemia in non-diabetic patients. Pulmonary hypertension, which is reversible after discontinuation of fenfluramine, can also occur.

The patient's usual medications such as cardiovascular drugs and steroids should be continued till the time of surgery. Antibiotic prophylaxis is important due to the risk of postoperative wound infection.

Preoperative DVT prophylaxis in the form of low molecular weight heparin should be started a day prior to surgery.

AIRWAY ASSESSMENT

Careful assessment of the airway will help anticipate difficulties. Assessment should include range of motion testing of atlantoaxial and cervical spine, mouth opening, thyroid and hyomental distance.[27,28,29] Excessive folds of tissue in the mouth and pharynx should be sought. A short, thick neck, suprasternal, presternal and posterior cervical fat are pointers towards a difficult airway. Ezri has said that ultrasound neck and circumference of the neck are predictors of a difficult airway.[34,35]

Peripheral and central venous access and arterial cannulation should be evaluated during the preoperative examination and the possibility of invasive monitoring should be discussed with the patient.

REPEAT BARIATRIC SURGERY

Patients coming for repeat bariatric surgery confront the anaesthesiologist days, months or years after the initial surgery. The anaesthesiologist should be aware of the possible metabolic changes in these patients. Common long term nutritional abnormalities include Vitamin B_{12}, iron, calcium and folate deficiencies.[2] Vitamin deficiency is uncommon in patients compliant with the daily vitamin supplements and following regular postoperative visits. With rapid weight loss, patients may be protein depleted. Electrolyte and coagulation indices should be checked before surgery, particularly if patient compliance has been poor or if the patient is acutely ill. Chronic vitamin K deficiency can lead to an abnormal prothrombin time with a normal APTT due to deficiency of clotting factors II, VII, IX and X.

PREOPERATIVE INVESTIGATIONS

A full blood count to exclude polycythemia, serum electrolytes, blood glucose, liver and kidney function tests are essential. An ECG along with X-ray chest and echocardiogram rules out arrhythmias, IHD, ventricular strain and hypertrophy. Lung function tests are important in preoperative assessment and any reversible pulmonary conditions should be treated. In our centre, measurement of neck circumference and an ultrasound neck are done routinely to assess the predictability of difficult intubation. Baseline arterial blood gas analysis is important as it tells the basal PaO_2 and $PaCO_2$ levels. It provides guidelines for perioperative oxygen administration and possible institution of and weaning from postoperative ventilation.[11,21-24]

PREMEDICATION

Preoperative assessment should guide premedication in the obese, but anxiolysis, analgesia, sedation (mild) and prophylaxis against pulmonary aspiration and deep venous thrombosis should be addressed.

Benzodiazepines are the most reliable for anxiolysis, but they should be used with caution in obese patients, especially in the ones associated with obstructive sleep apnoea. Intramuscular injections and opiates should be avoided, because injection into the adipose tissue gives an unreliable absorptive pattern.

Oral ranitidine 150 mg or 300 mg at bedtime and repeated in the morning before surgery increases gastric pH and in combination with 10 mg of metoclopramide reduces gastric volume. H_2 receptor antagonists effectively increases gastric pH and decreases gastric fluid volume if administered at least three hours before the anticipated induction of anaesthesia.[23,24]

Subcutaneous low molecular weight heparin administered preoperatively and repeated every 12 hours until the patient is ambulatory reduces the risk of DVT.[23,24]

INDUCTION OF ANAESTHESIA

The anaesthetic technique of choice for laparoscopic bariatric surgery is general anaesthesia with controlled ventilation.[1,2]

There is no role of spontaneous ventilation as it leads to hypoventilation. Carboperitoneum further compounds the hypoventilation in a spontaneously breathing morbidly obese patient. Regional anaesthesia alone is not enough as hypoventilation due to any cause cannot be tolerated.

It is desirable that two anaesthesiologists are present at the time of induction and that all appropriate equipment should be kept ready, which includes different types of laryngoscope blades, stylets, bougies, fibreoptic instruments, laryngeal masks and minitracheostomy sets. Difficult intubation trolley should be ready (Fig. 20.2).[1,2,10,37]

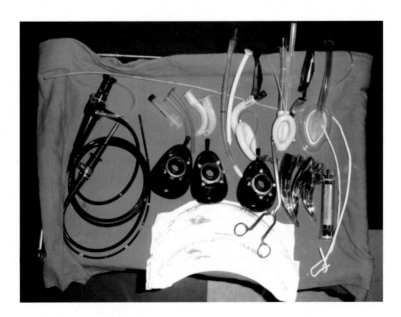

Fig. 20.2: Difficult airway equipment

PREOXYGENATION

Preoxygenation along with 10 cm H_2O PEEP during mask ventilation and after tracheal intubation reduces the incidence of post intubation atelectasis as assessed by CT scan and improves the arterial oxygenation i.e. PaO_2 of 457 ± 130 mmHg versus 315 ± 100 mmHg in the control group.[25] PEEP is safe and effective during induction of anaesthesia in patients with gastroesophageal reflux.[10,11]

CHOICE OF INDUCTION AGENTS [27]

The dose of induction agent should be increased in morbidly obese patients since blood volume, muscle mass and cardiac output show a liner increase with the degree of obesity. Lipophilic drugs, e.g. thiopentone and benzodiazepines have an increased volume of distribution and a longer elimination half life, but the clearance values are unchanged. Dosage of 7.5 mg/kg body weight of thiopentone has been suggested.[26] Greenblatt et al[27] found that midazolam elimination half life was prolonged significantly from a mean of 2.7 hours in control to 8.4 hours in the obese.

A comparison study with normal weight controls showed that administering doses of propofol on the basis of total body weight gave acceptable clinical results, unchanged initial volume of distribution, and clearance, with no accumulation of propofol when dosing scheme based on mg/kg of total body weight was used.[26]

The kinetics of fentanyl, alfentanil and remifentanil in the obese are somewhat unpredictable. Fentanyl kinetics is similar to those in the non-obese. Alfentanil and sufentanil have longer elimination half lives.[26,27]

Regarding volatile anaesthetic gases, two new drugs have become popular in morbidly obese patients in the last decade. Sevoflurane and desflurane offer lower blood solubility, which speeds up the anaesthetic after the drug delivery is terminated.[26]

Two studies comparing the effects of isoflurane and sevoflurane[27] in morbidly obese patients showed faster emergence after surgery with sevoflurane. A study comparing sevoflurane and desflurane in obese patients showed marginally higher oxygen saturation in patients treated with desflurane and more rapid emergence and therefore desflurane is the chosen agent. Sevoflurane offers clinical advantages in certain situations (mask induction) while isoflurane offers a long record of safety and very low administration costs.

MUSCLE RELAXATION

Rapid sequence induction is widely recommended and the use of a depolarising relaxant is mandatory.[27] Since pseudocholinesterase activity is increased in obese patients, succinylcholine 1.2 to 1.5 mg/kg ideal body weight with pretreatment with a non-depolarising relaxant (to avoid fasciculations) is appropriate.[1,2,10,37]

In a study by Weinstein et al,[36] the pharmacodynamic profiles of atracurium is superior to vecuronium as it has a consistent recovery time, due to non-organ dependent elimination. Neuromuscular blockade with vecuronium is prolonged since elimination is dependent on hepatic clearance. Complete muscular relaxation is crucial during laparoscopic bariatric procedures to facilitate ventilation and to maintain an adequate working space for visualisation and safe manipulation of laparoscopic instruments. Collapse of carboperitoneum may be an early indication of inadequate relaxation as muscle tone competes with the pressure limit set for the carboperitoneum.[2,4]

AIRWAY POSITION

Tracheal intubation in these patients is an anaesthetic challenge. The assessment of Mallampatti score is difficult in view of the cervical fat, large tongue size, and altered amount of soft tissue padding in the neck.[1,2,27-29] Frequently there is cervical immobility and inability to adopt the "sniffing the morning air position".[1,2] Difficult airway along with the physiological changes, i.e. increased oxygen consumption and carbon dioxide production coupled with a low FRC causes a rapid fall in oxygen saturation. Excessive large breasts render the laryngoscopy more difficult.[27,28]

To facilitate alignment of the oropharynx, mouth and vocal cords in a straight line for visualisation with the laryngoscope, a technique that has gained wide acceptance is to place the patient on a ramp of pillows with the head having many layers of support and the neck and shoulder having a fewer (Fig. 20.3).[27,28] This makes the chin higher than the chest, the breasts and shoulders to fall laterally, allowing flexion of the cervical vertebra and also increases the distance between the mandible and the chest thus making it easier to attain the proper sniffing position. Thus the anesthesiologist has to stand at a higher level so as to reach the patient to get a proper view. The use of a few rolled up sheets[27-29] or one rolled up blanket in the shape of a small log under and parallel to the thoracic spine lifts the trachea superior to the abdomen.[27,29]

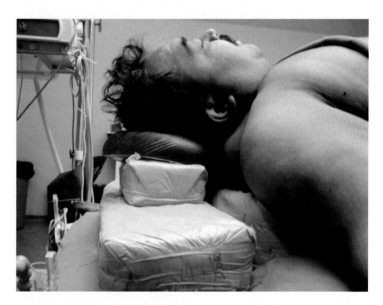

Fig. 20.3: Position for intubation

POSITIONING

Position of the patient for laparoscopic gastric banding is reverse Trendelenburg position with leg spread position (Fig. 20.4). Specially designed OT Tables are required as regular OT tables have a maximum weight limit of approximately 205 kg. Tables capable of holding upto 455 kg with a little extra width are available. Electrically operated tables facilitate maneuvering various surgical positions.[2] Bariatric patients are more prone to slipping off the OT table during the various position changes, thus, they should be well strapped to the OT table. The use of a bean bag is recommended, where the patient is positioned on the bean bag which is then moulded around the patient and a suction line is attached to it, creating a vacuum inside the bean bag which allows the outside atmospheric pressure to force the beads together so that the patient cannot move.[2]

After tracheal intubation, an intragastric calibration tube (Fig. 20.5) is inserted instead of a Ryle's tube. It is a bi-lumen tube with one port for suction and another port in which 15-20 ml of saline is injected to inflate the intragastric balloon. The balloon enables the surgeon to place the gastric band just below the esophagogastric junction which is then tightened and helps in deciding the size of the gastric pouch.

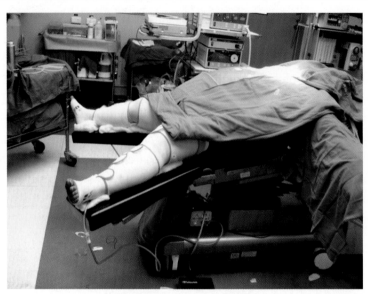

Fig. 20.4: Lloyd Davis position

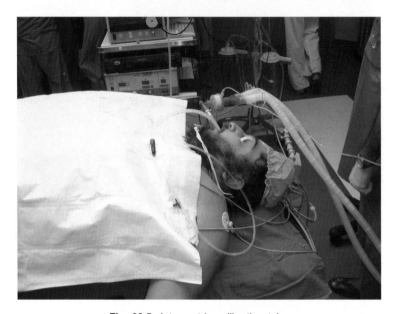

Fig. 20.5: Intragastric calibration tube

MONITORING (FIG. 20.6)

The standard monitoring includes pulse rate, ECG, NIBP, pulse oximetry, $EtCO_2$, temperature, urine output and intraabdominal pressure.

Due to the inappropriate fitting of the sphygmomanometer cuff in obese patients, invasive arterial blood pressure will be desirable. In addition, sampling of arterial blood for blood gas analysis becomes easier.

Respiratory monitoring with a respiratory module is a very useful monitoring in these patients as it given us the information regarding compliance of the lung, peak and plateau airway pressure work of breathing, etc. which helps us in adjusting the ventilatory settings.

CVP line is indicated in either superobese patients or in patients with difficult peripheral venous access. In addition it help us in assessing the fluid status of the patient.

The occurrence of intraoperative awareness is significantly increased in the morbidly obese patient as the pharmacokinetic and pharmacodynamic effects of anaesthetic agents are more unpredictable. In that regard, the use of a bispectral index monitor is recommended as an additional monitor that may allow the anaesthesiologist, the ability to ascertain intraoperative awareness.

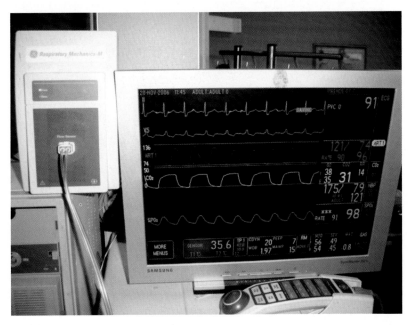

Fig. 20.6: Monitoring

INTRAOPERATIVE PROBLEMS

BLOOD PRESSURE MEASUREMENT

It is difficult to interpret blood pressure with a non-invasive cuff in morbidly obese patients, therefore a larger thigh cuff can be put on the arm and blood pressure taken. Obesity is not an absolute indication for placement of an arterial line.

MAINTENANCE OF ANAESTHESIA

Maintenance of anaesthesia is achieved with O_2 : N_2O and an inhalational agent sevoflurane / isoflurane along with a continuous infusion of non depolarising muscle relaxant, atracurium being the drug of choice.[38] Some centres prefer propofol infusion to maintain the depth of anaesthesia.[38]

FLUID REPLACEMENT

Classical evaluation of hydration and blood volume is difficult in the obese surgical patient. Although the total circulating volume is increased, it is less than normal on a weight basis as fat contains little water (6 to 10%). The technical difficulties of surgery may result in increased fluid and blood loss. The loss of fluids and blood must be meticulously recorded and replaced adequately.[38]

VENTILATION (FIG. 20.7)

In order to achieve higher levels of PaO_2, controlled mechanical ventilation with large tidal volumes (15-20 ml/ kg body weight) is recommended.[30] However the use of large tidal volumes may cause decrease in $PaCO_2$ tension and high inspiratory pressures which can cause parenchymal damage even in normal lungs. Gizella et al in his study says that 10-13 ml/kg body weight is ideal as higher tidal volumes do not significantly increase the PaO_2 levels.[30]

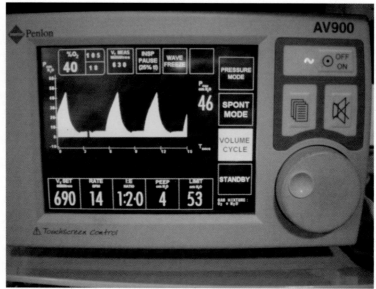

Fig. 20.7: Ventilatory settings

Application of moderate positive end expiratory pressure can improve oxygenation, but a high PEEP can reduce cardiac output. Thus, PEEP should be treated according to the SpO_2 values.[30,31]

TRACHEAL EXTUBATION

Residual effect of anaesthetics increases sensitivity to opioid analgesics and relative overdose of muscle relaxants may postpone tracheal extubation. Aspiration of gastric contents may be performed prior to tracheal extubation. Unless serious cardiopulmonary problems are expected, the trachea should be extubated in the operating room.

Montefire Obesity Surgery Score is used to decide where the postoperative obese should be transferred after surgery.

MONTEFIORE OBESITY SURGERY SCORE[32]

Class	Description	Disposition
I	< 40 years	If stable in PACU for
	No major respiratory problem	4 hrs postoperatively, can go to ward
II	40-50 years	Oximetry 24 hrs
	H/O asthma / snoring	HDU observation
III	> 50 years	Overnight HDU
	OSA, asthma, DVT	ICU if there are complications
IV	Pul. HTN, DVT, PE	Always to ICU
	Chronic resp. insufficiency	

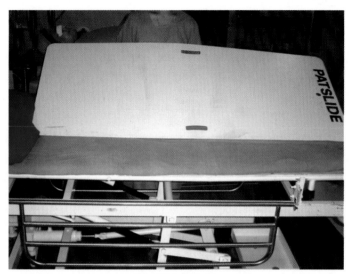

Fig. 20.8: Patslide

SHIFTING OF THE PATIENT

At the end of surgery a special patient transfer device (Patslide) (Fig. 20.8) is used. The operating table is raised higher than the patient's bed and tilted 20 to 30 degrees to the side where the patient's bed is positioned. The patslide is gently rolled under the patient which helps the patient to be safely and gradually rolled downhill into the bed.[2]

Ogunnaike et al use Walter Henderson maneuver instead of the patslide.[2]

POSTOPERATIVE CONSIDERATIONS

RESPIRATORY PROBLEMS

Morbidly obese patients are at great risk from postoperative respiratory insufficiency and supplemental oxygen should be given throughout the recovery period. Due to reduced FRC, they should be placed in semirecumbent position, i..e. upper torso elevated at 30° to 40° (Fig. 20.9).[32]

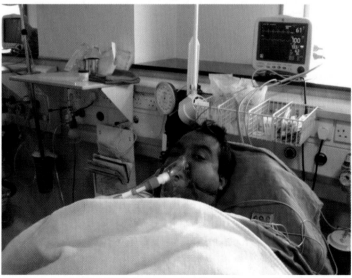

Fig. 20.9: Postoperative Recumbent position

Many of these patients may require bilevel positive airway pressure to reduce postoperative pulmonary dysfunction. Postoperative atelectasis is common due to effect of carboperitoneum. Prevention includes incentive spirometry, continuous positive airway pressure and a chest physiotherapy, which helps in alveolar recruitment during inspiration and prevents alveolar collapse during expiration.[32]

AMBULATION [32]

Thromboembolic complications contribute greatly to the increased morbidity and mortality in postoperative obese patients. Prolonged immobilisation must be avoided. Early ambulation is encouraged.

ANALGESIC REGIMES

Local anaesthetic infiltrated into the trocar sites during laparoscopy considerably reduces pain. Extreme caution is necessary when parenteral opioids are administered. Patient controlled analgesia (PCA) must be used very cautiously.[2,32]

The NSAIDS (non-steroidal anti-inflammatory drugs) are the drugs of choice as laparoscopic surgery requires less analgesics as compared to open technique.[37,38]

CONCLUSIONS

Though surgery in morbidly obese patients is associated with higher morbidity and mortality, the progress in the surgical technique and anaesthesia has substantially improved the safety of performing operations on them.

REFERENCES

1. Uberg L, Poulsen TD. Obesity : An Anaesthetic challenge – Review article. Acta Anaesthesiol Scand 1996; 40: 191-200.
2. Ogunnaike B, Jones SB, Jones DB, et al. Anesthetic considerations for bariatric surgery – review article. Anesth Analg 2002; 95: 1793-1805.
3. Brolin RE: Update: NIH consensus conference: Gastrointestinal surgery for severe obesity nutrition 1996; 12: 403.
4. Nguyen NT, Wolfe BM. The physiologic effects of pneumoperitoneum in the morbidly obese. Annals of Surgery, 2005; 241: 2.
5. Tan PL, Lee TL, Tweed WA. Carbon dioxide absorption and gas exchange during pelvic laparoscopy. Can J Anaesth 1992; 39: 677-81.
6. Demiroluk S, Salihoglu Z, Zengin K, et al. The effects of pneumoperitoneum on respiratory mechanics during bariatric surgery. Obes Surg 2001; 12: 376-79.
7. Dumont L, Maltys M, Mardisoff C. et al. Changes in pulmonary mechanics during laparoscopic gastroplasty in the morbidly obese patient. Acta Anaesth Scand 1997; 41: 408-13.
8. Ngurgen NT, Lee SL, Anderson JT, et al. Evaluation of intraabdominal pressure after open and laparoscopic gastric bypass. Obes Surg 2001; 11: 40-45.
9. Sanchez NC, Tenofsky PL, Dort JM, et al. What is normal intraabdominal pressure? Ann Surg 2001; 67: 243-48.
10. E. Peter Buckley. Anaesthesia for the morbidly obese patient. Refresher Course Outline. Can J Anaesth 1994; 41(5): 94-100.
11. Anthony N, Passannate, Peter Rock. Anaesthetic Management of patients with obesity with obesity and sleep apnoea. Anaesthesiol Clin N Am 2005; 23: 479-91.
12. Fried M, Krska Z, Zanzig V. Does the laparoscopic approach significantly affect cardiac functions in laparoscopic surgery? Pilot study in non obese and morbidly obese patients. Obes Surg. 2001; 11: 293-6.
13. Nguyen NT, HO HS, Fleming NW, et al. Cardiac function during laparoscopic vs open gastric bypass; a randomized comparison. Surg Endos 2002; 16: 78-83.

14. Sprung J, Whalley DG, Falcone T, et al. The effect of tidal volume and respiratory rate on oxygenation and respiratory mechanics during laparoscopy in morbidly obese patients. Anesth Analg 2003; 97: 268-74.
15. Jakimowics J, Stultiens G, Smulders F. Laparoscopic insufflation of the abdomen reduces portal venous flow. Surg Endos. 1998; 12: 129-32.
16. Nguyen NT, Braley S, Fleming NW, et al. Comparison of postoperative hepatic function after laparoscopic versus open gastric bypass. Am J Surg 2003; 186: 40-44.
17. Nguyen NT, Perez RV, Feming N, et al. Effect of prolonged pneumoperitoneum on intraoperative urine output during laparoscopic gastric by pass. J Am Coll Surg 2002; 195: 476-83.
18. McDougall EM, Monk TG, Wolf JS, et al. The effect of prolonged pneumoperitoneum on renal function in an animal model. J Am Coll Surg 1996; 182: 317-28.
19. Nguyen NT, Cronan M, Braley S, et al. Duplex ultrasound assessment of femoral venous flow during laparoscopic and open gastric bypass. Surg Endosc 2003; 17: 289-90.
20. Schwenk W, Bohm B, Fugener A, et al. Intermittent pneumatic sequential compression (ISC) of the lower extremities prevents venous stasis during laparoscopic cholecystectomy: a prospective randomized study: Surg Endosc. 1998; 12: 7-11.
21. Antonio Hernandez Conte, Robert T Marema. Innovations in Anesthesiology: New surgical procedures transalate to New Anesthetic Challenges. Anesthetic Challenges for the patient undergoing bariatric surgery. Seminars in Anesthesia, Perioperative Medicine and Pain 2003; 22: 1.
22. Farshal Abir, Robert Bell. Assessment and Management of the obese patient scientific reviews.
23. Shenkaman Z, Shir Y, Brodsky JB. Perioperative management of the obese patient. Anaesthesia 1993; 70: 349.
24. Ogunnaike BO, Whitten CW. Anesthetic Management of Morbidly obese patients seminars in Anesthesia, Perioperative Medicine and Pain. 2002; 21(1): 46-58.
25. Salihoglu Z, Demiroluk S, Dikmen Y. Respiratory mechanics in morbid obese patients with chronic obstructive pulmonary disease and hypertension during pneumoperitoneum. Euro J Anesthesiol July 2003; 20(8): 658-61(4).
26. Andrea Casati, Marta Putzu. Anesthesia in the obese patient: Pharmacokinetic considerations- Review article - J Clin Anaesth 2005; 17: 134-35.
27. Brodsky JB, Lemmens HJM, Brock Utne JG, et al. Anesthetic considerations for Bariatric surgery: Proper positioning is important for laryngoscopy. Anesth Analg 2003; 96: 1841-42.
28. Schmitt JH, Mang H. Head and neck elevation beyond the sniffing position improves laryngeal view in cases of difficult direct laryngoscopy. J Clin Anesth 2002; 14: 335-8.
29. Levitan RM, Mchem CC, Ochroch EA, et al. Head elevated laryngoscopy position: improving laryngeal exposure during laryngoscopy by increasing head elevation. Ann Emerg Med 2003; 41: 322-30.
30. Coussa M, Proutti S, Schnyder P, Frascarolo P, et al. Prevention of Atelectasis formation during the induction of general anaesthesia in morbidly obese patients. Anesth Analg 2004; 98: 1491-5.
31. Gizella I, Bardoczky, Jean Claude Yernault, Jean-Jacques Houben. Large tidal volume ventilation does not improve oxygenation in morbidly obese patients during anaesthesia. Anesth Analg 1995; 81: 385-8.
32. Levi D, Goodman ER, Patel M, Savransky Y. Critical care of the obese and bariatric surgical patient. Crit Care Clin 2003; 19: 11-32.
33. Fleming DRY, Dougherty TB, Feig BW. The safety of helium for abdominal insufflation. Surg Endosc 1997; 11: 230-34.
34. Juvin P, Lavaut E, Dupont H. Difficult tracheal intubation is more common in obese than in lean patients. Anesth Analg 2003; 97- 595-600.
35. Ezri T, Medalion B, Weisenberg M, et al. Increased body mass index per se is not a predictor of difficult laryngoscopy. Can J Anesth 2003; 50: 179-83.
36. Ezri T, Gewurtz G, Sessler DL, et al. Predictor of difficult laryngoscopy in obese patients by ultrasound quantification of anterior neck soft tissue. Anaesthesia 2003; 58: 111-4.
37. Loadsman JA, Hillman DR. Anaesthesia and sleep apnoea. Br J Anaesth 2001; 86(2): 254-66.
38. Brodsky JB. Anesthesia for bariatric surgery. ASA Refresher Course 2005; 49-63.

CHAPTER 21

Laparoscopy in High-Risk Cardiac Cases

INTRODUCTION

Laparoscopic procedures have rapidly gained popularity in the professional and lay people. The potential benefits are, the smaller incisions, shortened period of hospitalisation, decreased postoperative pain and cost-effectiveness. Attention is now focussing on extending established techniques to more extensive elective procedures, such as hernioplasty, bariatric surgery, gastrointestinal surgery and high risk patients as well as to emergency procedures like ruptured ectopic pregnancy and diagnostic laparoscopy for trauma. The issue of the effect of laparoscopic procedures on the cardiopulmonary status of patients is going to progressively become more important as the operative procedures being performed laparoscopically will increase in numbers and variety. Tuvla Kiviluoto et al studied laparoscopic cholecystitis in acute and gangrenous cholecystitis and found it to be safe and effective in experienced hands. Laparoscopic cholecystectomy did not increase the mortality rate, and the morbidity rate seemed to be even lower than that in open cholecystectomy. However he accepts a moderately high conversion rate. The postoperative hospital stay was significantly shorter and mean length of sick leave was shorter in the laparoscopic group than the open cholecystectomy group.[1]

It has been observed that the benefits of laparoscopic procedures are particularly important for patients with pre-existing cardio-pulmonary disease.[2] However the physiological stress of laparoscopy may be even greater than that of laparotomy, as significant alterations in heart rate, cardiac output, arterial and venous blood pressure and vascular resistance have been observed.[2,3] Early reports of laparoscopic cholecystectomy in patients with cardiopulmonary disease suggested the potential for worsening function, raising concerns about the safe use of laparoscopic techniques in this group of patients.[2] However these investigations focussed primarily on changes in systemic carbon dioxide levels because of peritoneal insufflation of CO_2, with considerably less attention paid to haemodynamic changes resulting from increased intra-abdominal pressure. In laparoscopy, the main trespasses to physiological haemostasis are insufflation of carbon dioxide, patient positioning and increased intra-abdominal pressure.[2,3] This chapter will address these issues and the anaesthetic management with specific focus on cardiac patients.

INSUFFLATION OF CARBON DIOXIDE

Carboperitoneum with an intra-abdominal pressure of 12-15 mmHg, is generally used during laparoscopy to provide adequate visualisation of intra-abdominal structures. Carboperitoneum is characterised by elevation of arterial pressure, an increase in systemic and pulmonary vascular resistance and fall in cardiac output. The decrease in cardiac output is proportional to the increase in intra-abdominal pressure and is well tolerated by healthy patients. Cardiac output which initially decreases during peritoneal insufflation due to decreased venous return subsequently increases due to surgical stress.[4]

Catherine M. Wittgen et al in1991, found that patients with preoperative cardiopulmonary disease demonstrated a significant increase in arterial carbon dioxide levels and decrease in pH during carbon dioxide insufflation compared with patients without underlying disease.[5] In this study, patients experienced an immediate, brief increase in heart rate and mean arterial pressure with the onset of insufflation. During the procedure when peritoneal distention with CO_2 insufflation had reached a steady state, patients in group 1 (no cardiopulmonary disease) experienced a decrease in heart rate and increase in mean arterial blood pressure, while patients in group 2 (patients with cardiac or pulmonary disease belonging to group II or III) demonstrated increased heart rate and mean arterial pressure. This was indicative of an increase in cardiac output. Patients in group 1 were able to increase cardiac output by increasing stroke volume alone, while patients in group 2 were more dependent on increased heart rate to increase cardiac output. Theoretically, in patients with impaired cardiac output, carbon dioxide transport from the peritoneal cavity to the alveolar bed might be slowed, permitting tissue levels to increase and the body to become a CO_2 sink.

Intraperitoneal CO_2 insufflation is inherently accompanied by an increase in MAP. Arterial blood pressure when used as one of the classical clinical parameters to assess depth of anaesthesia, may be misleading during carboperitoneum : its increase doesn't necessarily indicate an insufficient depth of anaesthesia. When MAP increases during surgery, it is a common clinical reaction to increase the concentration of inhalation anaesthetic. This reaction may be deleterious during CO_2 insufflation because it may lead to a depression of myocardial function especially in patients with heart disease. The administration of vasodilating drugs reducing specifically cardiac preload or afterload may be indicated in case of MAP increase during carboperitoneum.[3]

There is ventilation – perfusion mismatch during laparoscopic procedures. There is increased shunt and secondly increased physiological dead space. This is evidenced by a large increase in the $PaCO_2$ without such an increase in the end tidal CO_2. This phenomenon may be explained by collapsed alveoli from abdominal distension, an obvious sequelae of this procedure. In addition, increased dead space may occur when cardiac output is decreased. The problem of shunting can be minimised by two factors. One is minimising the insufflation pressure of carboperitoneum. Secondly the anesthesiologist can apply positive end- expiratory pressure (PEEP). Lastly increased dead space may have been related to decreased cardiac output. To reduce the dead space it would be ideal to have the patient's head up to get the maximum amount of diaphragmatic excursion.

In ASA III and IV patients, $PEtCO_2$ does not reflect changes in $PaCO_2$ during insufflation due to changes in alveolar dead space consequent to reduced cardiac output, increased ventilation perfusion mismatch or both.[6,7] Therefore, direct arterial $PaCO_2$ monitoring is recommended in patients with significant cardiorespiratory diseases. An arterial line is reasonable to monitor $PaCO_2$ in ASA III and IV patients for three reasons.

1. End-tidal PCO_2 is not a reliable index of $PaCO_2$.
2. The normal gradient of 3-5 mmHg between $PaCO_2$ and $PEtCO_2$ is increased

3. Even with normal PEtCO$_2$ achieved by increasing minute volume, PaCO$_2$ may be as high as 50 mmHg resulting in respiratory acidosis.

Patients with aortic outflow obstruction and left ventricular hypertrophy are extremely sensitive to changes in afterload, making the sequence of anaesthetic induction followed by peritoneal insufflation particularly hazardous. During induction, flow across the valve decreases, leading to a decrease in coronary and cerebral perfusion. The compensatory increase in HR leads to shortened diastolic filling time, further reducing the myocardial blood flow at a time when the hypertrophic left ventricle is increasing its work. Carboperitoneum then raises MAP, SVR and left ventricular wall tension, increasing myocardial oxygen demand; as well as the potential for myocardial ischaemia. With these conditions, careful afterload reduction becomes essential for unloading the left ventricle and controlling left ventricular stroke work. When managing these patients, it may be difficult to decide exactly when measured changes in haemodynamic parameters assume clinical importance.[2] From a practical standpoint, optimal intraoperative management involves anticipation of haemodynamic stress and early intervention. Mixed venous oximetry is useful for evaluating total body oxygen demand and delivery. A healthy patient under general anaesthesia usually displays a constant rise in SVO$_2$. Continuous assessment of mixed venous oxygen saturation, in surgery with little blood loss and preserved arterial oxygenation might directly reflect cardiac output. Therefore a decrease in SVO$_2$ during laparoscopic procedure should alert the surgeon and anaesthesiologist to the possibility of cardiovascular decompensation.[2]

HYPERCARBIA

The direct and indirect effects of hypercarbia on the cardiovascular system are dual and opposite. Directly hypercarbia dilates the arterioles and depresses the myocardium. Indirectly hypercarbia enhances the sympathoadrenal activity by liberating catecholamines. This causes abnormal inotropic and chronotropic cardiac effects and thus concomitant increase in myocardial oxygen consumption. In patients with heart disease, β adrenergic cardiac and vascular effects prevail. This results in hypertension, tachycardia, increased cardiac output and stroke volume and decreased systemic vascular resistance. These effects are due to two to three fold increase in plasma epinephrine and norepinephrine levels.

The physiologic effects of hypercarbia and respiratory acidosis are well known. Feig et al observed that hypercarbia stimulates the sympathetic nervous system resulting in tachycardia and vasoconstriction. Acidosis causes vasodilatation, which can counteract the vasoconstriction caused by hypercarbia. The combination of hypercarbia and respiratory acidosis results in a decrease in myocardial contractility and a lowering of the arrhythmia threshold. The haemodynamic changes observed in this study were ameliorated with the use of intravenous nitroglycerine (1 µg/kg/min). In those patients in whom the SVR reached 1500 (dyne. sec)/cm^5, the addition of nitroglycerine resulted in a rapid return of haemodynamic parameters to baseline levels. However PCWP which initially decreased in response to the infusion of nitroglycerin, continued to rise significantly as the insufflation period increased. This finding suggests that the haemodynamic effects produced by carbon dioxide abdominal insufflation are continuous and increase with time.[8]

Elevations in systolic and mean blood pressure, CVP, cardiac output and left ventricular stroke volume can all be observed in hypercarbic patients.[9] Cardiac oxygen demand is significantly increased, while coronary filling time is shortened. This signifies a relative myocardial under perfusion. Thus hypercarbia produces an unfavourable balance between myocardial oxygen consumption and supply.

Other investigators have observed that laparoscopy presents serious haemodynamic stress, but it can be performed safely in high-risk patients using aggressive intraoperative monitoring. There is an increase in MAP and SVR along with a decrease in cardiac output on insufflation of the abdomen to 15 mmHg with CO_2. A decrease in mixed venous oxygen saturation (SVO_2) after peritoneal insufflation was predictive of significant worsening of haemodynamic parameters, suggesting inadequate cardiac reserve.[4]

Hypercarbia and its attendant problems led to the discovery of alternative methods of carboperitoneum. Fred S. Bongard et al produced carboperitoneum with helium.[10] It does not cause respiratory acidosis associated with CO_2 and is stable in the presence of electrocautery and laser coagulation. Dissolved helium is rapidly and totally excreted from pulmonary arterial blood into the alveoli, with essentially none retained in systemic arterial blood. CO_2 has been the preferred agent because of its high aqueous solubility speeds the dissolution of gas bubbles in the blood stream. Although helium is less soluble in water than CO_2, it is more diffusible because of its low density: it thus enhances the dissolution of small helium emboli to a degree approaching that of CO_2. Therefore helium emboli behave similar to those of CO_2, because of their rapid diffusibility and minimal effect upon pulmonary mechanics. Increased $PaCO_2$ and $EtCO_2$ associated with CO_2 insufflation did not occur in the group that received helium. However decreased pH and HCO_3^- were noted. The decrease in pH was dependent on time and on the type of gas received. The decrease in HCO_3^- in both the groups was independent of the type of gas received and may have resulted simply from surgical stress. The exaggerated decrease in pH in the CO_2 group was accompanied by a continued elevation in $PaCO_2$. The abnormality was thus of respiratory origin and was produced by the CO_2 used for insufflation.

PATIENT POSITIONING

Dhoste et al used low intraperitoneal pressure (10 mmHg) and slow insufflation rates (1L/min) and observed that normal haemodynamic pattern was maintained in elderly ASA III patients. Marked cardiovascular depression occurred after anaesthetic induction, mainly because of decreased preload and increased afterload. Cardiac output was particularly dependent on venous return and any reduction in blood volume and in preload compromised myocardial function. An increase in afterload also resulted due to progressive reduction of arterial elastic properties. This study has demonstrated that loading conditions are not modified during laparoscopy when a moderate degree of headup positioning is imposed after progressive insufflation at limited IAP (12 mmHg).[4]

Gannedahl et al observed that the haemodynamic changes induced by the patient position during laparoscopy remain insignificant. Central blood volume and pressure changes are greater in patients with coronary artery disease with poor ventricular function, leading to potentially deleterious increased myocardial oxygen demand. In the headup position decrease in cardiac output and mean arterial pressure is observed secondary to the reduction in venous return. Venous stasis in the legs is compounded by lithotomy position and carboperitoneum.[11]

Joris et al reported that in young ASA I patients there is a marked decrease in cardiac index early after insufflation. It is explained by the marked decrease in cardiac preload because CO_2 insufflation was initiated when the patients were already in the headup position. Under these conditions blood pooling occured in the lower body and decrease venous return. This suggests that venous return can be affected to a greater degree when carboperitoneum is induced after head up positioning.[12]

Table 21.1: Management of patients with cardiac disease for laparoscopy[13]

1. Preoperative evaluation echocardiography
2. If LVEF < 30%
   Intraoperative monitoring
   - Intra-arterial line
   - Pulmonary artery catheter
   - TOE (Transoesophageal echocardiography)
   - ST segment analysis continuous
3. Intraoperative management
   - Slow insufflation – 1 L/min
   - Low intra-abdominal pressure (10 -12 mmHg)
   - Haemodynamic optimisation before carboperitoneum
   - Preload augmentation
   - Patient tilt after insufflation
   - Vasodilating drugs – nicardipine / nitroglycerin
   - Experienced surgeon and anaesthesiologist
4. *Postoperative care*
   - Slow recovery from anaesthesia

INCREASED INTRA-ABDOMINAL PRESSURE

Haemodynamic changes can also occur as a result of the acute increase in intra-abdominal pressure.[5] When right sided filling pressures were low high intra-abdominal pressure compressed the inferior vena-cava and impeded venous return, while at high right-sided pressures, venous return was augmented by the increased intra-abdominal pressure because of facilitated emptying of the splanchnic circulation.[2,6] In contrast when intra-abdominal pressure was only mildly elevated, although systemic pressure and arterial resistance increased, venous resistance remained generally unaffected, so that venous return was augmented irrespective of intravascular volume.

It is observed that during the laparoscopy procedure continuous adjustment of ventilatory rate and tidal volume settings is necessary based upon changing serum $PaCO_2$ or $EtCO_2$ levels during the operation. However patients undergo abrupt and frequently severe alterations in cardiac preload and afterload as a result of changes in intra-abdominal pressure. These changes are poorly tolerated by patients with severe coronary artery or valvular heart disease. These patients usually have an acute decrease in coronary perfusion pressure and increased left ventricular work and can have transient myocardial ischaemia and left ventricular dysfunction. Intravascular volume loading seems to be an important mode of myocardial protection because high central venous pressures are needed to overcome the increased venous resistance caused by the elevation in intra-abdominal pressure, permitting adequate right heart filling and left ventricular stroke volume. Unfortunately ischaemic heart disease patients are best maintained under conditions of reduced preload and after load. For them rapid increases in intravascular volume may result in left ventricular decompensation and heart failure, therefore meticulous monitoring is essential.[2]

CONCLUSIONS

Laparoscopic procedures can be performed safely in elderly ASA class III patients with increased cardiac risk since the haemodynamic changes induced by carboperitoneum are relatively benign and not different compared with healthy ASA class I and II patients. Monitoring of SVO_2^-, is an appropriate method of identifying haemodynamic tolerance in critical patients during laparoscopy besides the routine monitoring like pulse rate, non invasive blood pressure, SpO_2 and $EtCO_2$. Moderate IAP (12 mmHg) and 10° headup initiated after peritoneal insufflation preserves cardiac output; by minimally impairing ventricular loading conditions. Moderate haemodynamic variations lead to moderate consequences, on pulmonary blood flow and no major disturbance in V/Q ratios. However the potential benefits of improved postoperative pulmonary function and decreased hospital stay must be weighed against the risks associated with a longer procedure (in inexperienced hands) requiring general anaesthesia and the haemodynamic and pulmonary changes that are observed.

RECOMMENDATIONS (AS IN TABLE 21.1)

1. Induction and release of carboperitoneum should be slow smooth and progressive.
2. The problem of shunting can be minimised by reducing the insufflation pressure of carboperitoneum. Positive end expiratory pressure (PEEP)and increasing the inspiratory : expiratory ratio can be applied.
3. Mask ventilation before intubation can inflate the stomach with gas, which must be aspirated before trocar placement to avoid gastric perforation.
4. The bladder should be emptied before pelvic laparoscopy or prolonged procedures.
5. Gradual positioning (headup) helps to maintain haemodynamic status of the patient.
6. Venous return is affected to a greater degree when carboperitoneum is induced after headup positioning. Under these conditions blood pooling may occur in the lower body and decrease cardiac preload. Hence its recommended that slow carboperitoneum is done before positioning the patient.
7. The position of the endotracheal tube must be checked after any change in patient position.
8. Increased intrathoracic pressure interferes with interpretation of measured central venous and pulmonary artery pressure.
9. Preoperatively optimisation of the haemodynamic function.
10. Minimum monitoring standards along with radial artery and pulmonary artery catheter insertion.
11. Mixed venous oximetry may be useful for signaling myocardial decompensation during laparoscopy.
12. Preload should be augmented because volume loading seems to offset the effects of increased intra-abdominal pressures.
13. Vigilant attention must be given to haemodynamic changes that occur during the procedure, particularly at the time of insufflation; pharmacological support should be provided when perfusion deteriorates.
14. Hypercarbia should be avoided by using controlled hyperventilation with adjustment in respiratory rate and tidal volume. In line capnography is useful for continuous measurement of $EtCO_2$, to guide intraoperative changes in ventilator settings.
15. Use vasodilators instead of inhalation anaesthetic to counteract the increase in MAP due to increase in SVR.

REFERENCES

1. Kiviluota T, Siren J, et al. Randomised trial of laparoscopic versus open cholecystectomy for acute and gangrenous cholecystitis. Lancet 1998; 351: 321-25.
2. Safran D, Sgambati S, et al. Laparoscopy in high-risk cardiac patients. Surg Gynecol Obstet 1993; 176: 548-554.
3. Zollinger A, Kreiyer S, Singer Th, et al. Haemodynamic effects of pneumoperitoneum in elderly patients with an increased cardiac risk. Euro J Anesthesiol 1997; 14: 266-75.
4. Dhoste K, Lacoste L, Karayan J, et al. Haemodynamic and ventilatory changes during laparoscopic cholecystectomy in elderly ASA III patients. Can J Anaesth 1996; 43(8): 783-8.
5. Wittgen CM, Andrus CH, Fitzgerald SD, et al. Analysis of the hemodynamic and ventilatory effects of laparoscopic cholecystectomy. Arch Surg 1991; 126: 997-1001.
6. Feig BW, Berger DH, Dougherty TB, et al. Pulmonary effects of CO2 abdominal insufflation (CAI) during laparoscopy in high risk patients. Anaesth Analg 1994; 78 (Supplement) : S 108.
7. Monk TG, Weldon BC, Lemon D. Alteration in pulmonary function during laparoscopic surgery. Anaesth Analg 1993; 76 (Supplement) : S 274.

8. Feig BW, Berger DH, Dougherty TB, et al. Pharmacologic intervention can re-establish baseline haemodynamic parameters during laparoscopy. Surgery 1994; 116: 733-41.

9. Rosmussen JP, et al. Cardiac function and hypercarbia. Arch Surg Oct 1978; 113: 1196-1200.

10. Bongard FS, Pianim NA, et al. Surgery, Gynecology and Obstetrics. Helium insufflation for laparoscopic operation. Aug 1993; 177: 140-46.

11. Gannedahl P, Odeberg S, Brodin L-A, et al. Effects of posture and pneumoperitoneum during anaesthesia on the indices of left ventricular filling. Acta Anaesthesiol Scand 1996; 40: 160.

12. Joris JL, Noirot DP, Legrand MJ, Jacquet NJ, Lamy ML. Hemodynamic changes during laparoscopic cholecystectomy. Anesth Analg 1993; 76: 1067-71.

13. Joris JL. Anesthesia for Laparoscopic Surgery. In: RD Miller (ed). Anesthesia, Churchill Livingstone; 6th Ed, Vol 2, pg 2296.

CHAPTER 22

Pain Management after Laparoscopic Procedures

INTRODUCTION

Laparoscopic surgery presents several challenges for the anaesthesiologist. More than 70 per cent of laparoscopic surgical interventions are carried out as day-care surgery.[1] Inadequately controlled postoperative pain has undesirable physiologic and psychological consequences, such as, increased morbidity, delayed recovery and patient dissatisfaction.[2]

Pain following laparoscopic intervention is less intense and is of shorter duration compared to their open counterpart. However, the pain is most severe in early postoperative period,[3] which needs to be anticipated and addressed adequately. The reason for the above stated may be due to greater visceral than parietal (abdominal wall) component of pain.[4] Post-laparoscopic shoulder tip pain is more troubling than it seems as it may be a frequent occurrence after laparoscopy and can have prolonged persistence (upto 4 days) (Table 22.1).[3,5]

Table 22.1: Factors influencing post-laparoscopic pain

Age
Residual CO_2 – gas
Carbonic acid – auditory effects
Duration of pneumoperitoneum
Re-do laparoscopic intervention
Neuropraxia of phrenic nerve
Gas insufflation pressure
Surgery type – manipulation of viscera

Perioperative analgesia cover for patients undergoing laparoscopic surgery is largely similar to standard analgesia provided during a general anaesthetic, especially when short duration day care laparoscopy is being performed. It is for the prolonged laparoscopic interventions, a specified analgesia plan is warranted that varies with type of surgery. Interestingly, investigations are on in regard to pain relief in patients undergoing day care laparoscopic procedures in order to avoid delay in discharge time owing to algesic response attributable to laparoscopy itself, such as, shoulder pain, abdominal stretch pain and major trocar placement (> 10 mm diameter) pain. Following tabulated options are being otherwise considered to selectively handle analgesic profile of patients scheduled for laparoscopic surgery (Table 22.2):

Table 22.2: Methods for laparoscopic pain relief

Methods	Mechanism	Limitations
NSAIDs Diclofenac sodium Ibuprofen Etoricoxib/ Valdecoxib (COX-2 inhibitors) Tenoxicam[6]	↓ Secondary hyperalgesia	Modest relief (adjuvants only) Related side effects
Local Anaesthetics Intraperitoneal bupivacaine[6,7] Incisional infiltration Epidural local anaesthetics		

Opioids
Systemic Fentanyl
          Morphine
          Sufentanil
Intraperitoneal
          Tramodol[6]
Intrathecal morphine[8]
Extradural opioids (fentanyl, morphine)[9-12]
	Central / peripheral
	opioids effects
		PONV
		Itching
		Respiratory effects

Others CO₂ - gas warming[13]	↓ CO₂-induced Peritoneal irritation	Adjunctive only
Preoperative low dose ketamine[14]	Pre-emptive analgesia	Hallucination (If dose not adjusted)
Adhesionolysis Rectus sheath block (in gasless laparoscopy)	↓ Stretch pain Regional blockage	Only sometime helpful Accuracy, a must

SHOULDER PAIN

Carbon dioxide insufflation is the commonest means of achieving pneumoperitoneum and it is widely attributable for postoperative shoulder tip pain. In particular, shoulder-tip pain is presumed to be linked to carbon dioxide insufflation. The reported incidence of this variant of pain ranges from 35 to 63 per cent following gynaecological laparoscopic procedures[15] and between 30 to 50 per cent for laparoscopic cholecystectomy.[16,17] Pain following laparoscopy is thought to be due to peritoneal irritation by carbonic acid and also to the creation of space between liver and diaphragm.[18] Various efforts have made to reduce the shoulder tip pain, which is most frequent and severe after early mobilisation of the patient.

Simple measures like release of gas at the end of the operation, low pressure pneumoperitoneum, intraperitoneal local anaesthetic and the heating of CO₂ gas to 37°C during laparoscopy significantly reduces associated abdominal and shoulder tip pain.[13]

PRE-EMPTIVE ANALGESIA

'Pre-emptive' analgesia is an antinociceptive treatment that prevents establishment of and alters processing of afferent input that amplifies postoperative pain. The goal of pre-emptive analgesia is to prevent peripheral and central sensitization caused initially by surgical incision and by inflammatory injury later on.

There are many studies that support the effectiveness of pre-emptive analgesia[19,20] and some that do not.[21] The failure to demonstrate the advantages of pre-emptive analgesia may be due to an inadequate initial afferent blockade or inadequate treatment of the postoperative inflammatory response, which is equally responsible for postoperative pain. Low-dose ketamine has been utilised in the preoperative period to pre-empt post-laparoscopic surgery pain.[14]

PREVENTIVE ANALGESIA

It is believed that for effective relief of postoperative pain and for pre-emptive analgesia to be effective, consistent intraoperative analgesia must be maintained[19] and then followed by active management of pain in the postoperative period.[20] Intravenous NSAIDs are commonly used for preventing postoperative pain in patients undergoing laparoscopic surgery. Interestingly they have good opioids sparing effects and a modest decrease in pain scores.

LOCAL ANAESTHETIC

LOCAL ANAESTHESIA INCISIONAL INFILTRATION

Local anaesthesia (LA) is an efficient, non-opioid pharmacological approach to postoperative analgesia. It is a simple, safe and inexpensive pain management technique. It is even more effective in outpatients with surgical procedures of less magnitude in which fewer tissue planes are crossed during the surgery. Different infiltration techniques have been shown to be effective pain-reducing and opioid-sparing modality, especially after laparoscopic surgery, like, cholecystectomy.[22] Importantly, LA - infiltration (Fig. 22.1) needs to be administrated not only subcutaneously but also into subfascial planes to gain maximum benefit.

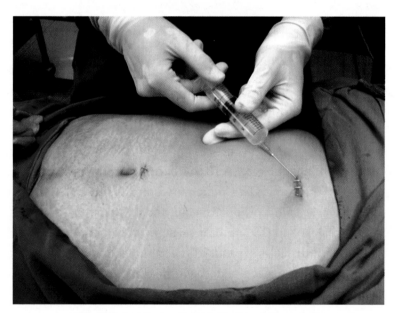

Fig. 22.1: Local anaesthetic infiltration of the port site

The role of the technique used for LA administration may be crucial. The relative contribution of different anatomical structures also needs to be evaluated, e.g., there is some evidence that subfascial lidocaine may be more effective compared to subcutaneous administration after inguinal hernia surgery.[23] Improved pain relief has also been noted if visceral structures are exposed to LA drugs in laparoscopic surgery.[22]

INTRAPERITONEAL LOCAL ANAESTHETIC

Intraperitoneal LA (Fig. 22.2) can be used during laparoscopic procedures to give effective postoperative analgesia. Many studies have demonstrated that LA used for intraperitoneal surgery can be effective in treating postoperative pain.

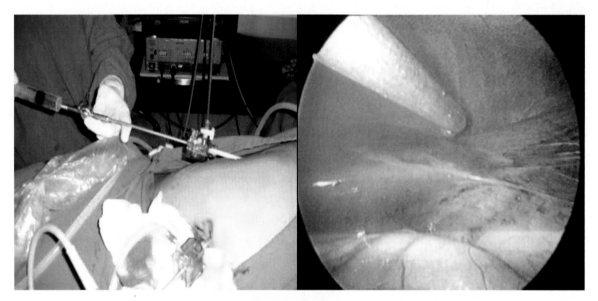

Fig. 22.2: Subdiaphragmatic instillation of local anaesthetic

Goldstein et al[24] instilled either LA (0.5% bupivacaine or 0.75% ropivacaine) or 0.9 per cent saline at the end of laparoscopic gynaecologic procedures and monitored pain at wake up and following 24 hours. They also monitored morphine sparing effect for the same time period. He found a large reduction in morphine, consumption in the patient treated with LA drugs compared with the saline group. Between the two LA drug groups, ropivacaine was found to be more effective.

Pasqualucci et al[25] compared intraperitoneal LA (0.5% bupivacaine) versus 0.9 per cent saline for patients undergoing laparoscopic cholecystectomy. The patients were divided into four groups, including saline preoperatively and postoperatively, saline preoperatively and LA postoperatively, LA preoperatively and postoperatively, and LA preoperatively and 0.9 per cent saline postoperatively. They found that all three groups that received local had lower pain intensity and reduced analgesic requirements postoperatively compared with the group that received only 0.9 per cent saline added. Of the three groups that received LA, two groups that received LA preoperatively had decrease in pain intensity and analgesic requirements postoperatively.

PHARMACOLOGICAL MODALITIES

ACETAMINOPHEN

Acetaminophen is a widely used over-the-counter analgesic and antipyretic drug. It is a weak analgesic suitable for the treatment of mild pain. Acetaminophen acts by the inhibition of the cyclo-oxygenase (COX)-3 isoenzyme with subsequent reduction of prostanoid release in the central nervous system. In addition, there is some suggestion that it acts on the opioidergic system and NMDA receptors.

Although it is generally considered safe, acetaminophen is associated with liver and gastrointestinal toxicity at high doses.[26-28] Interesting because of recent availability of suppository and injectable forms of acetaminophen has resulted in our better understanding of our knowledge of the pharmacodynamics of acetaminophen, such as the relationship between peak concentrations and clinical efficacy.[29]

The initial dose of injectable acetaminophen may be administered intraoperatively and may be followed by an oral administration after the patient is discharged. Compared with oral formulations, parenteral acetaminophen has a predictable onset and duration of action.[29]

NONSTEROIDAL ANTI-INFLAMMATORY DRUGS (NSAIDs)

NSAIDs play an important role in the management of pain in the ambulatory setting. With introduction of parenteral preparations of NSAIDs (ketorolac, diclofenac, and ketoprofen), these drugs have become more popular in the management of postoperative pain. NSAIDs produce analgesia by inhibiting COX enzymes and decrease prostaglandins production and thereby reducing sensitisation of nociceptors, attenuation of inflammatory pain response, prevention of central sensitisation, and thus improving postoperative pain relief. It has been increasingly apparent that, in an inflammatory model, the COX-2 enzyme plays an important role in peripheral and central sensitisation.[30]

Although the overall adverse events with nonselective NSAIDs are not increased in the perioperative period, the contraindications to their use are numerous.[31] Therefore, the limitations of nonselective NSAIDs prevent their use even when they would otherwise be desirable. The development of COX-2-specific inhibitors, a new group of anti-inflammatory and analgesic drugs, such as, valdecoxib and parecoxib, which selectively target COX-2 while sparing COX-I, were developed to obtain the therapeutic benefits of NSAIDs while overcoming their limitations. Although COX-2-specific inhibitors seem to have analgesic efficacy that is similar to nonselective NSAIDs, they may have an advantage over nonselective NSAIDs because they do not affect platelet function thereby reducing the risk of gastrointestinal ulceration.[32] The lack of antiplatelet effects and improved gastrointestinal tolerability, COX-2-specific inhibitors may be safely administered preoperatively.

OPIOIDS

Opioids are very effective analgesic in postoperative pain when the pain is of moderate to severe intensity. The use of opioid particularly in the day care setting is limited by their adverse side effects and may cause delayed recovery.[33]

In the ambulatory setting the choice of opioid is important. Fentanyl citrate remains the primary opioid for postoperative pain management because of rapid onset of action and easy titrability while morphine is very effective but associated with increased incidence of PONV.

Opioids reduce spontaneous pain but not very effective to control dynamic pain which may contribute to post-operative physiological impairment and development of chronic persistent postoperative pain.[34]

For postoperative pain relief it is now recommended that non-opioid analgesic and LA techniques be used as the first line of therapy and that opioid should be reserved for more severe pain not amenable to conventional nonopioids drugs.[35]

MULTIMODAL ANALGESIC TECHNIQUE

The concept of multimodal or "balanced" analgesia suggests that combinations of several analgesics of different classes and different sites of analgesic action rather than single analgesic or single technique provide superior pain relief with reduced analgesic related side effects.[31,36,37]

Use of multimodal analgesia technique(s), including, regional analgesic techniques, acetaminophen, nonspecific NSAIDs or COX-2-specific inhibitors, and opioids, have become standard practice. The choice of analgesic combinations should depend not only on their analgesic efficacy but also on the side effect profile of these combinations. Thus, even if a certain analgesic regimen provides superior pain relief, it may not be clinically beneficial if it is also associated with more adverse events.

Although it is clear that multimodal analgesia techniques improve postoperative pain relief, there are insufficient data on the optimal multimodal regimen for a particular patient undergoing a particular surgical procedure.

ADVANCEMENT IN SURGICAL TECHNIQUES

Changes in certain aspects of the surgical technique reduces the postoperative discomfort and hence pain. These advances includes

1. 'Needlescopic' approach which utilises ports smaller than 3 mm in diameter, has been associated with reduced incidence of postoperative pain and early recovery.
2. Incidence of shoulder tip pain after low pressure pneumoperitoneum (<9 mmHg) is less as compared those operated using normal pressure pneumoperitoneum.[38]
3. Reducing the size of epigastric port (5 mm instead of 10 mm) reduces pain scores, analgesia requirements and facilitates early recovery.[39]

CONCLUSIONS

CLINICAL PEARLS

- *"NSAIDs have a greater role in post-laparoscopic pain management."*
- *"The role of pre-emptive analgesia has not been fully realised."*
- *"Control and maintenance of carboperitoneum is essential for preventive analgesia."*

REFERENCES

1. McMohan AJ, Russell IT, Bexter SR, et al. Laparoscopic mini lap cholecystectomy: a randomised trial. Lancet 1994; 343: 135-8.
2. Liu SS, Carpenter RL, Mackey DC, et al. Effects of perioperative analgesic technique on rate of recovery after colon surgery. Anesthesiology 1995; 83:757-65.
3. O'Malley C, Cunningham AJ. Physiologic change during laparoscopic. Anesth Clin North Am 2001; 19: 1-19.
4. Joshi GB, Anesthesia for laparoscopic surgery. Can J Anaesth 2002; 49(6): pp R1-R5.
5. Joshi GP. Pain management after ambulatory surgery. Ambulatory Surgery 1999; 7:3-12.
6. Kareli B, Kanjakan M, Zorlu G, et al. the effects of intraperitoneal tramadol, tenoxicam and bupivacaine for pain relief after laparoscopic gynecological procedures. The Pain Clin 2003; 15 (3): 281-86.
7. Darwish AH, Zaheh H, lein EA. Intraperitoneal bupivacaine versus tramodol for pain relief following day case laparoscopic surgery. Gynecologic Laparosc 1999; 8 (3): 166-73.
8. Kong SK Onsiong MK. Chiu WKY, Lim KW. Use of intrathecal morphine for postoperative pain relief after laparoscopic colorectal surgery. Anaesthesia 2002; 51: 1168-73.
9. Kuvamochi K, Osupa Y, Yano T, et al. Usefulness of epidural analgesia in gynecologic laparoscopic surgery for infertility in comparison to general anaesthesia. Surg Endosc 2004; 18 (5): 847-51.
10. Bridenbaugh LD, Soderstrom RM. Lumbar epidural block anaesthesia for outpatient laparoscopy. J Reprod Med 1979; 23:856.
11. Bromage PR, Comporesi G, Chestnut D. "Epidural narcotics for postoperative analgesia. Anesth Analg 1980; 59: 473-80.
12. Luchetti M, Palomba R, Sica G massa G, Tufano R. Effectiveness and safety of combined epidural and general anesthesia for laparoscopic cholecystectomy. Reg Anesth 1996; 21(5): 465-9.

13. Slim K. Effect of CO_2 – gas warming on pain after laparoscopic surgery; a randomised double blind controlled trial. Surg Endosc 1999; 13(11): 1110-14.

14. Kwok RFK, Lim Jean, Chan MTV, et al. Preoperative ketamine improves postoperative analgesia after gynecologic laparoscopic surgery. Anesth Analg 2004; 98: 1044-49.

15. Dobbs FF, Kumar V, Alexander JI, Hull MGR. Pain after laparoscopy related to posture and ring versus clip sterilization. Br J Obstet Gynaecol 1987; 94:262-6.

16. Tsimoyiannis EC, Glantzounis G, Lekkas ET, et al. Intraperitoneal normal saline and bupivacaine infusion for reduction of postoperative pain after laparoscopic cholecystectomy. Surg Laparosc Endosc 1998; 8; 416-20.

17. Cunniffe MG, McAnena OJ, Dar MA, Calleary J, Flynn N. A prospective randomized trial of intraoperative bupivacaine irrigation for management of shoulder-tip pain following laparoscopy. Am J Surg 1998; 176:258-61.

18. Chamberlain G. The recovery of gases insufflated at laparoscopy. Br J Obstet Gynaecol 1984; 91:367-70.

19. Shir Y, Raja SN, Frank SM. The effect of epidural versus general anesthesia on postoperative pain and analgesic requirements in patients undergoing radical prostatectomy. Anesthesiology1994; 80(6): 1416-7.

20. Kissin I. Preemptive analgesia. Anesthesiology 2000; 93(4): 1138-43.

21. Moiniche S, Kehlet H, Dhal JB. A Qualitative and quantitative systematic review of preemptive analgesia for postoperative pain relief: the role of timing of analgesia. Anesthesiology 2002; 96(3): 526-7.

22. Alexander DJ, Ngoi SS, Lee L, et al. Randomized trial of periportal peritoneal bupivacaine for pain relief after laparoscopic cholecystectomy. Br J Surg 1996; 83: 1223-25.

23. Yndgaard S, Holst P, Bjerre-Jepsen K, et al. Subcutaneously versus subfascially administered lidocaine in pain treatment after inguinal Herniotomy. Anesth Analg 1994; 79:324-7.

24. Goldstain A, Grimault P Henique A, et al. Preventive postoperative pain by local anesthetic instillation after laparoscopic gynecologic surgery: a placebo-controlled comparison of bupivacaine and ropivacaine. Anesth Analg 2000; 91(2): 403-7.

25. Pasqualucci A, DeAngelis V, Contardo R, et al. Pre-emptive analgesia; intraperitoneal local anesthetic in laparoscopic cholecystectomy. Anesthesiology 1996; 85:11-20.

26. Ostapowicz G, Fontana RJ, Schiodt FV, et al. Results of a prospective study of acute liver failure at 17 tertiary care centers in the United States. Ann Intern Med 2002; 137; 947-54.

27. Garcia Rodriguez LA, Hernandez-Diaz S. Relative risk of upper gastrointestinal complications among users of acetaminophen and nonsteroidal anti-inflammatory drugs. Epidemiology 2001; 12: 570-6.

28. Rahme E, pettitt D, LeLorier J. Determinants and sequelae associated with utilization of acetaminophen versus traditional nonsteroidal anti-inflammatory drugs in an elderly population. Arthritis Rheum 2002; 46: 3046-54.

29. Holmer Pettersson P, Owall A, Jakobsson J. Early bioavailability of paracetamol after oral or intravenous administration. Acta Anaesthesiol Scand 2004; 48:867-7034.

30. Woolf CJ. Pain: moving from symptom control toward mechanism-specific pharmacologic management. Ann Intern Med 2004; 140: 441-51

31. Kehlet H,Dahl JB. Are perioperative nonsteroidal anti-inflammatory drugs ulcerogenic in the short term? Drugs 1992; 44 (Suppl 5): S38-41.

32. Gilron I, Milne B, Hong M. Cyclooxygenase-2 inhibitors in postoperative pain management. Anesthesiology 2003; 99:1198-208.

33. Wheeler M, Oderda Gm, Ashburn MA, et al. Adverse events Associated with postoperative opioid analogies: a systemic review. Pain 2002; 3:159-80.

34. Walder B, Schafer M, Henzi I, et al. Efficacy and safety of patient-controlled opioid analgesia for acute postoperative pain: a quantitative systematic review. Acta Anaesthesiol Scand 2001; 45: 795-804.

35. Kehlet H, Rung GW, Callesen T. Postoperative opioid analgesia: time for reconsideration? J Clin Anesth 1996; 8:441-5.

36. Kehlet H, Dahl JB. The value of "Multimodal" or "balanced analgesia" in postoperative pain treatment. Anesth Analg 1993; 77:1048-56.

37. Kehlet H, Werner M, Perkins F. Balanced analgesia: what is it and what are its advantages in postoperative period? Drugs 1999; 58:793-7.

38. Sarli L, Costi R, Sansebostion S, Trivially M, Roncoroni L. Prospective randomized trial of lowpressure for reduction of shoulder-tip pains following laparoscopy. Br J Surg 2000; 87: 1161.

39. Golder H, Rhodes M. Prospective randomized trial of 5 mm &10 mm epigastric Port in laparoscopic cholecystectomy. Br J Surg 1998;85:1066.

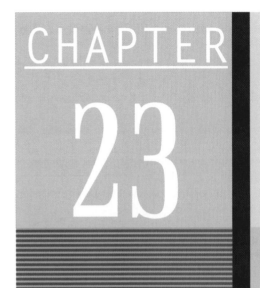

CHAPTER 23

Anaesthesia for Thoracoscopy

INTRODUCTION

Thoracoscopy is the insertion of an endoscope, through a very small incision in the chest wall (Fig. 23.1).

The first series of thoracoscopic cases was reported in 1921 by the Swedish physician Jacobaeus, who used the technique to diagnose and treat pulmonary tuberculosis and pleural effusion.[1]

Thoracic surgery and thoracic anaesthesia evolved significantly in the last century. In the 1930s, techniques were developed for endobronchial intubation and placement of bronchial blockers, enabling ventilation of a single lung. During the 1940s, use of neuromuscular blockers and controlled ventilation was introduced while in the 1950s and 1960s, use of double lumen tubes (DLT) was started.

With the introduction of video endoscopic surgery the approach to surgery of the thorax has been revolutionized and video-assisted thoracoscopic surgery (VATS) is now increasingly being used in clinical practice.[2]

VATS has many advantages over open thoracotomy including decreased postoperative pain, less pulmonary impairment and respiratory depression and reduced hospital stay.

Patients undergoing thoracoscopy range from healthy patients scheduled for minor diagnostic and therapeutic procedures of brief duration to high-risk patients in whom thoracotomy could result in significant postoperative morbidity.

INDICATIONS OF THORACOSCOPY[2,3]

I. *Diagnostic*

a. Lung and Pleural disease

    Biopsy, staging (malignancy) biopsy

    Trauma evaluation

    Infection : Tuberculosis

    Interstitial fibrosis

b. Esophageal disease

    Biopsy, staging (malignancies)

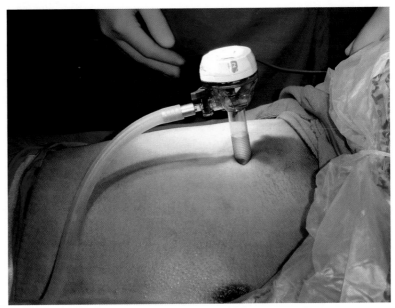

Fig. 23.1: Right Thoracoscopy (Left lateral position)

c. Mediastinal masses

    Lymphoma, metastatic diseases

d. Cardiovascular

    Biopsy of pericardium

    Pericardial effusion

II. Therapeutic

a. Lung and pleural disease

    Pneumonectomy

    Lobectomy

    Wedge, subsegmental, segmental resection

    Resection of pulmonary metastasis

    Excision of blebs and bullae

b. Pericardiocentesis

    Pericardiectomy

    Insertion of implantable cardioverter-defibrillator

c. Esophageal disease

    Esophagectomy

    Repair of esophageal perforation

    Fundoplication

d. Excision of tumors/cysts in thorax

e. Transthoracic endoscopic sympathectomy

f. Truncal vagotomy

g. Thoracic spine disease

Disc herniation

Deformity correction

Abscess drainage

Although thoracoscopy is used extensively for above mentioned conditions there are certain contraindications as well.

CONTRAINDICATIONS OF THORACOSCOPY[3]

ABSOLUTE

1. Extensive pleural adhesions: since a potential space between visceral and parietal pleura must exist so that the lung can collapse and structures can be seen adequately.
2. End-stage pulmonary fibrosis: since a thoracoscopic biopsy of a honeycomb lung may result in bronchopleural fistula.
3. Haemodynamically unstable patient: since the patient is unable to tolerate collapse of the ipsilateral lung.

RELATIVE

1. Respiratory insufficiency which requires ventilatory support
2. Unstable cardiovascular status
3. Hypoxemia unrelated to pleural effusion
4. Pulmonary arterial hypertension
5. Uncorrectable hypocoagulation profile

The choice of anaesthesia requires a meticulous understanding of, both, the underlying pathology and the pathophysiological changes associated with thoracoscopy e.g. differential lung ventilation and capnothorax.

ANAESTHESIA TECHNIQUES FOR THORACOSCOPY

The recommended anaesthesia technique for thoracoscopy is general anaesthesia with controlled ventilation however local anaesthesia and regional techniques are also used in certain situations.

LOCAL ANAESTHESIA

During thoracoscopy under local anaesthesia, collapse of lung on the nondependent side occurs allowing good visualization of pleural space.[4]

Historically, thoracoscopy was performed frequently under local anaesthesia, with the patient breathing spontaneously. The procedure was usually short and the ipsilateral lung was deflated only for a brief period. Patient showed little changes in arterial oxygen and carbon dioxide tensions and cardiac rhythm.[1] However, there may be impaired gas exchange and mediastinal shift so supplemental oxygen must be given and the procedure should be short and simple.[4]

REGIONAL ANAESTHESIA

VATS may be performed under regional anaesthesia if specific conditions are met. It requires an extremely cooperative patient, the procedure should be short (<1hr) and the surgical staff should be gentle and quick.

Regional anaesthesia consists of a combination of intercostal nerve blocks and ipsilateral stellate ganglion block (to block cough reflex associated with manipulation of the hilum). Other techniques include paravertebral blocks, thoracic epidural block and local field block.

With any of these techniques, complete anaesthesia of port sites and operating area must be ensured prior to incision to prevent cardiopulmonary compromise caused by pain and anxiety.

Patients breathe spontaneously with an open chest, therefore, the risk of developing hypoxaemia and hypercapnia from paradoxic respiration and hypotension from mediastinal shift persists. Thus, there should be provision of securing the airway in case of an emergency. Intraoperative shortness of breath can be managed by application of positive pressure with a mask.

Insufflation with CO_2 into pleural cavity (capnothorax) is not recommended because this can contribute to further hypercapnia and shift of mediastinal structures. Procedures involving apex and pleura should be performed under general anaesthesia since these areas are poorly blocked by regional techniques.[3]

Mechanism of Mediastinal Shift and Paradoxical Respiration[5]

When the nondependent hemithorax is open, the atmospheric pressure in that cavity exceeds the negative pleural pressure in the dependent lung and causes a downward displacement of the mediastinum into the dependent thorax. During inspiration, the caudal movement of the diaphragm increases the negative pressure in the dependent lung and causes still further displacement of mediastinum into the dependent hemithorax.

During expiration, as the diaphragm of dependent lung moves cephalad, the pressure in the dependent hemithorax becomes relatively positive and the mediastium is pushed upward out of the dependent hemithorax. Thus, the tidal volume in the dependent lung is decreased by an amount equal to the inspiratory displacement caused by mediastinal movement. This phenomenon is called mediastinal shift. It can cause decreased venous return to the heart and sympathetic activation that may mimic shock.

Similarly when the pleural cavity is exposed to atmospheric pressure, during spontaneous ventilation, the lung collapse is accentuated during inspiration and lung expands during expiration. This reversal of lung movement with an open chest during respiration is termed paradoxical respiration.

GENERAL ANAESTHESIA

The recommended technique for most VATS procedures is general anaesthesia with controlled ventilation (Fig. 23.2). The anaesthetic goals are satisfactory levels of anaesthesia, adequate muscle relaxation and rapid reversal with spontaneous ventilation at the conclusion of surgery. It also allows for rapid elimination of CO_2.[6-8]

Subcutaneous infiltration with local anaesthetic prior to placement of ports reduces stress response to surgical stimulation and postoperative pain.

Maintenance of anaesthesia with a volatile anaesthetic provides several desirable effects like bronchodilatation in patients with reactive airway disease. A high inspired oxygen can be useful in patients with one lung ventilation.

The various ventilatory techniques used during general anaesthesia for thoracoscopy are spontaneous respiration with single lumen tracheal tube, controlled ventilation with single lumen tracheal tube (SLT) and controlled ventilation with double lumen tracheal tube (DLT).

Spontaneous Ventilation

Since pulmonary pathologies (e.g. large bullae) can be worsened by PPV, thoracoscopy is performed with the patient breathing spontaneously through a standard tracheal tube.[8]

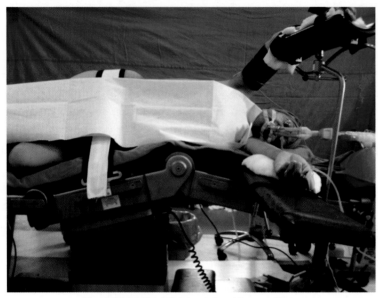

Fig. 23.2: Patient in lateral decubitus position

A pneumothorax is created by exposing the operative hemithorax to atmospheric pressure. Use of 5-10 cm H_2O CPAP after lung collapse prevents the lung from reexpanding, due to high critical opening pressure. This technique is associated with good surgical exposure.

Although it decreases the incidence of barotrauma, spontaneous ventilation during thoracoscopy has physiologic implications (Table 23.1).

It is the preoperative condition of the patient which determines the cardiovascular and pulmonary compromise faced by the patient.

General anaesthesia depresses alveolar ventilation and may cause atelectasis resulting in V/Q mismatch and hypercapnia. In order to counter this effect an increase in minute ventilation is desirable, but, this causes expansion of the operative lung and decreases the surgical vision. Another way to increase minute ventilation is to increase the respiratory rate, which can be achieved with light anaesthesia but this causes haemodynamic instability due to mediastinal flap and interferes with surgical exposure.

In patients breathing spontaneously, adequate oxygenation is maintained with administration of 100 per cent oxygen. Since N_2O cannot be administered, anaesthesia is maintained by use of drugs like opioids which may cause central respiratory depression resulting in hypercapnia and respiratory acidosis.

Therefore, spontaneous ventilation for thoracoscopy is used in very limited conditions like other diagnostic procedures of short duration.

Table 23.1: Spontaneous respiration by a single lumen tracheal tube.[5]

Advantages	Disadvantages
1. No positive-pressure ventilation	1. V/Q mismatch
2. Barotrauma↓	2. 100% inspired oxygen required
3. Hypoxic pulmonary vasoconstriction+	3. Hypercapnia
4. Intrapulmonary shunt↓	4. No nitrous oxide
5. V/Q relationship+	5. Hypercapnia
6. DLT insertion not required	6. Mediastinal flap
7. Less trauma	
8. CO_2 insufflation not required	

Use of LMA or facemask for airway management in spontaneous ventilation

When spontaneous ventilation by LMA was compared with one-lung ventilation using a double-lumen endobronchial tube, SpO_2 was significantly higher in LMA group.[3,9,10] Similar results were obtained when a tight fitting facemask was used.

This was because one-lung ventilation is associated with V/Q mismatch and shunting, therefore, two-lung ventilation by LMA or facemask resulted in improved oxygenation.

Controlled Ventilation with Single Lumen Tracheal Tube[3,11]

During two-lung ventilation CO_2 is continuously insufflated into the pleural space until the conclusion of surgical procedure.

CO_2 insufflation (Capnothorax)

CO_2 is insufflated intrapleurally to enhance collapse of lung and improve visualization. Caution should be used when insufflating CO_2 in spontaneously breathing patient under local or regional anaesthesia. CO_2 insufflation can be performed safely during one-lung ventilation without haemodynamic compromise if insufflation pressure is maintained below 10 mm Hg and flow limited to 1.2L/min.[3,10]

Controlled Ventilation with Double Lumen Tracheal Tube

Techniques of lung separation[4]

The use of double lumen endobronchial tube has evolved as the technique of choice for most cases of one lung anaesthesia (Fig. 23.3). Bronchial blockers are typically the second choice for one lung anaesthesia but may be necessary in children and small adults (< 50 kg). Bronchial blockers have high pressure, high-compliance cuff, which can get dislodged and obstruct the trachea while the distal lumen is too small for effective suctioning and ventilating the lung distal to the blocker.

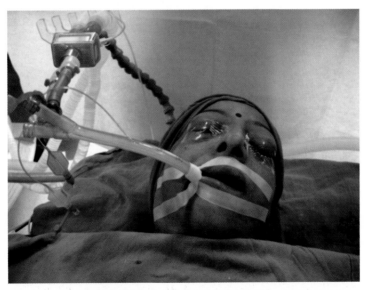

Fig. 23.3: Double lumen tube *in situ*

Physiology of one lung ventilation[4,12]

When the nondependent lung is nonventilated, as during one lung ventilation, any blood flow to the non-ventilated lung becomes shunt flow, in addition to whatever shunt flow might exist in the dependent lung.

One-lung ventilation creates an obligatory right-to-left transpulmonary shunt through the nonventilated nondependent lung. Consequently for the same FiO_2, haemodynamic and metabolic status, one-lung ventilation results in a much larger alveolar-arterial oxygen tension difference [P (A-a) O_2] and lower PaO_2. The ventilated lung removes CO_2, keeping the alveolar carbon dioxide tension ($PACO_2$ - $PaCO_2$) gradient small. The ventilated lung cannot take up enough oxygen because of the shape of the oxygen-haemoglobin dissociation curve, and thus does not allow compensation for the nonventilated lung.[12]

Both passive and active mechanisms operate during one-lung ventilation which minimize the blood flow to the nondependent, nonventilated lung thus preventing a fall in PaO_2. The passive mechanisms are gravity, surgical interference with the blood flow and extent of disease in the nondependent lung,[4] while the active mechanism is vasoconstriction known as hypoxic pulmonary vasoconstriction. The selective increase in the pulmonary vascular resistance of the atelectatic lung diverts blood flow towards the ventilated lung.

Management of patient on one lung ventilation (Fig. 23.4)[12]

Since one-lung ventilation carries a definite risk of systemic hypoxaemia ventilation should be managed optimally. The FiO_2 should be increased, since high FiO_2 in a single lung ventilation increases PaO_2 from arrhythmogenic and life threatening levels to safer levels. The FiO_2 should be increased, even to 1.0, to maintain arterial oxygen saturation greater than 90 per cent. Despite theoretical possibilities of absorption atelectasis and oxygen toxicity, the benefits of 100 per cent oxygen far exceed the risks.

The dependent lung should be ventilated with a tidal volume of 10 ml/kg and the respiratory rate adjusted to maintain $PaCO_2$ at 37-42 mm Hg. Continuous monitoring of ventilation and oxygenation is necessary in this setting.

If hypoxaemia persists, differential lung positive end-expiratory pressure (PEEP) to dependent lung or continuous positive airway pressure (CPAP) to nondependent lung or both should be instituted. Low levels of

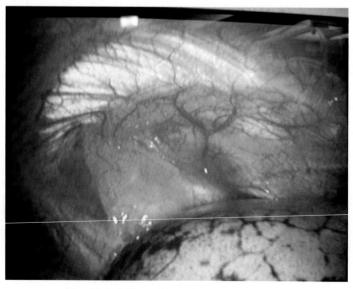

Fig. 23.4: Collapsed lung during thoracoscopy

CPAP (5 to 10 cm H_2O) maintain patency of nondependent lung airways allowing some distention of the gas-exchanging alveolar space without affecting the pulmonary vasculature and thus increase the PaO_2. However PEEP induced increase in lung volume can cause compression of the small dependent-lung intralveolar vessels diverting the blood to the nonventilated lung increasing the shunt and decreasing PaO_2. Therefore, dependent lung PEEP should not be the first line maneuver by itself.

If oxygenation does not improve with 5-10 cm H_2O CPAP delivered to nondependent lung, 5-10 cm H_2O PEEP should then be added to the dependent lung. If severe hypoxaemia persists, then nondependent CPAP is increased to10-15 cm H_2O. In this way, a differential lung PEEP and CPAP is used in search for maximum compliance and a minimum right-to-left transpulmonary shunt.

The resumption of two-lung ventilation is the fastest way to improve oxygenation and should be used if severe hypoxemia persists.

ANAESTHETIC MANAGEMENT FOR THORACOSCOPY

Preexisting lung disease increases the risk of pulmonary complications in the perioperative period.

PREOPERATIVE EVALUATION

Preoperative evaluation is same as for patients undergoing noncardiac thoracic surgery. Detailed history, physical examination, workup for respiratory and cardiovascular systems are necessary. The anaesthesiologist must be familiar with laboratory results, ECG and radiologic studies of the chest. PFT and their predictive value on the patient's postoperative pulmonary function are the integral part of preoperative evaluation.[3]

Preoperative optimization of reactive airway disease and treatment of infection minimizes postoperative complications.

PHYSICAL EXAMINATION

Patient's inability to tolerate supine position has multiple ramifications, including possibility of a compromised airway, poor cardiac function or decreased pulmonary reserve all of which affect perioperative anaesthetic plan.

Along with a routine examination of the airway and cardiovascular system, the presence of clubbing and cyanosis, the respiratory rate and pattern and the type of breath sounds on auscultation provide an insight into the pulmonary reserve of the patient.

Evidence of arterial hypoxaemia can be established by the presence of central cyanosis in which case the arterial saturation is usually 80% or less and indicates a limited margin of respiratory reserve. Peripheral cyanosis must be distinguished from central cyanosis (poor circulation). Clubbing of fingers indicates chronic hypoxia, malignancy, congenital heart disease with right to left shunt. In patients with arterial hypoxaemia and hypercapnia, pulmonary artery hypertension and cor pulmonale are likely to develop and therefore signs of right ventricular failure and pulmonary hypertension should be sought. [3]

The rate and pattern of respiration can distinguish obstructive versus restrictive disease. Deviation of trachea can signify presence of haemothorax, pneumothorax, empyema or mediastinal mass.

Wheeze, rales or rhonchi usually indicate abnormalities which should be managed preoperatively. Institution of bronchodilator therapy, chest physiotherapy and adequate hydration of patient is a useful approach to facilitate mobilization of secretions and reduce infection of the airway.

INVESTIGATIONS

Complete blood count, urinanalysis, prothrombin time, partial thromboplastin time, serum electrolytes, blood urea nitrogen and creatinine, blood sugar and chest radiograph are mandatory tests. Polycythaemia reflects prolonged smoking and hypoxia. Leucocytosis can be due to an active infection. The ECG may show an ischaemic pattern, heart strain or rhythm abnormalities.

Review of chest radiograph indicates a possible difficult intubation (e.g. tracheal deviation, mediastinal mass), need for invasive monitoring (e.g. pleural effusion, cor pulmonale), risk of pneumothorax with positive pressure ventilation (e.g. bullous disease) and need to separate the two lungs (e.g. abscess) (Fig. 23.5).

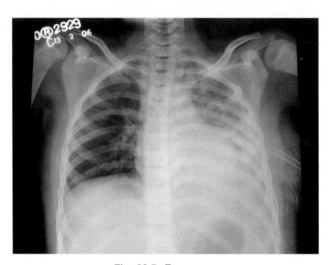

Fig. 23.5: Empyema

Thoracoscopic procedures tend to be less stressful than thoracotomy with fewer cardiopulmonary sequelae. However, one-lung ventilation, lateral decubitus position, longer duration of surgery, need for extensive lung resection necessitate knowing the pulmonary functional reserve of the patient.

PFTs are performed for evaluation of lung volume, total lung function and assessment of ventilation and perfusion of each lung separately. Differential lung function tests simulate postoperative physiology by temporarily eliminating vascular supply to the lung being resected. The PFTs value may indicate high-risk for postoperative pulmonary complication (Table 23.2).

PREOPERATIVE PREPARATION

Preoperative respiratory preparation is directed towards optimally managing any pre-existing pulmonary disease. It includes cessation of smoking, dilating airways, loosening and removing secretions and increasing patients motivation and education to facilitate postoperative care.

These patients are at a high risk of postoperative pulmonary complications.

1. The incidence of postoperative respiratory complications is correlated with the degree of preoperative respiratory dysfunction.
2. While nondependent lung function may be impaired by resection of functional lung or trauma to the remaining lung, the dependent lung function may be impaired as a result of atelectasis and oedema formation.

3. The third cause of increased pulmonary complications relates to postoperative pain. These patients resist deep breathing and coughing leading to retained secretions, atelectasis and pneumonia.

MONITORING

Monitoring includes pulse oximetry, noninvasive blood pressure, capnography and ECG.

Pulse oximetry detects problems of oxygenation, capnography detects the problems with ventilation such as airway disconnection, apnoea, hyperventilation and significant changes in ventilation- perfusion mismatch.

Other monitoring devices include precordial or oesophageal stethoscope for detection of wheeze, rales, rhonchi or bronchospasm, while measurement of lung compliance gives information regarding lung compliance.

The need for invasive monitoring should be individualised, based on patient's cardiovascular and pulmonary status and complexity of the procedure.

Arterial blood gas analysis helps in measuring $PaCO_2$ in patients with significant pulmonary disease when $EtCO_2$ reading may be unreliable. It is also helpful in patients with significant coronary artery disease, left ventricular dysfunction, severe emphysema or COPD.

Placement of central venous access should be limited to patients with significant cardiac disease who require restricted infusion of fluids or placement of pulmonary artery catheter.

Table 23.2: Pulmonary function test predictors for postoperative pulmonary complications.[3] (PFTs)

Parameter	Value
Forced expiratory volume in 1 second (FEV$_1$)	<50% of FVC or 2L
Forced vital capacity (FVC)	<50% of predicted
Maximum breathing capacity (MBC)	<50% of predicted or 50 L/ min
Residual volume to total lung capacity ratio (RV/TLC)	>50% of predicted
Lung diffusion capacity for carbon monoxide	<50-60% of predicted

COMPLICATIONS

Each procedure has a potential for general or systemic complications. The complications may be minor or life threatening depending on their extent.[8]

Pulmonary

Pulmonary complications are common in patients given a general anaesthetic and usually are minor and not life threatening (Table 23.3).

Table 23.3: Complications of thoracoscopy[8] (Pulmonary)

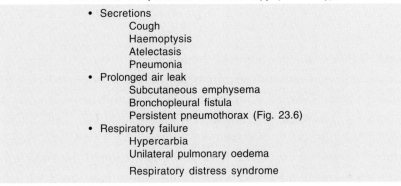

- Secretions
    Cough
    Haemoptysis
    Atelectasis
    Pneumonia
- Prolonged air leak
    Subcutaneous emphysema
    Bronchopleural fistula
    Persistent pneumothorax (Fig. 23.6)
- Respiratory failure
    Hypercarbia
    Unilateral pulmonary oedema
    Respiratory distress syndrome

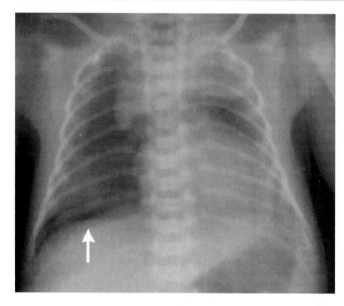

Fig. 23.6: Pneumothorax

To reduce the incidence of prolonged air leak, partial pleurectomy, minimal manipulation of the remaining lung to avoid tears and punctures, proper pleural apposition, avoidance of air space and direct control of air leak with suture or staples have been recommended.

Multiple small perforations or one large perforation can result in formation of bronchopleural fistula.

Subcutaneous air, puffiness and emphysema upto the eyes or down to the toes, may develop and may create speech difficulties.

Control of air leak is important in preventing respiratory failure, hypercarbia and respiratory distress syndrome specially in patients on pressure or high volume respiratory support.

Unilateral life threatening pulmonary oedema can develop in patients where high volume pleural effusion is evacuated. The lung when expands rapidly develops pulmonary oedema. These patients then require long term respiratory support or recollapse of the lung with slow expansion.

Increased secretions, atelectasis and pneumonia can develop postoperatively, known as 'down lung syndrome'. Its diagnosis should be considered in the event of respiratory deterioration or development of productive cough.[13,14] It may be ipsilateral or contralateral and particularly develops if bleeding occurs with tracheal intubation. Ventilation and removal of secretions should be adequate in the postoperative period to avoid hypoxia, hypercarbia and respiratory acidosis.

Cardiac

Under local anaesthesia, tachycardia, dysrhythmia, hypoxia and vasovagal stimulation may develop with hypertension and bradycardia. Appropriate use of oxygen, atropine and sedatives may help. Any shift in mediastinum may cause hypoxia.[3] Cardiac complications like arrhythmias, ventricular tachycardia and atrial asystoles have been reported.[14] Hypertension in association with hypercarbia, mediastinal shift, blood losses and removal of large pleural effusion resulting in pulmonary oedema have been reported.[15] (Table 23.4)

Acute myocardial infarction and cardiac arrest have also been reported. Monitoring of patient's vitals signs and provision of oxygen and appropriate preoperative evaluation reduce the chances of complications.

Table 23.4: Complications of thoracoscopy (Cardiac)

- Blood pressure
    Diminished venous return
    Hypotension
    Hypertension
- Arrhythmias
    Bradycardia
    Atrial - including atrial fibrillation
    Ventricular tachycardia/ extrasystole
- Hypoxia
    Hypotension
    Myocardial ischaemia or infarction
    Cardiac arrest

Technical

One of the most common problems is the inability to locate a free pleural space in case of fibrosis and to locate the lesion specially those tucked behind the adhesion.

In case of a malignant lesion the problem may be of recurrence of tumour. It is due to a partially removed persistence of tumour and to spread of primary tumour if it is taken out through the wound or incision without placing a bag or protective device.[16] While inserting the trocars, the surgeon must be careful not to injure the intercostal artery, lung or diaphragm(Table 23.5).

Table 23.5: Complications of thoracoscopy[16] (Technical)

- Bleeding
    Intercostal artery
    Lung
    Hilum
- Inability to locate the lesion
- Spread of the malignancy
    Carcinoma of lung- primary/secondary
    Sarcoma
    Mesothelioma
- Inadequate resection
- Neurologic
    Injury to nerves
    Pain

Other Complications

- Fever, wound infection and empyema
- Thoracoscopic failure with conversion to open procedure
- Intra- abdominal injuries, liver and spleen
- Oesophageal injuries
- Horner's syndrome
- Air embolism
- Mortality

The complications related to DLT are similar to those seen whenever a DLT is used in thoracic surgery. Pharyngeal trauma and pain, traumatic laryngitis, balloon rupture and malposition of DLT leading to impaired gas exchange, difficulty in ventilation dependant / nonoperative lung, unsatisfactory collapse of nondependent/

operative lung, tension pneumothorax and barotrauma. (Contamination of unaffected lung with blood, tumour particles, infectious organisms and lavage fluids.) Tracheobronchial tree disruption and disruption of posterior membranous wall and bronchus may result.

Ischaemia of tracheobronchial wall and incorporation of DLT into surgical site are some rare complications.

POSTOPERATIVE PAIN MANAGEMENT

Analgesic requirement and length of hospital stay are less for uncomplicated thoracoscopy. Most healthy patients with a simple thoracoscopy procedure can be discharged in 1 to 2 days and the procedure may be performed on an outpatient basis.

Since most pain is attributed to chest tube, comfort can be achieved with intercostal nerve blocks or field block around the tube.[17,18]

POSTOPERATIVE MANAGEMENT

Although patients undergoing thoracoscopy have reduced pain and respiratory dysfunction compared with those undergoing thoracotomy, there is need for aggressive pulmonary therapy. The use of incentive spirometry is ideal to reduce postoperative pulmonary atelectasis. Sitting upright in bed and early ambulation augments FRC. Mobilisation of secretions with chest physiotherapy (e.g. percussion and postural drainage) and administration of bronchodilators help in reducing the incidence of postoperative respiratory complications.

THORACOSCOPY IN PEDIATRIC PATIENTS[19]

Although mainly used to biopsy an intrathoracic neoplasm, thoracoscopy in paediatric population is also now applied to treat empyema, ligate PDA and for anterior spinal fusion.

PREOPERATIVE EVALUATION

The preoperative history and physical examination should be aimed at identifying acute problems and previously undiagnosed problems that can place the patient at an increased risk intraoperatively.

The preoperative laboratory evaluation depends more on clinical status of the patient than the procedure itself. Although rarely needed, blood should be readily available. Pulmonary function testing and electrocardiogram are not routinely indicated.[18,19]

Child with an anterior mediastinal mass requires careful preoperative evaluation. Preoperative computerized tomographic (CT) scan of chest is helpful. Compression of greater than 50% of cross-sectional area of the trachea on CT imaging indicates high risk in whom general anaesthesia with loss of spontaneous ventilation can lead to total airway obstruction.[19,20]

PREMEDICATION AND TECHNIQUES OF ANAESTHESIA

In healthy patients without signs of airway compromise, oral premedication with midazolam (0.5-0.75 mg/ kg) 45 minutes prior to anaesthetic induction provides anxiolysis and allows for easy separation from parents and acceptance of anaesthesia mask for gentle inhalation induction. H_2 antagonists or motility drugs (e.g. metoclopramide) may also be added for decreasing gastric secretions and increasing gastric motility respectively.

Anaesthetic induction techniques include either inhalation with sevoflurane or halothane in nitrous oxide and O_2 or use of intravenous anaesthetic drugs. This is followed by administration of nondepolarizing muscle relaxant to facilitate tracheal intubation and maintenance of anaesthesia. Adequate venous access should be secured. Central venous access is generally reserved for cases in which an adequate peripheral intravenous access is unavailable.

If a central venous access decided it should be on the side of thoracoscopy. Standard perioperative monitoring include pulse oximetry, end-tidal CO_2 monitoring, noninvasive blood pressure monitoring, continuous ECG, esophageal stethoscope and continuous temperature monitoring. As $EtCO_2$ monitoring can be inaccurate during thoracoscopic procedures due to alteration in dead space and shunt fraction, transcutaneous CO_2 monitoring can be considered.[18]

PERIOPERATIVE ANAESTHETIC CARE

Local and Regional Anaesthetic Techniques

In older adolescents, local anaesthesia or regional anaesthetic techniques are possible. These techniques are usually reserved for brief procedures without involving intrathoracic surgical manipulation specially in children with severe systemic illness that can be associated with an unacceptable risk of perioperative morbidity or mortality following general anaesthesia. A combination of intravenous sedation and local anaesthetic infiltration is an option.

The regional anaesthesia techniques that can be used for thoracoscopic procedures include thoracic epidural anaesthesia, thoracic paravertebral blockade, multiple intercostal blocks and intrapleural analgesia.[19]

CONCLUSIONS

Although minimally invasive thoracoscopic surgery has obvious benefits, the physiological changes associated with it present multiple challenges. There is a conflict of interests between the need to maintain normal pulmonary and cardiovascular physiology. As a result an understanding of anaesthetic—surgical technique and patient physiology is essential.

Careful attention to patient selection and understanding the complications associated with one lung ventilation and VATs can help to anticipate and prevent complications.

RECOMMENDATIONS FOR THORACOSCOPY

- General anaesthesia with DLT (one lung anaesthesia) and controlled ventilation
- 100% O_2 before deflation of lung
- Lumen of the bronchial tube should be opened to atmosphere
- Slow insufflation of CO_2 at 1 L/min (capnothorax)
- Low pressure insufflation (<10 mmHg)
- Another source of O_2 1 L/min to be available
- Maintain $EtCO_2$ limits (35-45 mmHg)
- Complete removal of CO_2 at conclusion of procedure

REFERENCES

1. Jacobaeus H. Cauterization of adhesions in pneumothorax. Treatment of tuberculosis. Surg Gynaecol Obstet 1921;32: 49.
2. Allen M. Video-assisted thoracic surgical procedures: The Mayo experience. Mayo Clin Proc 1996;71: 351.
3. Shah JS and Bready LL. Anesthesia for thoracoscopy. Anesthesiol Clin N Am 2001;19(1): 153-73.

4. Brian Fredman. Physiologic changes during thoracoscopy. Anesthesiol Clin N Am 2001; 141-53.
5. Mark M, Aronoff R, Acuff T, et al. Present role of thoracoscopy in the diagnosis and treatment of diseases of the chest. Ann Thorac Surg 1995; 54: 402.
6. Pyng L, Hensi GC. Using diagnostic thoracoscopy to optimal effect: Technical know-how is key. J Crit Illness, 2003; 18(6): 244–51.
7. Robinson RJS, Slinger P, Mulder DS, et al. Video-assisted thoracoscopic surgery using a single-lumen tube in spontaneously ventilating anaesthetized patients: An Alternative anaesthesia technique. J Cardiothorac Vasc Anesth 1994; 8: 693.
8. Dieter RA Jr., Kurvez GB; Complications and contraindication of thoracoscopy: Int Surg 1997; 82(3): 232-9.
9. Sakuraba M, Masvda K, Hebisawa A. Thoracoscopic pleural biopsy for tuberculosis pleurisy under local anaesthesia. Ann Thorac Cardiovasc Surg 2006; 12(4): 245-8.
10. Lieou FJ, Wang JJ, Liu MY, et al. Total intravenous anaesthesia with O_2 mask in thoracoscopy. Chring Hau I Tsa Chih Taipai 1993; 52: 398.
11. Wong RY, Fung ST. Use of Single lumen tube and continuous CO_2 insufflation in thoracoscopy. Acta Anaesthesiology, Singapore 1995; 33(1): 21-6.
12. Senturk M. New concepts of management of one lung ventilation. Curr Opin Anaesthesiol 2006; 19(1): 1-4.
13. Lamb JD. Anaesthesia for thoracoscopic pulmonary lobectomy. Can J Anesth 1993; 40(11): 1073-5.
14. Kodali Bhavani Shankar. Haemodynamic effects of CO_2 insufflation during thoracoscopy: Capnography in thoracics.
15. Woler RS, Krasna MJ, et al. Haemodynamic effects of CO_2 insufflation during thoracoscopy. Ann thorac Surg 1994; 58; 404-8.
16. Paige Latham, Kimberlie K, Dullye. Complications of thoracoscopy. Anesthesiol Clin N Am, 2001; 187-201.
17. Furrer M. Thoracotomy and thoracoscopy postoperative pulmonary function, pain and chest wall complaints. European Journal of Cardiothoracic Surgery, 1997; 12: 82-7.
18. Landreneau RJ, Weichmann RJ. Effect of Thoracoscopy on acute and chronic postoperative pain. Chest Surg Clin N Am 1998; 8(4): 891-906.
19. Cooper MG. Bronchial blocker placement: A technique and some considerations. Pediatr Anaesth 1994; 4: 73.
20. Hammer GB, Brodsly JB. Methods for single-lung ventilation in paediatric patients. Anaesthesiology 1996; 84: 1503.

Index